The Cherokee Herbal

The Cherokee Herbal

Native Plant Medicine
from the Four Directions

J. T. GARRETT

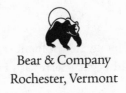

Bear & Company
Rochester, Vermont

Bear & Company
One Park Street
Rochester, Vermont 05767
www.InnerTraditions.com

Bear & Company is a division of Inner Traditions International

Library of Congress Cataloging-in-Publication Data

Garrett, J. T., 1942–
    The Cherokee herbal : native plant medicine from the four
directions / J. T. Garrett.
        p. cm.
    ISBN 1-879181-96-7
        1. Materia medica, Vegetable—United States. 2. Cherokee
Indians—Medicine. I. Title.

RS171.G375 2003
615'.321'0899755—dc21

        2003040388

Printed and bound in the United States.

10 9 8 7 6 5 4 3 2 1

Text design and layout by Rachel Goldenberg
This book was typeset in Legacy Serif with Frutiger and Neuland as
the display typefaces

Contents

A Note on Cherokee Language and Pronunciation

The use of Cherokee words in *The Cherokee Herbal* is intended to add a cultural and historical dimension to this book. Although some direct translations of Cherokee words have been lost over the past several hundred years, I wanted to preserve words in the original language as provided by the elders themselves, and by old documents that otherwise end up collecting dust in some archive. Common names of plants in the Cherokee vernacular local to North Carolina, Oklahoma, and Arkansas would be based on the plant's use in a formula, so some plants would be referred to by more than one name.

This book is not intended to teach the Cherokee language or to record every Cherokee word. I simply want to offer the reader a taste of this unique cultural dimension to the plant world and the uses of plants as helpers from a Cherokee perspective. A Cherokee language dictionary can be used to find many words not mentioned in this book. I also realize the importance of keeping certain words and plant uses sacred. Some of what I learned from the elders therefore does not appear in this book.

A list of syllables from the Cherokee syllabary follows, along with the corresponding sound in English that will assist in the Cherokee pronunciations.

a	ah	*di*	dinner
da	doc	*do*	doe
de	day	*du*	due

e	egg	*se*	say
ga	goggles	*si*	see
ge	gay	*so*	sew
gi	gift	*su*	sue
ha	hop	*sv*	suck (nasal sound)
he	hay	*ta*	tom
hi	it	*te*	tail
hu	hoot	*tla*	clock
i	Italy	*tlu*	clue
ka	call	*tsa*	jock
la	lollygag	*tse*	hay
li	lee	*tsi*	pig
lo	low	*tso*	jock
lu	lue	*tsu*	jewel
me	may	*u*	hue
na	knot	*wa*	wah
ne	neighbor	*we*	weight
ni	knee	*wi*	wheel
no	no	*wo*	Iwo Jima
nu	new	*ya*	yah
o(o)	Ohio	*ye*	yes
qua	quad	*yi*	yield
qui	quiver	*yo*	yoyo
s	say	*yu*	you
sa	sock	*yv*	young (nasal sound)

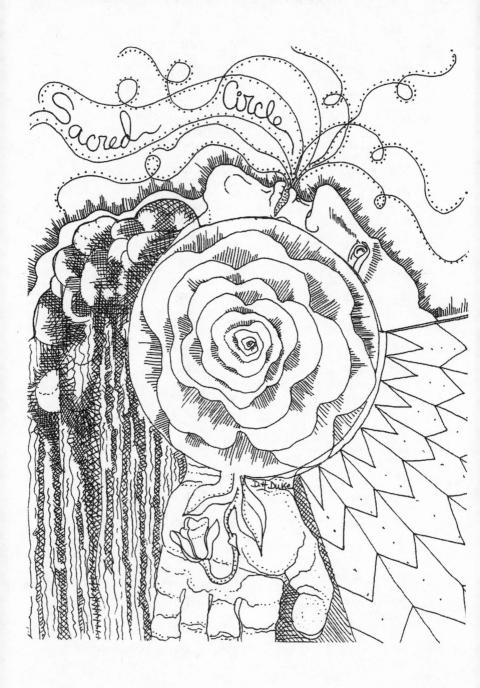

1

The Medicine Way of Life

A Cherokee elder puts his hand on a plant at the edge of the Oconaluftee River at Toe String on a cool fall morning. "This is a plant that the old ones used for thrush in the mouth and sore throat," he says. "This is the one you can take for that hoarseness that keeps bothering you." He is pointing to yellowroot *(Xanthorhiza simplicissima)* as he continues. "Some of the old people used this in a formula for easing childbirth. Here, scratch the bark with your knife. You see the yellow stem? That's how you recognize it." He cuts a piece. "Just chew on this, and it will help your throat."

As I write the plant's Cherokee name in my notebook the old man asks, "Why are you writing that down?" I replied that I could not remember all he was telling me about the plants. "In the old days you had to remember because you didn't have paper to write on. Besides, some folks would wonder why you are writing it down. You just gotta' remember and learn the hard way."

It is with the support of several Cherokee and other elders that I share the plant-healing teachings I am putting forth in this book. As with my elder guide at the river, others have encouraged me not to write teachings down on paper, nor to use my computer to sort and store this information. Said one elder: "It is another's way to share with words; it is the Indian way to share with feelings."

"Others have recorded these things and they were not respected— nor were we for our way," as another elder put it. "It was like when Mooney was doing the work here in Big Cove. He was taking the

1

stuff he learned back to Washington. Why did the government need to know about the story of Rabbit, or about how we used the plants for Medicine?" Since the Indian Removal Act of 1830 and the Cherokees' forced relocation on the "Trail of Tears," in which the U.S. Army transported the Cherokee to Oklahoma Territory, there has been a deep mistrust of the U.S. government on the part of the Cherokee for all the broken treaties and promises.

Only a couple of elders were willing to have their names referenced in this book. One of those elders was Doc Amoneeta Sequoyah, a Cherokee Medicine Man of the Eastern Band of Cherokee Indians. I highly respected Doc for his willingness and determination that others should see and learn respect for the "old ways." Doc, one of my teachers of Cherokee Medicine, did not mind speaking out to the non-Indian public. He was always curious about what was written in what he called my "black book." He even warned me that others would "steal everything and call it theirs, like so many have done in the past to Cherokees." Doc's wife, Ella Sequoyah, and his children were very encouraging to me.

My mother, Ruth Garrett (nee Rogers), was concerned that my writing would be an issue with those tribal members who believe that "we should just keep things the way they are, because people would not understand the way of things on the boundary" ("the boundary" being the Cherokee Indian Reservation in Cherokee, North Carolina). My promise to the elders was to not share those things that were considered sacred and meant to be kept secret for the "keepers of the way, the teachings of the ancestors."

LEARNING FROM OUR ELDERS

Like many others of the Eastern Band of Cherokee Indians, I am a mixed blood: White and Cherokee. I felt fortunate to be chosen to learn the way of Cherokee Indian Medicine. I share Doc Amoneeta Sequoyah's vision that others will appreciate the teachings and the values of the "old wisdom."

This book is about the teachings in Indian Medicine related to the plants and natural "Medicine" of the Cherokee and other southeastern American Indian tribes. Unless otherwise mentioned, notes on the plants and their use are from Cherokee Medicine men and women. There is reference to a Natchez-Cherokee, Archie Sams from Oklahoma, who I met in the 1980s when I was administrator of the Cherokee Indian Hospital in Cherokee, North Carolina. Reference to "mountain folks" in this book is in keeping with the way Cherokee refer to the "friends of the Cherokee," those people of European descent who settled in the Appalachian and Smoky Mountains of eastern North America. These were hardy people respected by the tribes for their values and for their willingness to live in harmonious cohabitation with the environment. There is a wonderful body of knowledge and understanding in communities in Appalachia and along the Blue Ridge Mountains, from New York down to North Carolina. This knowledge also extends into Canada, where I have friends who helped me verify indigenous uses of plants in the north.

My first experiences with the Cherokee Medicine was as a youngster. My mother remembers me being interested in studying the plants and flowers beginning at the age of twelve. My early interest in plants eventually led me to study biology and botany. Unlike students who would simply make their leaf and flower books by pressing and drying, I wanted to learn more about where the plants came from and how they were used as "helpers." I wanted to grow plants too. My science projects became ways to test how plants could be improved using different mixtures of plant nutrients and common things people would throw away, such as coffee grounds.

I had very little time to learn about plants from my grandfather, Oscar Rogers. His passing while I was young meant that other grandfathers in the tribe would teach me the Medicine. Our Cherokee family connection is through the name of Walkingstick, which goes back to Polk County, Tennessee (as it is called today), as well to Union County, Georgia, and Marble, North Carolina. My Cherokee ancestors were quite independent. They farmed the land, and their way of life depended on a few neighbors, both Cherokee and "friends of the Cherokee." My closest teacher was my mother, Ruth Rogers Garrett. Her sister, my aunt Shirley Arch, shared much with me about the myths and stories. There were many others. Ed George helped me with the language of the plants, as did Sampson Lossiah. A master elder with the plants was William Hornbuckle. Ann Bradley and William took me on trips in the mountains to learn about the plants in their natural habitat. Doc Amoneeta would go with me to hunt certain plants that were considered sacred and to share with me how they were used in ceremonies. I am very thankful to others who helped me with plants and stories, and who influenced me to write: Annie Sherrill, Chief John Crowe, Mary Chiltoskey, Myrtle Driver, Abe Lossiah, Freeman Owl, Francis Reed, Chief Ed Taylor, Richard Teesatuskee, Oscar Welch, Tom Underwood, Edmond Youngbird, Jerry Wolf, and others in Cherokee who encouraged me to learn and share.

Cherokee Medicine is a way of life for me, for my family, for the Cherokee, and for other American Indians. It is my vision that others will come to better know and understand this way of life that shows respect for every living thing here on Mother Earth, how each has its own beauty and is a helper to us. My vision is that we will learn to respect Mother Earth more each day and come to know how we can be a protector for the resources that our ancestors have called "the Medicine Way."

In a very practical sense, early human use of tree barks and plants were a Medicine Way for the tribe to take care of its members. Using plants as medicine has always been an exact natural science based on experience of many generations. As an example, earlier Cherokee used willow bark *(Salix alba)*, or white willow, in the same way that meadowsweet *(Filipendula ulmaria)* was used by another culture of people for pain. Willow bark is a natural source of salicylic acid, the active ingredient in aspirin. While we have no written record of willow bark's properties, the world has the writings of the early Greek physicians

Hippocrates and Dioscorides, who both recorded willow's use for pain and fever. As a matter of fact, native people in other countries used it for pain in the joints and muscles and to relieve arthritis, fever, headaches, and toothaches. Today, except for knowing that salicin is an active ingredient in the inner bark of white willow, we really do not know enough about white willow's chemical actions. Yet white willow is still used by American Indians, along with dogwood, laurel, and other plants, as a pain reliever and an anti-inflammatory. It takes approximately 3 grams of the dried willow powder as an extract, standardized to contain approximately 50 milligrams of salicin, to be effective. A standard aspirin contains 325 milligrams of the synthesized acetylsalicylic acid. Of course, synthetic nonsteroidal anti-inflammatory drugs, such as naproxen, also relieve pain and inflammation; they cost about $50 per month and come with potential side effects, such as nausea, constipation, ulceration and bleeding, liver damage, headaches, rashes, drowsiness, fluid retention, and ringing in the ears.

As a society we have become used to risking such side effects and bearing the costs of medical insurance. We also have one of the finest medical systems in the world—this is the Western Medicine Way today, and it works well, just as plant Medicine did for American Indians of yesterday—and still does for some contemporary Indians.

There is a story to tell about the Medicine Way as a way of life based on choice, time, and culture. The Medicine story helps us to better appreciate how the term *Medicine* with a capital *M* is used in Indian teachings in reference to a Medicine bundle or Medicine way of life. A Medicine "object" is anything that we have been gifted or learn that we keep in a special place, physically and mentally, and that is special to us or guides our lives and our memories. The story here is a traditional means for better understanding the "Cherokee Way."

THE MEDICINE STORY

A Natchez-Cherokee from Oklahoma and a Cherokee elder from Carlin, Nevada, visited me in North Carolina in 1981. The purpose of the visit was to speak with other Eastern Band of Cherokee Indian elders about the story of Indian Medicine. The story has been told in many different ways based on specific tribal teachings and relative to where the tribe was located. For example, the Medicine story of the Alaska Natives has the ocean and fish or a large water species as main figures that bring Medicine to the people. The White Buffalo Woman brings the Medicine pipe to the Lakota (Sioux) people; and the eagle and the hawk, or the owl, bring messages to the Cherokee.

There are several versions of a story in Cherokee about the beginning of Medicine. Sometimes these stories have been considered sacred and not to be shared outside of the individual tribe. It was important to respect these very old traditions. However, this story was permitted to be told.

A Cherokee elder who lived near Bryson City, North Carolina, shared a story about the Tuckasegee River that runs through what is known as Governor's Island in North Carolina. He said that the spirits of the mountains knew there would be a time when strange beings would come from the stars as light beings. The spirit of the mountains knew that these beings, who had no hair (unlike the animals), would not be able to survive the cold of the mountains, even with their warm, star-borne light. They would need shelter and warm pelts from the animals to survive.

A council was called. At this early time in Earth's history animals could speak a common language with each other and with the spirits of the mountains. The animals were vocal about not sharing their skin pelts, yet even as they protested they also knew that "things were to be as they were intended by universal plan," as the elder said. The animals knew that as spirits they could teach other animals how to stay in harmony and balance in the circle of this world. They would also become teachers of the new beings, who would be called humans.

Therefore, the animals agreed to gift the light beings with their skin pelts, as long as these new humans would agree only to take of these skin pelts after following ceremony and getting permission from the animals to share.

The spirits of the mountains were satisfied. All was well. The spirits of the mountains began to carve a trail with the help of the Thunder Beings, the spirits in the sky who bring us thunder, lightning, and rain. With the Thunder Beings' help, the mountains opened themselves to the hard rains that created what is now called the Tuckasegee River valley, a place for the humans to live and care for Mother Earth and all the animals.

The mountains surrounding the Tucksagee River valley, the Great Smoky Mountains are some of the oldest mountains in North America (what many American Indians call Turtle Island). According to the Cherokee elder telling this origin story, the people we now call the Cherokee existed as small bands of humans who came from the Four Directions in the star-filled sky, long before any recorded dates regarding human existence here on Mother Earth. These beings were called *no lun see,* or the Star People who came from the land of the north sky. The Tuckasegee River valley was always their place on Mother Earth.

I heard another story that mentioned a people who lived here long before the Cherokee came to this part of the mountains; they were called Turtle People. They got their name because of the strange shells they wore as protection. Some even said they were actually manifested spirits of the turtles, which were plentiful at one time.

I do not believe that anyone today knows much about the people who made their home near the banks of the Tuckasegee before the Cherokee made this their sacred and ceremonial home.

The old Cherokee who made their home near the Tuckasegee River were the Kituhwa, or *kah doh wah,* people. According to the elder, the Kituhwa were the true light people, while the *tuc wa ge* people were a mix of animal and human who may have been some of the first to have the animal spirits share with them. They could have been the first human beings to truly survive within the animal world. While their Medicine Way may seem primitive compared to ours today, they understood the connection with Mother Earth, the animals, the plants, and everything in their circle of life. It is said that they did not fight the first intruders because they knew they were coming to make the river valley their village, which would be sacred and with ceremony. It is also said that these beings eventually disappeared into the caves of Deep Creek in what is now Bryson City, North Carolina. These are the ones known as the Little People. The elder said that the old Cherokee referred to these people as dwarfs who had shapes just like the humans. They had the ability to take on the shape and even the personalities of the humans, but somehow they also had the quality of the earth and the animals around them. They held the secrets of nature and survival in this harsh climate and mountainous region of North America and carved out a unique way of life based on traditions, the way of the ancestors, and survival.

The Medicine of that earlier time started with learning to track the animals and to become skilled hunters and fishermen. Certain values were learned for survival. For example, fire was used for cooking the meat, but it was also used for ceremonial purposes. Tobacco was offered as a clearing-way, a ceremony of forgiveness for taking the life of the animal and giving thanks for the meal and the sharing. The animals were plentiful: rabbit, groundhog, deer, and wild turkey. The women were good hunters as well, and some of the best cooks of corn dishes were men. It has been said that women learned what aromas and smells the deer liked in the wild, including wild onions and certain other wild plants, which they used to attract the deer. Medicine was learned from the plant helpers for treating cuts, the stings and bites of insects, and for treating the upset stomachs of children and the full bellies of the adults. While life was simple, there were mystical events and occurrences that required special forms of Medicine as well.

The earlier Cherokee were a hardy people who enjoyed the outdoor way of life. As the elder said, "The story of Cherokee Medicine begins with nature, ends with man, and begins again with nature. Mother Earth gives us life, and all life goes back to her so that life can begin again. The spirit of the mountains, the animals, the stars all tell us of our beginning and how to survive here on Mother Earth."

PAST AND PRESENT: A CIRCLE JOURNEY

Cherokee Indian Medicine is an interesting and confusing subject, even to those of us who have had the opportunity to study it for a lifetime. As a member of the Eastern Band of Cherokee Indians, I understand how sensitive this subject can be and how important it is to treat some things in a sacred and traditional way. My purpose in writing this book is to provide information that might otherwise be lost, like so much of our culture and traditions. I also want others to better appreciate the value and benefit of the old art and science of Indian Medicine. Using plant and animal helpers was a way of life for the survival of tribes and people, long before de Soto and Columbus stumbled onto what some American Indians call Turtle Island, or North America.

An elder said, "Today we talk of the past and the present, but to earlier Native people the present was an extension of the past, with our ancestors here to guide us. The present crosses over to tomorrow that is a part of today, as we are the ancestors. It is a different way to look at life." This helped me to realize how important it is to follow the "right path," or the way of right relationship. The earlier American Indian way of life was about the way of right relationship. While it seems more difficult these days to live the way of right relationship, as American Indians and "mixed ones" we understand that we are on a journey. This journey is in a circle of the Four Directions, which is the Indian way of life.

THE MEDICINE: AN INTERPRETATION

There is an inherent risk in my trying to interpret much of the information gathered from the work I've done since 1960. It was my original intent that only firsthand interviews would be used in my book on Indian plant Medicine. Early on I concluded that a combination of interviews and information gathering would be necessary for me to validate the use of many of the plants. Therefore, several reference books were used, which I have listed in the bibliography. Information was also gathered from the National Archives, where I found a lot of incomplete information in the Cherokee language—notes in Cherokee that were supposedly taken from a "black book" kept by a Cherokee who recorded the Medicine and sacred chants. Interpretation of the old language was very difficult; interpretation can create opportunity for error. As an elder put it, "Just admit up front that you did the best you could. Besides, you were not there two hundred years ago, and this is the way you see it now."

James Mooney's fieldwork in the 1880s in Cherokee villages for the Bureau of Ethnology in Washington, D.C., resulted in the publication of two books that provide some historical reference for our study: *Sacred Formulas of the Cherokee,* published in 1891, and *Myths of the Cherokee,* published in 1900. Mooney missed some of the value of the plant remedies as sacred formulas.

Rather than being an intentional effort on his part to mislead the public, it seems that his omissions had more to do with his agenda for being in Cherokee country—to record specific plant uses. Mooney found that many of the plant uses were inconsistent with the pharmacy knowledge at that time. As an example, eyebright *(Euphrasia officinalis)* and pennyroyal *(Hedeoma hispida)* were European herbal remedies for conjunctivitis in Mooney's time. Conjunctivitis is an inflammation of the eyes that affects the blood vessels, causing redness or bloodshot eyes that burn and itch. Both eyebright and pennyroyal were also used to clear up the pus discharge from a bacterial eye condition.

At the time that eyebright was introduced by the English to the Cherokee, the Cherokee were using other plants that were felt to be more effective for eye conditions, especially for bacterial infections. The Cherokee formula included bilberry *(Vaccinium myrtillus)* as an eyewash and astringent; blue flag or snake lily *(Iris versicolor)* as an eyewash, with the addition of chicory *(Cichorium intybus)* in recent years; chickweed *(Stellaria media)* for eye infection; oak *(Quercus prinus)* for inflammation; pansy *(Viola tricolor)* to lower blood vessel pressure in the eye; raspberry *(Rubus odoratus)* to ease soreness and inflammation; a formula of spleenwort *(Aspenium platyneuron)*, sycamore maple *(Acer pseudo-plantanus),* and evening primrose *(Oenothera biennis)* as a juice for eye conditions related to asthma or allergic reactions; and for eye pain, a formula that includes feverfew *(Chrysanthemum parthenium)* in more recent years. There were other plants and barks used by different Medicine people that included maple *(Acer rubrum)* for soreness of the eyes and infection; fireweed *(Epilobium angustifolium)* for asthma-related conditions and infections; and barberry *(Berberis vulgaris),* goldenseal *(Hydrastis canadensis),* and mullein *(Verbascum thapsus)* as a mild sedative and anti-inflammatory that was especially gentle for children.

As you can imagine, it becomes a matter of interpretation as to who is right and who is more right. This is one of the many reasons I am thankful to the elders for being willing to share the Medicine Way.

THANKS TO THE ELDERS

My interest in natural plants and their use as food and medicine started as a child. My mother, Ruth Rogers Garrett, would teach me about plants and tell stories about their values as helpers. While working for the Cherokee Historical Association in the early 1960s, one of my responsibilities was to share the Cherokee culture in a positive way with visitors to the museum. I had a chance to speak with many Cherokee elders, including Medicine elders. My interest in the early use of plants evolved into listening to the stories told by many of these elders. They emphasized the values of plants as helpers, not as medicinal remedies for specific conditions of illness. Eventually, I did study with several of these Medicine men and women. Of course, the memory of my grandfather, Oscar Rogers, was always with me in studying the Medicine. He encouraged me whenever he placed me on his broad shoulders as a young boy and told me stories and talked about the plants as we sat together on the rocks at the edge of the Oconaluftee River.

Serving with the U.S. Public Health Service provided the opportunity to visit many other tribes. I was hospital administrator in Cherokee, North Carolina, from 1980 to 1984. That wonderful experience provided many opportunities for me to talk with elders. We established a Traditional Cherokee Medicine program to allow the Medicine to be respected and used under patient rights and the American Indian Religious Freedom Act. It was always a special day when an elder would come into the hospital and say, "I bet you don't know about the use of this plant."

There is a wonderful and fascinating world still to be learned about plant-derived medicines from American Indians and all other indigenous people of the world. As one elder put it, "The elders are a bridge to the future and cross over to our ancestors as we follow the teachings of the Medicine and live this way of life."

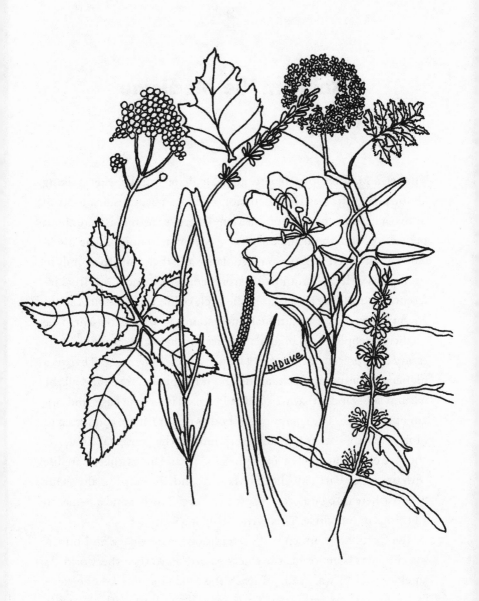

2

Being in the Medicine

The term *Medicine,* or reference to a Medicine bundle when talking about plants, frames the discussion of those natural substances in terms of healing and prevention. Many Cherokee formulas were about prevention and about making "good Medicine" choices. The Medicine also involved seeking spirit guidance and including the family in healing, as well as examining environmental influences, spiritual inference, and all that affects us in the circle of life. As life itself is about energy, there was a traditional understanding with early Cherokee Medicine people that a higher awareness of the plant or tree was necessary to appreciate how it was a helper. As one elder said, "There is a higher and deeper understanding about the plants, trees, and all the natural substances that we call Medicine." This is the basis and origin of Medicine. The energy of our bodies and spirit are connected to Mother Earth, Father Sky, and everything in the Universal Circle. As another elder put it, "We are connected to all things that share life with us on our Earth Mother. She is alive, and She keeps us alive. Our purpose here is to be a protector to our Earth Mother and a helper to all things in our circle. This is the Medicine way."

Unfortunately, much of this traditional knowledge and understanding has been lost as the elders passed on to the otherworld. As an elder said, "I was ready to teach the Medicine, but no one came forward to listen and learn. They were all too busy with television and sports to listen, as we did in the old days." Then he looked at me and, laughing, said, "Well, you are here. I guess you will have to do." Fortunately, much has been preserved by researchers like James

Mooney, who likely had no idea how important the information he collected would be in the future to those of us seeking to preserve plant Medicine knowledge. Many of those researchers were non-Indians who could see the value of the Medicine. As an elder put it, "Some of the people who wrote the words about what we do in the Medicine were just doing it for history. In fact, they preserved not just the past, but they preserved for the future as well." Another elder said, "I knew that it would be the White man that would bring the Medicine back to the people, because it was the White man that tried to take it from us Cherokee."

A Natchez-Cherokee elder from Oklahoma once said to me, "The Medicine will always be here, 'cause the ancestors and spirit ones will provide for the Indian people."

THE WAY OF RIGHT RELATIONSHIP

A Cherokee elder once told me, "The Medicine did not just start in the beginning of life. It begins again with every new generation. It is our purpose as 'keepers of the secrets' to share and teach, to preserve not just our past, but the future. The Medicine is about our relationship with Mother Earth, the Great One, and all things in our Universal Circle." The elder taught me that every green plant is much more than a live cellular structure that reaches to the sun for photosynthesis. It also reaches into the depths of Mother Earth for nutrient life, and every mineral or rock has energy too. This was a concept that seemed foreign to my instructors in botany, especially when talking about organic plants that draw on inorganic or nonlive elements from the earth. It was difficult for them to relate to the Cherokee teaching that Mother Earth was alive, and that she gave us life. As an elder said, "There is a way of right relationship. This is true with nature, and it is the same for humans. Everything in this creation is kin to us. We cannot live without these kin, but they can live without us."

My mother taught me to respect nature, with its trees, plants, and creatures that share this circle of life with us. She taught me about ecosystems and synergy long before I discussed these ideas in college. She and the elders taught me Cherokee stories, poems, and prayers to learn respect for the trees and plants. I understood about the process of photosynthesis—carbon dioxide combining with water to produce nutrients for the plant in the form of carbohydrates—much earlier than when it was taught to me in school. As a youngster I understood the process of transformation of inorganic molecules into organic molecules of life, with oxygen produced as a by-product. I recognized the sacredness of the Sun as a catalyst, as told in several Cherokee stories. While I did not know these processes by their scientific names, I did know that *na wa te* was the energy of life coming together, in the same way that carbohydrates are precursors to sugars with enzymes, the building blocks of life. Earlier Cherokee taught that the humans share the world with the plants, which act as phytomedicines to sustain life. I knew more about ferns and fungi and saprophytes than many of my teachers. This was part of the Cherokee way of life, to understand the "underworld" as being a part of our beginning-again. We were taught the way of right relationship through the stories and teachings of nature.

Since my grandfather had to leave Mother Earth early in his life, he had others guide me in order that I might learn from the "old ones," the respected elders of the tribe. Respect for elders as teachers and "keepers of the secrets" is a way of life in my tribe. There were many who helped me through some thirty years in learning the Medicine that is shared here. Myrtle Driver, a good friend from Big Cove in Cherokee, was always willing to help me interpret some of the old language. Aunt Shirley Arch helped me to identify plants. William Hornbuckle helped me to learn the names and uses of "nature's gifts." Edmond Youngbird taught me to better appreciate nature and everything around me as having a purpose. He would talk about making baskets and using some of the same plants that were sacred as Medicine to the early Cherokee. Ann Bradley helped me to contact elders and go to the places where the "real Medicine" is—in the mountains.

These elders I have named and many others are the Cherokee people who "know these things," while I continue to be the student of nature. I also learned from writers and travelers in earlier years who braved the elements to record what they could learn about the land of the Cherokee and its indigenous people. While these early travelers may not have been able to truly understand the Cherokee way of life, they did record things lost in the changes and adaptation of the Cherokee culture. They were the true pioneers, often called "restless spirits" by earlier Cherokee.

THE CONTRIBUTIONS OF TRAVELERS

The limited literature on the subject of Cherokee herbal knowledge leads any researcher to the travel documents of John Howard Payne and William Bartram and the work of James Mooney on the Qualla Boundary in North Carolina. These documents provided important verification of the many plants by earlier generations of Cherokee. Their contribution is to be admired and appreciated when one considers what they did and the risks they took to provide their contributions to the literature and to the living history of the Cherokee.

William Bartram was a well-respected naturalist known for his travels through the Georgia barrier islands, the bayous of the Mississippi River, the savannas of Seminole country in Florida, and into the mountain home of the Cherokee. He published his findings in *Travels* in 1791, which has become a classic for botanists and naturalists. His drawings and plant identifications provided a valuable resource; while difficult to read, the book confirmed several plants that existed at that time. It also helps to distinguish some plants that were naturalized from Europe but are nonetheless very popular even today as plant remedies.

John Howard Payne provided documentation on early Cherokee ceremony and rituals in existence when the Europeans were first "discovering" the land of the Cherokee and other Native people here in North America. The documented use of pine needles and other plants as sacred drinks in ceremonies helped me verify uses of some plants that had been lost to contemporary Medicine elders. Payne, born in 1791, was an actor and songwriter and was honored as a playwright, for which he achieved his fame. Because he was in Georgia in 1835, Payne knew firsthand of the Cherokee plight. He managed to gain information from Chief John Ross that led to several published articles in that same year. Until his death in 1852, Payne wrote about the government-mandated evacuation of the Cherokee from their ancestral lands. An article by Payne that appeared in the *Quarterly Register and Magazine* in 1849 was entitled, "The Ancient Cherokee Traditions and Religious Rites." This and other writings by Payne were most helpful to me as a secondary reference.

James Mooney, in Cherokee in 1887 and 1888, documented extensive information on plants, formulas, and remedies. The syllabus created by Sequoyah in 1821 finally gave the Cherokee "paper writing" to preserve the sacred formulas for Medicine, love, hunting, fishing, foretelling the future, conjuring, and ball playing (friendly competition). These were important topics of concern among the Cherokee of that time. The Cherokee learned to read and write their own language and even had their own newspaper, the *Cherokee Phoenix*.

While working for the Cherokee Historical Association I had the opportunity to see many of these travel and research documents, catalogued by the Bureau of Ethnology and maintained in the National Archives in Washington, D.C. I was careful to use Mooney's work only as a secondary source of information or reference. His conclusions regarding the effectiveness of plants used by the Cherokee were erroneous and unfounded. However, his collection of information from the brief period he was in the Qualla Boundary region is valuable.

Mary Chiltoskey, a retired teacher from the Cherokee High School on the reservation, helped me to understand that Mooney's work had many flaws and was not well accepted by many on the reservation. When conducting my own interviews I would ask the person I was speaking with if he or she had spoken to Mary. Mary was respected by everyone, but especially the elders. Like Mary, I was quite surprised how many of the plants and their uses were remembered by the elders, and even which ones were learned or gifted from other tribes. Mary Chiltoskey was a wonderful human being, teacher, and friend of the Cherokee.

Many on the reservation have encouraged me to write this book, especially with the passing of so many of the elders who were interested in Cherokee Indian Medicine. Being a student of the Medicine for so long, it is nevertheless difficult for me to realize that now I am the elder teaching others.

RESPECT FOR THE MEDICINE VISION

Respect is a valuable Cherokee lesson to learn as a student of the Medicine. Respect for the traditions, the elders, and the Great One is foremost in the hearts and minds of Cherokee. Unlike many searchers and researchers, I had an entire lifetime to dedicate to Cherokee Medicine.

In 1960 I met several Medicine men who helped me to "seek my vision" about the Medicine. In the Cherokee tradition one does not just decide to learn the Medicine. There must be an event that leads one to the Medicine. It started for me when I had a vision at the age of twelve. Then I met Doc Amoneeta Sequoyah and his family while working at the Methodist Mission in Big Cove. Like the pieces of a puzzle, my vision came in successive moments while working for the church and going to college. My vision was to learn and to teach the Medicine. In a way the vision helped me to understand how my Irish heritage from the paternal side of my family would be so very important to my work. My father encouraged me to learn from the Medicine elders, primarily because his family lost so much of their culture after several generations away from the "motherland." As an elder put it, "You are who you are, that is for a reason. You've got to let it happen the way it's supposed to. The ancestors will decide those things when it is time. Listen to the elders. When you get through their aches and complaints, they will share a secret with you that will guide you the rest of your life. Sometimes it will come in bits and pieces, but then one day you will wake up and see what the Medicine is really all about."

I also realized that the way of right relationship is a key to many of life's secrets for harmony and balance. This was the beginning of my true understanding about the Medicine. The relationship of plants, trees, and minerals connect us to health, harmony, and a positive relationship with our environment and the Universal Circle. While this may seem trite, it is a truth in the way of Medicine.

True respect for the Medicine vision came when an elder stopped me on the road late one evening coming out of Big Cove. He said his name in Cherokee, then began speaking to me in perfect English. He said, "It is not enough to listen with your ears. You must listen with your heart. The Medicine is sacred because the Indian people keep it sacred. The people will respect you if you respect the Medicine. Look in the Four Directions for the Medicine, instead of following the way of those who brought their ways to the land of the Great One. We are a people born of the Earth Mother. We can hear her heartbeat in the drum, and we can learn more by giving thanks than by asking questions. You don't learn the Medicine, you are the Medicine."

This event changed my life. No one seemed to know the old man, nor had they ever heard of him by name. One elder just smiled when I was asking about the old man. He said, "Maybe you don't need to ask so many questions. Just listen to the messenger."

CHEROKEE INDIAN MEDICINE

What is Indian Medicine? While there are many variations in answers, the meaning of the term *Medicine* is much broader than "treatment," "health," "self-care," or "prevention." The traditional idea of Medicine is based on the earlier meanings of the four cardinal directions and the Universal Circle. When the sacred pipe was shared in the Four Directions in earlier years, each of the directions had its own prayer of thanks.

I frame the meanings of the Four Directions as spiritual in the East, natural in the South, physical in the West, and mental in the North. These broad aspects help to describe the importance and the sacred influence of each of the directions in our lives. The lines that cross from North to South and East to West represent harmony and balance. Thus, one direction in our lives does not exist without the opposite energy. Of course, everything exists within the Universal Circle of life, energy, influence, and relationship that makes up our Medicine. The phrases "Medicine bundle" or "Medicine bag" are ways of describing all that exists that influences or assists us in the circle of life.

In earlier Cherokee times the Medicine was based on formulas, and ceremony and rituals included the family, clan, and tribe. These Medicine formulas were traditional values that guided and helped the individual and family to find healing. A key in understanding Cherokee Indian Medicine is to accept that within our circle of life are influences and interferences that upset our balance and harmony as an individual and part of the family, clan, and tribe. Unlike the prevailing thought of today, the individual is not the center of the circle; he or she is an integral part of the circle. When a person fails, abuses drugs, or becomes diseased, it affects the entire circle of life. As an elder said, "Disease or illness affects all of us, not just the individual person." The Medicine is to prevent such occurrences, or to bring that harmony and balance back to the circle. The formulas and remedies respect this harmony and balance for the benefit of all in the circle.

As I stated earlier, the Cherokee formulas were more than just an herb or mixture for treating a sore or cut. There were formulas for love potions, for clearing the way to safe journeys, for seeking your own vision, for good hunting, and for planting foods. Earlier Cherokee Medicine people were well known and respected for their "strong" Medicine that attracted new relationships or resolved a relationship going on the wrong path, for finding things that were missing physically or in a person's life, for understanding the future, blocking influence or interference, influencing or conjuring in a positive and helpful way, and for being a helper in tribal decisions involving ceremonies for survival of the tribe. Of course, the listing of trees and plants in this book will only provide information for the cuts, bruises, and prevention or wellness from disease or illness as taught by the earlier Cherokee and other American Indians.

In this book, Cherokee Indian Medicine is presented according to the Four Directions. This is to facilitate understanding the manner in which the plant and natural helpers were used in an earlier time. Taken together, the Four Directions are sometimes referred to as a Medicine Wheel or Medicine Shield. Designs used on warrior shields signified one's family, animal protectors, and spirit connections. The Medicine Wheel connects us with our family, the ancestors, the Universal Circle of life, the Great One, and the guides who are special to us. Every culture's people has some form of shield that portrays who they are and what is important to them.

THE BASIS FOR CHOOSING PLANTS FOR MEDICINE

The sacredness of the numbers 4 and 7 greatly influenced almost everything in an early American Indian's life. The sacredness of the circle also figured prominently in ceremonies and even in the socialization of the families, clans, and tribes. This tradition has been brought forward today. One sacred manner of teaching and learning the Medicine was based on the four cardinal directions and their importance to American Indians. The choosing and using of plants was determined by these sacred teachings, even down to which plant was picked when out in nature. This manner of learning included asking for guidance from the ancestor spirits to have a vision of what to choose in nature for healing. Healing was not based on a treatment; it was based on a way of bringing a person into harmony and balance with their environment, keeping in mind the tremendous influence that plants, animals, birds, and everything in the environment had on early American Indians.

Unfortunately, many earlier travelers seeking to learn from the Indians were looking at the use of plants from their own approach to medicine at that time. American Indians did not have dictionaries of plant use, nor was there an Indian pharmacopeia. From a Cherokee perspective it was important to understand the relations of plants as helpers in bringing the circle into harmony and balance. The Four Directions help in describing and learning the value of plants and trees as Medicine.

MEDICINE OF THE FOUR DIRECTIONS

Framing the plants, trees, and natural substances in the Four Directions provides a guide for us to follow. Then we ask the plants to direct us on how and when to use them as helpers.

I can almost hear the reader saying, "Listen to the plants?" That takes more time and training that can be shared in this book, so I will just talk about the Medicine of using these plants as helpers in the Four Directions. The sacred formulas themselves will not be included.

Unlike in some cultures, for the Cherokee the shape of the leaves or the color of the plant does not indicate how the plant is used. We need to understand the "life values" in each of the Four Directions in order to better understand the use of certain plants. This is the way I learned the Medicine from the Cherokee elders, and I'm sharing with you here my interpretation of those teachings.

The "life values" in each of the Four Directions are as follows.

The direction of the East, or East Medicine, values the importance of family life; the importance of women as Mother Earth, those who give life; and the importance of the heart in relationships and life. The color of the East Medicine is red or yellow to represent the Sun. The key is spiritual.

The direction of the South, or South Medicine, reminds me of a child who gets a cut or sting or is exposed to the elements of nature while out playing. As an adult in earlier years working in the planting field or hunting, the outdoors exposes our exterior body and skin to many risks and harmful elements. The color of the South Medicine is white or green. The key is nature.

The direction of the West, or West Medicine, is about internal conditions and diseases that can influence the physical body and its endurance to compete in games or in life. The color is black to represent sacredness and the "darkening land"—the setting of the Sun and the protection of the Moon. The key is physical.

The direction of the North, or North Medicine, would always in early years refer to the four winds, cold weather, and calm. If the South is the child who learns, then the North is the adult who teaches. The color is sky blue, dark blue, or purple, and sometimes white to represent the sky and the snow of the North. The key is calm.

For this study of Cherokee plant Medicine it is also critical to understand what I call the Rule of Opposites. The eagle feather has two distinct colors—black and white—but in between are the variations of brown found in the eaglet's feathers. The Cherokee didn't differentiate between energies of good and bad, as all things and events in nature are related to the balance in life. As an example, it was (and still is) a strong tenet of the Medicine that a person's health and well-being is based on the balance of work and play, or ceremony. A good competitor or a peak runner understands that running as a "deer rider" exercises his physical body (West) and his spiritual body (East), and is the greatest way to succeed in his endeavor. The Rule of Opposites relates to intense energy coupled with the calm and cool to rest the body and spirit. The Chinese recognized this balance as the interplay between *yin* and *yang*. As one elder put it, "If you spend too much time being alone in the cold North, then go play in the warmth of the South. If you think too much about winning or losing the game in the West, then go join the family or have a spiritual experience in the East."

The Rule of Opposites is used in the choice of plants and their Medicine for keeping things in harmony and balance. Plant effects are referred to as stimulating or calming, and cleansing or tonifying. The energy, or *na wa te* in Cherokee, and the *chi* in Asian traditional teach-ings are similar. The teaching of the Rule of Opposites is about this movement of life force and the magnetic energy that polarizes our bal-ance in the circle of life and in the Universal Circle.

The science, art, and skills of the Medicine are very difficult to learn to apply or practice. The values of opposition and harmony were included in the formulas, prayers, and ways of practicing the Medicine. The Medicine people are to be honored and respected not only for the remedies they developed and the healing they encour-aged, but also for the traditional way of life passed down from gen-eration to generation.

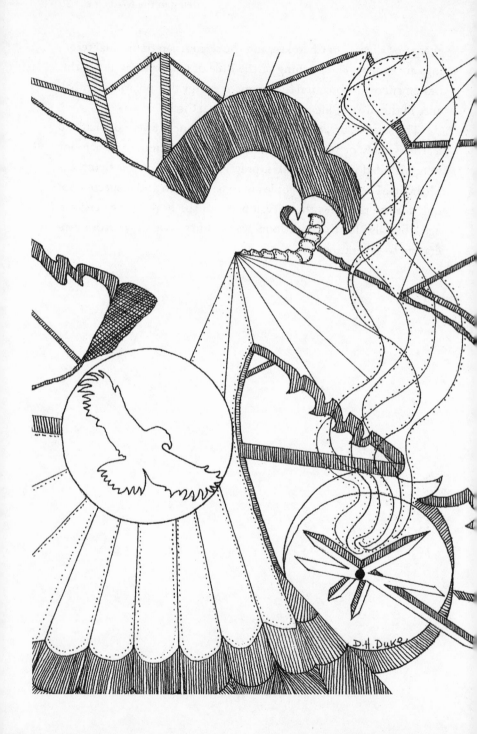

3

The Origin of Cherokee Medicine

As is the American Indian tradition of teaching with stories, the reader is asked to consider some stories about how and why some of the plants, trees, and substances came to be. As I often say, I know these stories to be true because my grandfather told them to me. After all, he always told the truth and taught me to tell the truth, so I know the stories to be true myths of the Cherokee. Several of these stories have never been shared, but "The Origin of Disease and Medicine" was recorded by James Mooney in the *Myths of the Cherokee*, his now-famous work from his time with the Eastern Band of Cherokee Indians.

A modified version of "The Origin of Disease and Medicine" will begin our story of Cherokee Medicine. As the Cherokee elders have shared and as passed down from our ancestors, the beginning always starts with a time when all the animals, birds, fish, plants, and all things on Mother Earth could speak a common language and understand each other. As the story goes, Turtle Island became crowded after the human being came to this planet. In a quest to be skillful in hunting, the human beings made spears, bows and arrows, knives, blowguns, and hooks. These were used to take the lives of the animals for their skins, and the lives of the fish and the birds. In our early traditions, a council was always called for special concerns and resolution. As was lamented in a special council, even the grubs and worms were complaining to the Great One about being crushed and stepped on by the disrespectful humans.

The bears were the first to speak in council. Old White Bear, the chief, complained about how the humans had killed their friends with disrespect. The bears called for revenge, that they should make bows and arrows to shoot back at the humans. But of course the bears knew that the string on the bow would surely get caught in their large claws, so that idea was scrapped. All the bears wanted is that the humans ask for pardon and that they give thanks when taking one of their fellow bears or their little animal friends for the meat and the skins.

Little Deer, as chief of the Deer Clan, was the next to speak in council. While the deer were certainly willing to share their beautiful skin for sacred uses and for ceremonial attire, the humans were tracking and hunting without asking permission. The deer decided that every time one of them was killed without the proper respect from the humans, they would follow the hunter in spirit and give the hunter rheumatism and pain for the rest of their lives. Of course, Little Deer was also willing to teach the humans a special prayer-chant they could use to properly hunt deer to ask for a pardon and to give thanks for the meat they would share.

The fish or "water ones," and the snakes, the "crawling ones," came forward to complain of the hooks used for fishing and the cruel treatment of snakes and worms. The snakes said they would come into the dreams of the humans to make them sick. The fish said they would give off a toxin to make the humans sick if the humans didn't treat them properly. As the rattlesnake said, "I will give them a warning, but then they must allow me to go my way." The copperhead said, "I will strike them anytime they come near me!"

The birds flew into council, with the Great Eagle leading the way. The Great Eagle also supported the worms and insects. The grubworm spoke as chief of the insects. Eagle said they had to build their nests very high to be far away from the humans, but they were concerned for the little birds whose task it was to spread flowering fruit seeds. Grubworm wanted to call for a "vote of seven," which would make the human an enemy. Even Grandfather Frog hopped in to say that the humans had stepped on his back so many times the sores were hurting him. The little birds said they were tired of the humans burning their feet in the fire.

Grubworm was so pleased with the long list of diseases the animals were concocting that he laughed so hard he fell on his back with his feet in the air. He had to crawl away on his back, which he still does today.

As the animals continued creating diseases for their human predators, the squirrel spoke up for the humans, saying, "Even though he shoots me just for fun, the humans will only pick the acorns from the ground and not dig in the special winter storage places." This displeased some of the other animals.

The plants and trees had Sunflower and Pine Tree speak as a friend to the humans. Even the mosses spoke with regard to being a helper to the humans for the diseases conjured to harm them.

Of course, the Great One wanted to be assured that the world would live in harmony and balance. The suggestion was for the humans to give thanks in the Four Directions as they prepared and shared the meal of meat, fish, fowl, and plants. It was agreed that the plants would make themselves known to the humans for protection and for ailments. To this day there are those we call upon the plants and those familiar with the plant helpers for healing and protection. For every ailment there is a healing agent among the plants that is known in spirit. This is called the Medicine, and this is the story of the Medicine, or *na wati*.

THE STORY OF THE RABBIT MEDICINE

In early Cherokee teachings the rabbit was the trickster, but he usually ended up tricking himself. The lesson of the rabbit was to listen to your own gut feeling about things. One elder said that the rabbit was an easy animal for the conjurers to enter in spirit, but they also were fearful that the rabbit would be scared to death, literally. He remembered seeing a rabbit scared so badly by a bear that the rabbit died in his tracks. When the elder looked away and looked back again he saw a glimpse of an old friend in spirit looking in fear.

The next day the elder went to see his friend, and none of the family knew where he had gone. The elder said that, to this day, his friend has not been found. Some say that he conjured his spirit to be in the rabbit that disappeared on that frightful day. These stories, while seldom heard, are nonetheless considered part of the Medicine teachings.

What can we learn from the rabbit story about Medicine? First, we can realize that fear can destroy us by literally killing our spirit. Second, that fear always shows itself, so to speak, in our actions. Even if we try to hide fear, it is still our enemy and it can still trigger anxiety reactions. As the elder said to me, "Sometimes, like the rabbit, we think we can hide the human spirit. When faced with a great fear, such as the enormity of the bear, we find ourselves unable to move from our tracks. We must learn to react quickly and experience fright and flight both!" As far as his friend goes, we learn from this story that we can project ourselves to be the trickster, or we can simply want to hide our spirit. However, there may come a time when we are revealed and have nothing to "hang our hat on," and then we are caught in another world.

So we learn from this story that the Medicine is more than just plants and herbal combinations. The Medicine is also formulas for life.

THE STORY OF ANT MEDICINE

The simple little ant was said to bring "Big Medicine" to the Cherokee. This story would have been lost if it weren't for an elder who remembered it. One cool fall morning in the mountains, the elder saw me looking down at a row of ants moving tiny bits of chicken feed from the wooden deck. He said, "Let's follow them. They go long distances from their home just to please a female in their clan. Do you think there is a lesson here for the Medicine?"

My first response was that we could learn patience from the ant. The elder responded, "Yes, but there is much more to learn about Ant Medicine." I can just imagine what someone from the outside might have thought seeing this young guy and an elder man crawling around in the dirt, the chicken feed, and whatever else there was on the ground.

We followed the ants around a post at the end of the porch and under the back edge of the house, up an ant trail to the base of a Black Jack oak tree. The elder said, "This must be over two hundred ant miles. How do you suppose they know to come all that distance to find food. Why not just take what nature provides?"

"There certainly must be a lesson here somewhere," I thought, although my belly was hungry for some lunch and my attention was growing short.

The elder went on to share a story about a simple ant who had big plans. The ant did not want to just follow the other ants—he wanted to find his own trail. One of the elder ants told Little Ant that he was being foolish, that he had much to learn about patience.

Well, the young ant decided to slip away to find some pleasure in just being free to roam the vast countryside. He found so many things to see and experience. Little Ant spoke to Rabbit as they met along a beaten path in the mountains. Rabbit said, "What are you doing, Little Ant. Why are you not with the ant troop carrying food?"

Little Ant replied, "I decided to go out on my own to see what nature is really all about, to experience life! I want to honor my clan by finding something special to share with them on my return home."

As he plopped his big hind feet on the ground, Rabbit said, "Oh, my mother told me to only stay on the trail because of the twisted laurel branches and the briars of the berry plants." Then Rabbit continued so fast that Ant could not keep up with him.

"Rabbit, where are you going?" asked Little Ant.

In a faint voice Little Ant heard Rabbit say, "I am going to find my Medicine." Suddenly Little Ant realized that that was what he was doing too—trying to find his Medicine. He was happy and excited to continue his journey to find his Medicine!

A mountain rain started to fall, a light rain that trickled through the leaves of the trees as it struck the ground. Of course, you have to imagine how a splash of a small raindrop must feel to a little ant on the ground. Little Ant was not worried because he knew to just hide under a strong leaf until the rain subsided. The rain fell harder and harder until it was coming down in "buckets full," with a flash flood occurring. Little Ant crawled onto a piece of tree bark that started to flow down the mountain on the water. Little Ant was getting scared. Oh, how would he ever get back home to his clan family and friends?

As the hard rain stopped and the sun appeared through the trees, Little Ant realized that he was far from home. What would he do now? With nothing to eat he started to nibble on the inner sides of the tree bark that had been his protector during the storm.

Ant heard a troop of ants coming in the near distance. "Rump, rump, ah hey ya hey, rump, rump. . . ." The troop of ants came nearer. As Little Ant looked closer he thought he recognized Old Elder Ant, the leader of his clan troop. "Where have you been and what have you been doing?" asked Old Elder Ant. Little Ant told him he had been looking for his Medicine. He told him of finding a protector piece of bark that had a sweet taste, and he showed Old Elder Ant the leaf. Immediately Old Elder Ant said, "That leaf and tree are not to be eaten because they will make your belly swell, according to the old ones."

Little Ant showed Old Elder Ant that he could eat it and that it was good. The others quickly started to nibble, with permission of course. Finally Old Elder Ant tried the bark too. To this day, ants will do almost anything to enjoy the taste of black cherry or wild cherry bark.

Little Ant found his Medicine, but he never again wandered away from the troop of ants.

The Cherokee elder looked at me and said, "I bet that Little Ant is now Old Elder Ant leading the troop back to the clan home." The elder said, "Like Little Ant, sometimes we have to get away from the troops to find our Medicine."

THE STORY OF DEER MEDICINE

There are many stories in the Cherokee teachings. This particular story is relatively recent in that it goes back to the early 1800s. It was passed down by my great grandfather, who was a farmer near present-day Marble, North Carolina. Many of the Rogers family still live on the old farmland on Vengeance Creek, where everyone has a story to tell and knows how to tell stories "in the old way."

This story is dedicated to Uncle Jim, who told me: "In the olden days the animals and even the plants could talk to each other. There is always a story about a plant that got its name from a special event in life." As Uncle Jim told me the story I began to realize how much we have lost in just one generation. My mind wondered a bit as he was sharing the story. I felt so grateful to have had the opportunity to learn from Uncle Jim and from several in the Rogers family.

Uncle Jim said a young deer was looking for his horns while he made friends with a young Cherokee. "Youngdeer was his name," said Uncle Jim. Unlike other adolescent deer, Youngdeer went out on his own to find his Medicine. Youngdeer thought that if he could find his Medicine he would also find his horns. Then he could be an adult and win the favor of a particular young doe.

"Well, that is another story," said Uncle Jim. Many of the stories would blend into other stories, but this one focused on a plant and how it got its name.

A young Cherokee was watching at a distance as a beautiful young woman went to the river each day to retrieve water for cooking. She had long black hair that would flow with the wind as she slowly made her way to the edge of the Oconaluftee River. The young man knew it would not be proper to just talk with the girl without getting permission from her brother—besides, he was too shy to say anything.

The young man was talking to himself when Youngdeer came by. Youngdeer asked, "Are you talking to the shrub?"

The young Cherokee, named Nip, was startled by Youngdeer's presence. As they shared names Youngdeer could not help but wonder how the young Cherokee got his name. "Well, when I am anxious about things I nip at a pine needle or a plant's leaves."

Youngdeer noticed that Nip was busy nipping at the leaves of the shrub he was obviously hiding behind.

They both saw the young woman coming down the trail. She had a beautiful round face that seemed to glow with a radiant smile. It was getting near evening. As the young woman went by with a smile on her face she lit up the dusk.

"Why don't you talk with her? I can see that you are smitten by her," said Youngdeer. Nip explained that it was the Cherokee way to be respectful and to talk with your eyes and heart.

Youngdeer continued to share with his new friend as they hunted for berries in the woods.

Youngdeer told his friend all about his search for his horns. The young Cherokee told him that his dad said that the young maiden was destined to be something special, so all he could do is enjoy her glow and presence from a distance.

It was finally time for the young deer, who noticed a nub starting to appear on his head, to continue his journey. Before leaving he wanted to share his name with the young Cherokee, which was gladly accepted.

To this day some believe this is the way that the name Youngdeer came to the Cherokee. Of course, there is also another story of how a young Cherokee became a great hunter and earned the name Youngdeer. I happen to believe that the young deer out to find his horns taught the young Cherokee the secrets of hunting for deer in the woods, how to ask for permission, and how to give thanks.

Uncle Jim went on. "Well, I almost forgot about the plant that the newly named Cherokee, Youngdeer, used to hide behind. It was a beautiful shrub about ten feet high near a stream that was fed by the Oconaluftee River. It has flowers that can hardly be seen in the summer, like the young Cherokee who hid behind the shrub. In the early autumn bright red pods appear and burst open, which have bright red to orange seeds. While it goes by many names—wahoo, arrowwood, strawberry bush, and swamp dogwood—the Cherokee call it 'hearts-a-bustin'" and "pretty by night" (*Euonymus americanus*). As this naming story goes, Youngdeer was a Cherokee who got his name because he was observed talking to a deer. His heart was busting with love for the young maiden, but he saw her for the last time on the trail carrying water, her long black hair trailing in the wind. His love was certainly "pretty by night," as she became the bright glowing moon that we see each evening, smiling down at her young lover. Some say that if you look closely behind the shrub called hearts-a-bustin' at dusk you can catch a glimpse of a young Cherokee waiting to see his love as she lights up the night sky, pretty by night. Sgi!

THE STORY OF SNAKE MEDICINE

The snake was considered a friend by the early Cherokee people. The snake was thought to have conjuring ability and could make its way into your dreams if you did the snake any harm. Early plant and natural medicine information from both the American Indians and the Europeans who moved to the Smoky Mountains includes much about snakebite remedies.

American Indian myths include stories about giant snakes that eat everything in their path, and about snakes that are invisible. Plants like the cocklebur (*Xanthium spinosum*) rattled, making the sound similar to a rattlesnake. The plant was used to mimick the sound of a snake in a chant "to awaken the spirit of the snake to go on his way." Flowers called *ou gu gu ski*, with white centers similar to an owl's eye, were used to alleviate snakebites. There was even a plant with roots that supposedly smelled like a snake. Called *ah yu ta wi gi*, or snakeroot, it was also used as a remedy for bites. (Of course, I never wanted to get close enough to a snake to smell it.) Certain young plants and roots, called *ku ne li tu*, usually a single long branch with a flower, were used for treating snakebites as well. Other snakebite remedies commonly used by American Indians include Senega snakeroot

(Polygala senega) and Virginia snakeroot *(Aristolochia serpentaria)*. The Medicine man or woman chewed the root and spit it on the bite before sucking out the poison.

When I first learned the Medicine, knowing all about Snake Medicine seemed very important to the Medicine elders who taught me. Later I understood the sacredness of the snake and how Snake Medicine would be used for treating more than just the physical bite of a snake. Pain remedies would sometimes refer to the spirit of the snake. Snake Medicine included the dogwood tree *(Cornus florida)* or basswood tree *(Tilia americana)* that was struck by lightning. The poplar tree, or tulip tree *(Liriodendron tulipifera)*, that had been struck by lightning was also considered sacred for use in Snake Medicine. Most of this knowledge has been lost; it was my desire to preserve this little understanding of Snake Medicine learned while studying Indian Medicine. The story of Snake Medicine has meaning for us today.

A young Cherokee hunter was hunting for deer. It was very cold, and the brave young Cherokee went out to get food for his family. He had heard the story of the large snake named Ou ka ti na that ate everything in its path, but he was brave and unafraid. It was cold and dark this particular evening when Youngbrave dozed off to sleep. He awoke to a slithering sound and the rustling of leaves and small twigs on the ground. Could this be the large snake that so many had spoke of but none had seen?

Youngbrave hid behind a large oak tree with bow and arrow in the cocked position. The movement stopped. Youngbrave walked around searching the area but did not see or sense anything. A hunter is taught to be sensitive to smells and sounds and to the spirits of all things in nature. Youngbrave sensed nothing, so he slowly fell back into a night slumber.

Youngbrave awoke the next morning to the rustling of leaves. A deer came onto the path only a few steps away. As taught, Youngbrave offered tobacco to Mother Earth and called upon the spirit of the deer to let him know if this was the meal and the warm deerskin for his family. The deer looked directly at him with what Youngbrave perceived as a clear signal that it was all right to shoot his swift arrow into the cold morning stillness. The arrow was perfectly on target, and the deer quietly slumped to the ground.

Youngbrave prepared to harness the deer after cutting the hind-leg muscle and tendon when he again heard the sound of rustling leaves and twigs on the ground. Youngbrave knew the sound was coming from something large, but still he could not see through the early-morning dew in what is now called the Smoky Mountains. Youngbrave hoisted the deer up onto his broad shoulders and moved quickly to a nearby clearing. Still he heard the sounds of something large slithering near him.

Youngbrave hid behind a large rock. As he lay quietly under the weight of the deer Youngbrave felt a large presence move over the top of the rock and the deer but he could see nothing. It seemed a very long time until all was quiet again. Now Youngbrave was afraid to look for fear that the face and fangs of a large snake would be looking at him. As he peered toward a bluff that led down the mountain Youngbrave saw what appeared to be a large tail moving from side to side in the cold morning dew. Then it was gone. Youngbrave ran over to the bluff, slowly looking over the edge to see what he knew would surely frighten him, but he saw nothing. He quickly put the deer back on his shoulders and moved as quickly as possible down the mountain, back to the village of his people.

Youngbrave told his story when he arrived home but everyone said that it was a myth. Besides, they said, if it had been the large snake it would have eaten him. Nobody believed Youngbrave. An elder Medicine man saw Youngbrave's downward-pointed chin and the disappointment in his eyes that no one believed him. The elder said, "You need not be sad, because I believe you. I have seen the large snake from a distance, and I hid quietly so as not to draw its attention. It had a tongue that stuck out at least twelve feet and fangs that were at least four feet long. Just be glad that you did not see the large snake because you would have dreamed about it for many moons. The reason the large snake did not eat the deer, and probably you as well, is because you sent your prayers out to the spirit of the deer to feed and clothe your family. The spirit is the same spirit that protects us all, as long as we live the right way in harmony with all the animals and Mother Earth."

With that the young Cherokee brave smiled and started sharing his experience with the Medicine man.

While neither Youngbrave nor Uncle Jim is around to share his story, some Cherokees still believe there is a large snake, or Ou ka ti na, in the mountains of North Carolina. Uncle Jim reminded me that the poisonous snake had some powerful Medicine for us while he kept things in natural order on Mother Earth. He also taught me that we could shed our skin like the snake to change ourselves with the passing of each twelve moons. "There are lessons to learn from all the four-legged ones, the winged-ones, and even those with no legs that move on our Earth Mother in their own way."

PLANT MEDICINE: A STORY OF NAMING

Now we are ready to learn how before there were scientific names of plants there was a way to "talk to the plant and to listen to how it is a helper for our Medicine bag," as one elder put it. The early Cherokee had many stories of how plants became Medicine and how each plant got its name. Naming was a very important ceremony in earlier years, and even the plants had to earn their names. There are a few plants, such as "pretty by night," that have a special story in the early Cherokee Medicine teachings. There are certain plants in each of the Four Directions that receive special recognition in ceremonies. These were names given to plants by some story or event that characterize their use or value to early American Indians. For example, Adam and Eve root, or puttyroot (*Aplectrum hyemale*), has special significance in the Medicine of the East, with the dried bulbs used in ceremony for the "joining" of two people. The bulb of this orchid is still used by some in the mountains of Appalachia for treating bronchial illness. Certain Cherokee were the keepers of the formulas. This formula for bronchial relief was passed down by Jimmik, and the story by Tanasky. While I did not know these members of my tribe, who were from different clans than my own, I felt that I knew them through the stories that were passed down.

Angelica plant, or *e me nah* (also the Cherokee expression for "Amen"), is a "prayerful plant that does as much good for the spirit as it does the body." This information was passed down by a Cherokee elder by the name of White Path. Today angelica is used as a digestive aid, but it was also mentioned by the name of watch when used for female menstrual concerns.

These elder Medicine people have passed on, and my concern is that the stories and uses of plants could be lost forever if not shared now.

There are certain plants, such as bear's foot and bear grass, that are mentioned in East Medicine as having special use that is considered sacred and not to be shared. I am comfortable that a Cherokee family will continue to be the keeper of its use. However, the common use of bear's foot in earlier years was for expelling afterbirth. While bear's foot is not used today, there may be an agent in the plant that will have special medicinal value to us in the future. Bear grass, or yucca as it is called today, was used with the North Carolina longleaf pine as a ritual drink in the Green Corn Ceremony. As far as I know, bear grass's use and "value" have been lost. I feel that someone out there must have heard something about this plant and its ceremonial use from a member of his or her family, as a kind of oral knowledge passed down from generation to generation. Maybe someday these old formulas and their "value" teachings will be revived and preserved for tomorrow.

The cardinal flower listed in the East Medicine, like the cardinal itself, has stories about its value and use with Indians in North

Carolina. The flower is very distinctive in the Appalachian Mountains, as it stands nearly three feet high with lance-shaped leaves and a beautiful crimson flower. Somehow the earlier Cherokee knew it was a cousin to the great blue lobelia with its purplish blue flowers. The other cousin was Indian tobacco, which was used for sacred purposes and when saying prayers or giving thanks to the Great One.

Mistletoe has been used in many cultures for stealing a kiss from a sweetheart. To the early Cherokee and for many tribes in the Southeast, mistletoe was an important East Medicine used in ceremonies. While this use is considered sacred and therefore will not be described, mistletoe was also commonly used in Appalachia for nervous conditions, especially in women. Its uses for improving blood vessels and healing infections probably deserve more attention, especially in regard to conditions of irregular heartbeat and tension. Mistletoe is of synergistic value to the trees, a fact that has intrigued both Indians and non-Indians alike in North America. A Cherokee elder agreed that the "kiss and tell" feature of mistletoe was certainly a good use learned from non-Indian visitors to these shores, but "mistletoe's value to calm the nerves of the female may be a better use," although, as the elder admitted, "kiss and tell was more fun."

Burdock as a South Medicine seems to be universal in its early use as a poultice for treating skin irritation and sores, as well as a natural antiseptic. Doc Amoneeta Sequoyah taught me to enhance burdock's value as a Medicine by including chamomile, comfrey, crowfoot, dock, evening primrose, and goldenseal as a mixture of seven sacred plants. This was considered an ultimate natural-healing formula. With all those powerful agents, burdock was respected as "the one that makes them work best as Medicine."

An elder told the story of once being chased by a black bear in the mountains. As he was running through the weeds his hands and arms got scratched all over. He finally got away from the bear, who found a honey pot in a nearby tree. The elder sat there aching from running and from the cuts and scratches. He looked around for some plantain, but there was none to be found. Removing all the burrs and brambles that had gotten stuck to his pants he was reminded to pick some burdock leaves for making a wash to soothe the aching cuts and to gather some willow bark for the pain. While he did not learn the lesson to leave a mama bear and her cubs alone, he was thankful for being a Cherokee and knowing how to take care of himself in the mountains.

Indian tobacco is a South Medicine plant that was used in early years to treat ringworms and insect bites. "A Cherokee would not be in the woods without his tobacco, because you might want to pray with it or put it on a sting or insect bite," said an elder. There is a sacred story about how Indian tobacco came to be a gift from the Great One as a special Medicine for Indian people. Indian tobacco, or *Lobelia inflata,* is valued for an alkaloid called lobeline that has been used in anti-smoking preparations. The Indian way to use the plant was to crush the leaves to make a formula for treating intestinal problems and diarrhea, as well as for asthma and severe coughs. The Cherokee enjoyed Indian tobacco for use against insect bites, sores, and ringworm.

A very old formula listed mullein leaves as Indian tobacco. An old Cherokee story referred to Indian tobacco as a means for opening the lungs in order to "run in spirit" for competitions, such as Indian ball, and for running messages to and from Cherokee villages.

Passionflower is a South Medicine that is also an East Medicine. As an elder put it, "It [passionflower] can heal a bruised body or a bruised heart." As a South Medicine the leaves were crushed and used as a poultice for bruises and injuries. Some folks thought it to be a special Medicine "for making you stronger in love." Another elder said, "It won't spark your fire, but it will calm your flames." The plant was also mixed with peppermint leaves and used as a calming tea.

Ga ni qui li ski, or self-heal, and seven-bark shrub (also called wild hydrangea) were old remedies mixed in a formula as South Medicine. Wintergreen and sometimes willow bark were added to make a special

Medicine. With much antiseptic and antibacterial value, this formula had to be a good remedy for "whatever ails you with the skin."

Certain plants received their names from humans observing the plant's use by animals. While not mentioned in this book, rabbit pea was used in a formula for treating both intestinal worms and chronic cough. The plant, also called Virginia tephrosia *(Tephrosia virginiana),* or "devil's shoestring" by mountain folks, has been used to treat bladder problems. The Indian name comes from the pealike pod that grows in open and dry fields and woods. The pod is "like the rabbit that eats it as a special food." As the elder said, "You can see the young rabbits hopping around in a field of 'rabbit pea' just having a ball, hiding in the plants while eating the pods."

Racoonberry, or Indian apple, another plant with animal associations, is mentioned under the South Medicine. It was used by American Indians to treat warts and moles. The mountain folks called it "mandrake"; the plant is more commonly known as mayapple *(Podophyllum peltatum).* Racoonberry received its name from "several raccoons playing in a very wet and covered part near Ivy Log. As they grabbed the yellow plums they would throw them to each other as though they were playing catch." While there may be other stories for how mayapple got a local name, the resin from the plant was used for getting rid of warts. As one elder said, "There is a story about how the frog was looking for 'Indian Apple' to cure its back of the warts, or just give warts to the people who would get in his path or handle him."

There are numerous stories about plants used by animals for cures and for improving competition in "the games that animals play with each other." These stories are found in the Medicine of the West, or "Animal Medicine." There is a story of the tree squirrels living high in the balsam fir trees. "Being sticky, the other animals and even the birds did not like resting or nesting in the balsam fir and the tall pine trees. There used to be a small black squirrel, called *sa lo li,* who lived and hid there. When someone would come nearby the squirrel would throw the small cones to scare the person away. These small cones would sometimes cause cuts and scratches. One day a young Cherokee was trying to get some of the live needles from the balsam tree to use in a sweat, 'cause back then they would use them on hot coals for inhaling, to treat colds and a bad cough. Well, the squirrel was going to have none of needle collecting so he started throwing the cones down on the young Cherokee, who they now call Squirrel. The young man was so cut and scraped that he sat down and rubbed some of the resin on the cuts. Lo and behold, the abrasions started to go away. To this day balsam resin is used for sores and cuts, and it is even used in a poultice for the back and chest, while the needles are still used in sweats."

The North Medicine, or "Wind Medicine," included many trees in the Appalachian region. The inner bark of the trees was used in formulas for lung conditions and colds. There is one story about Bear and Rabbit discussing "a good smoke to clear the lungs." Rabbit said that he found what he called "rabbit tobacco" to be the best for clearing the lungs by a smoke in the early morning. Bear said that "bearberry," which is listed in the North Medicine, would take the edge off the bitter tobacco that Rabbit smoked and it would relax the spirit as well. They both knew that the wild tobacco, or Indian tobacco, was good for the lungs, but it was also so strong that it would sometimes make you sick.

Bear was climbing a black cherry tree one early morning, just trying to find a good place to sit and have a smoke. As he was climbing the tree he happened to notice Youngbear in the distance. "She was a fine-looking bear, just strutting as she was walking briskly through the woods." Bear lost his composure and slipped on the cherry tree. His tobacco got lodged in the strips of bark as his paws scratched through the inner bark. Bear continued up the tree to find a good spot to have his smoke and to catch a glimpse of Youngbear when she strutted back through the woods.

"Hum," said Bear. "What is this unusual taste with my tobacco?" He thought maybe something had been planted too close to the tobacco plant; then he remembered holding the tobacco in his mouth and claw as he was climbing. The taste was sweet and the aroma was very nice.

While Bear could not wait to share his newfound "smoke" with the other animals, he did not know that Rabbit was watching him. Rabbit immediately tried some of the wild cherry bark with his tobacco, and it tasted very good. He hopped down to where the council was in session to share that he, Rabbit, had a new tobacco. The council members tried the smoke and all loved it. Here came Bear as he lumbered in to council with his new find. Rabbit said immediately that Bear was sitting high in the black cherry tree while Rabbit was trying different inner barks with his tobacco.

Well, the council told Bear that he better go back to his bear-berry. Some say that Bear was so upset that he started using the bearberry for urinary tract problems, and that is how we got the common expression used today to describe our condition when we're really upset ("pi--ed off"), as well as a good remedy for urinary tract problems.

Another plant listed in the North Medicine that had a story of interest to me is pleurisy root. When Little Butterfly was just a small larva he noticed the white silky strands on the seeds that seemed to glow in the sunlight. He knew that was something he wanted to investigate when he was able to fly. He didn't have much fun being enclosed, but there were those birds out there who would be glad to have him for a meal.

The other insects and animals seemed to not pay attention to Little Butterfly. He decided to show them something that would be important to them—the plant he had his eye on while hiding inside the cocoon.

Suddenly it was time for him to come out of the cocoon and fly as a beautiful yellow butterfly. Several of the animals and humans had colds, and they could not seem to "shake the winter's edge." Little Butterfly noticed they had coughs so he told them about this beautiful plant with silky fuzz on a stalk with long narrow leaves and bright orange flowers, and with seeds with silky hairs.

At first the animals and the humans said, "Ah, you just noticed the fuzzy hairs because you were a larva in a cocoon, because that's what kept you warm. The plant you speak of is just a weed." One human was tired to the point of coughing and hacking, so he tried Little Butterfly's suggestion and boiled the entire plant as a drink. To the human's surprise his condition started clearing up and the cough was going away. Little Butterfly was given the Cherokee name of *ka ma ma,* and the plant was given the name of butterfly weed.

Each of the plants and natural substances has its origins and is a member of a family. It may be possible that each has its own tribe, and possibly were able to communicate with animals and humans in another time. As you read through the Medicine in the Four Directions in the next part of this book, consider all the possibilities of how plants were named for their use and that many of them are also related to animals.

We will start with the East Medicine, which is a helper to us in our coming into this world and supports our spirit life "by the wind from the north greeting the Sun, that generates life." Then we will spiral to the South Medicine, where we will grow from the natural foods and Medicine helpers "for competition as ball players and dancers," coming into the West Medicine, where we "learn our limitations and experience our youthful challenges." Then we will spiral to the North Medicine, where we will learn and teach the Medicine as adults. Finally, "we will share the wind of life with others in the spirit world as we move to our place in the universal tribal council."

Being in the Medicine is a way of being in harmony and balance within your own circle of life, and within the Universal Circle as a helper of all beings and a protector of Mother Earth. Enjoy your journey into plants as Medicine in the Four Directions.

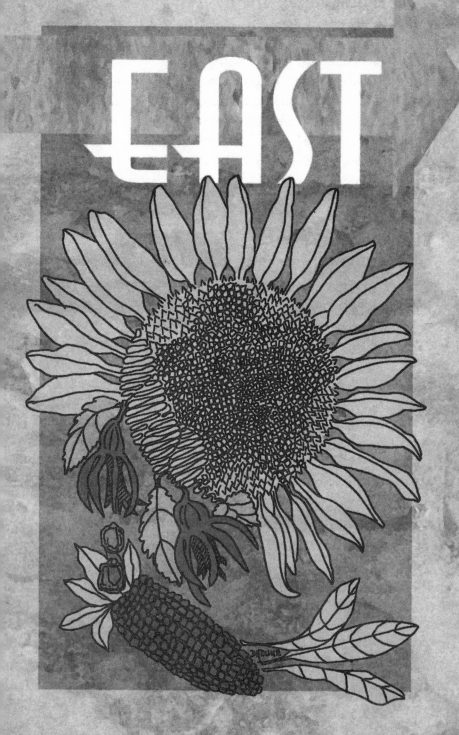

EAST

4

Plant Medicines of the East

East Medicine focuses on the viability of the heart and of the energy within the body relative to the Universal Circle, the environment of our lives. It also includes plants and natural agents used in the seven traditional ceremonies of the Cherokee. (These ceremonies included the Green Corn Ceremony, Fall Festival, Summer Planting, Friend-making Ceremony, Great New Moon, First New Moon of Spring, and Seventh Year Ceremony.) Fire is the "center" of the Four Directions, with the direction of the Sun (East) being paramount in Cherokee sacred ceremonies (as it is for most American Indian tribes).

The elders were considered keepers of the universal knowledge—the teachings or sacred ways, and the secrets passed down from the ancestors. While some might say the old ways are lost, there is a body of knowledge that is alive in every tribe. As an elder said, "It [sacred teachings] is alive in every cell of our body and in every living and nonliving thing we see here on Mother Earth."

The East Medicine teachings begin with a story of the beginning of life, which starts with the center, the sacred fire. East Medicine is our spirit connection to the otherworld. The elders would say that the East is the beginning and the spiritual basis of the family, clan, and tribe. We are here for a purpose—to be protectors of Mother Earth and helpers to all living things. This is the first and last statement of our covenant with life, according to the old wisdom.

The color associated with the East is red, or yellow for some tribes. These colors represent the power of the Sun, sent by the Great One to look over us while also providing warmth and nourishment for the plants and trees to bear food and fruit.

East is considered the direction of the beginning of life, of ceremonies, and of sacred teachings for preservation of the tribal way of life. Little is said openly about the East Medicine except by the Medicine men and women, or by the elders as keepers of the wisdom. In earlier years only certain tribal members were chosen to learn the East Medicine, the sacred ways of ceremonies.

In the old Cherokee stories there were "apportioners," such as the Sun and the Thunder Beings, who were assigned the tasks of overseeing life here on Mother Earth. Certain members of the tribe were chosen to "learn and understand these sacred things" and to commune with the apportioners. This was similar to a minister receiving "the calling" to preach, or a person finding herself in a critical position in life where a decision was made for her to be a special leader or helper.

The East was considered the "open door," the direction we are born into in this life to meet the Sun. Conversely, the West, the direction of death and passing from this world to the otherworld of our ancestors, was considered the "back door," with spirit guides as the gatekeepers to the "darkening land." The sacred teachings taught us that life and death were experiences of the spirit moving through a doorway or a portal, from which we continue our journey.

The plants, we are taught, are our allies and helpers for preservation of life in their serving as food and Medicine. Certain plants were considered sacred and had a special place beyond food and Medicine. The sunflower *(Helianthus annuus)* was one of those special plants that represents humility and power, its bright yellow color being "the spirit of the Sun that is always in the planting fields of native people everywhere in the world," says an elder teacher. The sunflower is a reminder to us that everything on the planet has value for survival and energy. As an example, sunflower oil was used in cooking and the seeds were used to thicken the mush and dough for bean bread as a food. The elders would say that sunflower seeds were "good for the body and the spirit."

As one teaching elder said, "The sunflower stands in the crossroad between us and the mighty mountains of Peru, while it is the rainbow connection between native people in the East and the sacred people of the West." Some elders say the sunflower was the first plant to greet the newcomers to the shores of North America, while other elders said it stood as a sign to let all know they were on sacred ground. The many petals and seeds of the sunflower represented the fertility of this land and its way of life that will always survive, as long as we save four seeds during the winter months to plant again in the spring.

The East also represents the female and male energies and the gift of birth, or "beginning-again." Female energy focuses on producing life, while male energy is directed toward serving and protecting life. Many elders say that the female energy is the strongest energy in life. To the elders, birth was a special event deserving of ceremony, a time to give thanks to the Great One for the gift of life. It was considered a beginning-again, another opportunity to follow the "way of right relationship." In this way birth not only meant bringing a child into the world but could also refer to embarking on a new path or opportunity, or renewing commitment to a well-traveled path.

Much of the plant Medicine of the East is focused on females, birthing, and the physical challenges of being female. As a Natchez-Cherokee elder said, "All the Native peoples knew of the love Medicine of the Cherokee. It was powerful, and they knew of the formulas gifted by the Great One to resolve the problems of women. We were taught from an early age that as American Indians we were the keepers of Mother Earth. We were told that we could speak to the plants in an earlier time, so we knew what to do about these things. We know these things today!" The Medicine of the male was mostly about ceremony, strength, endurance, and protection. Together as male and female we are one.

Cherokee Medicine in earlier years consisted of formulas made of plants and other natural substances. The natural substances included water, considered sacred when used in healing; ashes from certain woody trees; minerals from shells and rocks; and nature's gifts, such as a bee's wing. The focus in this book will be plant-derived substances used in formulas, called *remedies* by the non-Indians who settled in North America. Formulas usually consisted of four plants or barks, or as many as seven for certain sacred formulas. Few plants were used alone except as a "first-response" remedy, such as holding a root on an aching tooth or using a plant to stop the bleeding at a wound. When two plants were mixed it was usually to balance each other, such as a calming agent mixed with a stimulant. Mixtures of three plants were considered a "special Medicine" for "calling on the Sky Vault spirit ones to drive away bad spirits." Mixtures of four helpers were the usual formula remedy. Five plant helpers would be a ceremonial mixture and six would be for "spirit work." Mixtures of seven substances were usually used for sacred Medicine and tonics.

The direction of the East is associated with family, clan, one's support circle, and protection of the circle of family and friends. The East Medicine is about the heart; herb formulas of the East Medicine include blood-building tonics and tonics for energy, as well as plants and substances that are purifiers, "for cleansing and clearing the body and the blood for Good Medicine." Earlier Indian people understood the heart as an organ of special strength. The blood was thought of as similar to the water that flows through Mother Earth. The heart was considered as having a separate spirit, a life of its own within the physical body. The heart was much more than just a physical muscle and a pump. While the blood supplied life to the rest of the body, the spirit energy of the heart connected the physical body of a human to Mother Earth and to the Great One. The plants associated with the heart are considered "special Medicine."

The plants and formulas of the East Medicine offer protection energy. When the family was protected the members could come together in ceremony, to share and enjoy activities together. When you feel the protection energy of the East you can face the Sun and give thanks, recognizing the power of plants and natural substances as "helpers" protecting and preventing disease or harm, or restoring balance. Many of the formulas of the East are cleansers, intended for detoxifying the body. Often referred to as "blood purifiers," these formulas protect us and bring us into balance.

The Sun provides heat and light energy to the Earth Mother to grow plants and trees for food, shelter, and Medicine. The formulas of the East provide this same kind of nurturance and balance. In the East Medicine there are formulas for slowing down the body and others for stimulating the body or increasing energy. In addition to the use of plants, many formulas also included minerals and animal or insect parts. In this book I will include no mention of these additional ingredients, because they were considered sacred and only to be known by the keepers of the formulas. I honor that sacredness.

In relation to the heart, in the East Medicine there were also special Medicines, potions for love or for "catching the right person," as one elder put it. Myths and Medicine came together sometimes for influence and interference—depending on the practitioner's focus, conjuring was either considered a form of "good Medicine" or "bad Medicine." I suspect that the terms *good* and *bad* came into the Medicine vernacular with European and religious influences. An elder related, "There was no 'good' and 'bad' before the White man; Medicine was a matter of choice and influence."

These formulas referred to as "good" and "bad" Medicine were only known to the tribal "keepers of the secrets." For example, the power of the Cherokee love Medicine was well known by other tribes. It was a spirit influence meant to favor a relationship, to keep people together, or to help people find each other. The healing formulas were "power Medicines" to positively affect a person, family, or tribe, and especially to guard against negative influences.

Many of these old Cherokee formulas were kept in what one elder referred to as the "old black book." This reference was confusing, as the Bible was also sometimes referred to as the "black book." However, a few books of formulas written in Cherokee do exist. As an elder said, "The words were finally printed in the old Cherokee language, 'cause we didn't have the old meeting or coming-together like we used to." In earlier days the Medicine men and women would get together and visit with each other, and would even invite visitors from other tribes. It was a time of celebration and sharing, and a time of learning about new formulas, or *doh de wah wi ski huh*.

The elders who remembered these gatherings fondly recalled the power that showed itself when everyone met in a circle with drumming, songs, and sharing. I suspect that after about 1920 the Cherokee Medicine Society and its gatherings were discontinued. With the loss of these gatherings we also lost a way of life. Fortunately, there is a new energy and interest that is recapturing this old way.

While in this book I am willing to share information on the uses of many plants employed in Cherokee Medicine, I cannot share the sacred formulas and prayer-chants. However, there is much richness in the teachings about the plants. Indian Medicine has much to offer the world in teachings about preserving health and about healing of the body, mind, and spirit using the plants and trees that are gifts to us all. Many herbal reference books provide remedies and formulas that are known in different cultures of people here on Mother Earth. My purpose in writing this book is to preserve Cherokee knowledge and to educate, not to provide any form of treatment modality or therapy. In this respect, my role is as a keeper of the Medicine. It is my hope and vision that the information shared about the plants and trees, and the stories, will encourage the reader to learn more about our helpers in the natural world.

This next part the chapter provides a listing of plants of the East Medicine, including the plants' common and scientific names. The Cherokee name for the plant is also included when known or able to be shared. Coming from a mixed (Indian and non-Indian) heritage, I truly respect and appreciate the gifts from all those who settled here on Turtle Island. My father, Jasper Garrett, would always say, "Mountain folks know these things."

Instead of referring to people as Indians or non-Indians, I prefer to use the term *mountain folks* to reference the non-Indian people of the Smoky Mountains, the Appalachia, and the ridge of mountains covered by the Blue Ridge Parkway from North Carolina to New York. I truly respect their survival knowledge passed down from their European (or other) ancestry.

It has been my intent to share Cherokee knowledge about plants as related by elders, using references only to verify certain uses. The information in this book has been collected over the course of more than four decades from conversations with elders. The elders did not want to be treated as informants but as teachers of nature and experience. Actually, I believe that those elders created this document as a summary of their real-life experiences. The information spans many generations of the ancestors.

I hope the reader can appreciate the enormous costs that would have been associated with showing pictures of all the plants discussed. Some wonderful illustrated books that can be used for reference are listed in the bibliography. Well-known herbal references include works by James A. Duke, Ph.D., and Arnold Krochmal. Also helpful is the *Physician's Desk Reference for Herbal Medicines,* and a more recent book by Fetrow and Avila entitled *The Complete Guide to Herbal Medicines.* Cherokee elders and others provided valuable information on plants and stories that would absolutely have been lost without their transmission. Mary Chiltoskey was able to validate much of what I learned on the traditional uses of many plants. Unfortunately many of the incantations and prayer-chants used with the plants for healing have been lost. Thankfully elders such as Geet Crow and Walter Calhoun have kept many songs, dances, and ceremonial chants alive.

While in this book I am less concerned with noting chemical constituents and active components of the plants discussed, I do make note of such substances as tannins in plants, which are astringents. I do feel it is critical for students of herbology to understand a plant's chemical actions and reactions in the body for safe use of plants as agents of health and healing. For instance, components such as flavones or flavonoid glycosides have varying diuretic and circulatory effects in the body; while milk thistle's flavonoid can aid the liver, the standardized content is critical. Chemicals such as saponins, which have a strong anti-inflammatory action, are also related to the synthesis of sex hormones. Such is the case with wild yam and red clover; both have some estrogenic ability. Some commonly used plants, such as goldenrod and mullein, have anti-inflammatory value.

There is mention here of such plants as foxglove and lily-of-the-valley, but caution is a must with these cardiac glycosides—it is advised that these be administered only by a physician or those trained in the safe use of herbs. The volatile oils commonly found in aromatic plants, such as lavender or passionflower, have been marketed as perfumes. The aromatic oils of garlic and thyme are also antiseptics, which enhance the immune system. I tend to think of these plants as relaxing for the nervous system. Plants that contain volatile oils must be stored in sealed containers to keep the oils from evaporating.

While I have not mentioned anything here about the principles of bitters and other chemical contributions of plants, the reader will want to consider these and all other valuable effects of a plant in creating her own Medicine bag. The point is this: *Do your research and refer to the experts before using anything listed in this book for any purpose.*

Now we are ready to take our journey through the Medicine of plants as helpers to us in the East. Some plants listed here are not commonly used today, but there are probably some Medicine people or "keepers of the knowledge" who still have these plants in their Medicine bag. From the chemical actions of plants and their precautions to the building of formulas, we must remember that for many generations American Indians have specially trained some tribe members to better understand plants in regard to their actions and effects. The information presented here is given as a starting point for the reader to search other resources and to begin a relationship with the plants of the East. As my grandfather Oscar Rogers said, "Learn to respect the plants, use them in the way of right relationship, give the proper thanks, and they will be healing helpers to you and me."

The following is a listing of plants and their uses as East Medicine.

Adam and Eve root *(Aplectrum hyemale)*. Commonly known as putty-root, or *ta li, tsi ge yu i* in Cherokee, Adam and Eve root was used in ceremonial Medicine for joining a man and woman. This element of the wedding ceremony is still used today. The elder who taught me this ceremony said it was used to see if the couple would stay together. The dried root would be placed in the right hand of the Medicine man or beloved elder. The Medicine man would shake that hand. As the tradition is described, the couple will stay together if the root pieces come together in the Medicine man's hand. If the root pieces did not come together, one of the seven chosen counselors would work with the couple, or the man and woman "would be separated until they find their love."

If the root pieces joined in the Medicine man's hand, the larger corm would be given to the woman to keep in her Medicine bag, and the smaller corm was given to the man in the joining ceremony. The corms would be placed in a wedding bowl, a pottery vessel with two openings, with prayers for the coming together and staying together. The ceremony was intended to be a reminder that it takes both corms, or two people, "to make up Adam and Eve, just as the Eagle feather has two energies for balance," as one elder put it. Adam and Eve root is a member of the Orchid family.

Adam's needles (see Bear grass).

Agrimony *(Agrimonia gyposepala* and *A. parviflora)*. Also called tall Harry agrimony, or *a la s ga lo gi* in Cherokee, this plant was used in a formula as a blood purifier and tonic. Agrimony *(Agrimonia)* is not to be confused with tansy *(Tanacetum vulgare)*, which is colloquially called wild agrimony. An elder called agrimony "speckled," or *u nv tsa dv*.

Agrimony was used by the ballplayers in "little wars," or games of competition, each day for seven days before the game. Several plants for strength and clarity were used for four days prior to the competition. An elder described agrimony as "a sticky shrub burr that sticks to clothing or the fur of animals to ride anywhere."

Also called "liverwort" by people in Appalachia and "cocklebur" or "beggar lice," it is a member of the Rose family. One elder remembered agrimony leaves used as an astringent to stop bleeding. My father called it "church steeple," probably because of the plant's towering spires of flowers. Agrimony is still popular as a mild astringent that has antifungal and antibacterial properties.

Alder (*Alnus serrulata* and *A. glutinosa*). Known as alder, red alder, or tag alder, the bark of this small tree is called *gi ga ge i* in Cherokee. European settlers used alder for its shade and for ornamental purposes. The Cherokee used the inner bark of the black alder as an astringent to stop bleeding.

Common alder *(A. serrulata)*, a member of the Birch family, is also known as hazel alder and tag alder. Common alder was used in a tea for the pains of birthing, for treating swelling and fever, and as a blood purifier and tonic when combined with Indian root. An elder mentioned its use as a helper for high blood pressure and "for those with weak hearts."

Another elder, who called the tree "tag alder," or *tsa ta na* in Cherokee, described it as "water Medicine," because it grows near rivers. Common alder acts as a hemostatic to stanch or reduce bleeding. It was used as a tonic in a formula given to all participants at ceremony. Alder and black walnut were used to make brown dye for baskets and ceremonial masks.

Alfalfa (*Medicago sativa*). Alfalfa, or buffalo plant, was called *so qui li* in Cherokee. Alfalfa was a gift from the Europeans, who used it in a tonic to improve energy according to one elder. Tribes would put it in their formulas for ballplayers, runners, and other competitors, who took the forumula every day for seven days before an event. It was probably introduced to Indians by the Spanish, but the word *alfalfa* is Arabic. One elder called it *ya na s gi*.

Alfalfa is a member of the Pea, or Bean, family. The leaves may have estrogenic value when taken as a tea; alfalfa sprouts have been found to contain phytoestrogens. Alfalfa sprouts can be crushed and spread on salads or used in a salad dressing. It is a mountain remedy for diabetes and postbirthing problems associated with thyroid ailments. Saponin, an active compound of alfalfa, acts on the cardiovascular and nervous systems.

Allspice or pimento tree (*Pimenta dioica*). Allspice is the fruit of the pimento tree. The pimento tree was called *e tsi* or *eg sig*. This plant helper is used by women to control discharges when the monthly bleeding is especially profuse. It was used as an astringent and stimulant with other plants in a very old Cherokee formula. It was probably traded in early years for furs and other plants, the spice being recognized by Alabama tribes as a special flavor in cooking. An elder said that early Cherokee enjoyed using spices when cooking deer meat and fish, adding sweet berries and leaves for flavor. Today allspice is more popularly used for indigestion, similar to the way papaya was used on the Pacific Islands.

Alumroot *(Heuchera americana)*. Alumroot is an old remedy to "stop the bleeding for women giving birth, as well as for cuts in the skin." A formula used alumroot, wild geranium (also called alumroot), purple coneflower, and other plants. Formulas usually contained three, four, five, or seven plant helpers based on sacred chants in the formula. A typical chant would start with "Hey ya, hey ya, hey he . . ." and then the plant would be mentioned as a helper, giving thanks to the Great One for healing. Wood or common avens *(Gerum urbanum)*, a member of the Rose family, was used in one of the old formulas with alumroot. While difficult for me to identify, common avens has three lobed leaves and a bright yellow flower of five petals with unique green spines between each petal. An elder pointed out that alumroot has a clovelike smell, an indication of its tannin properties and essential oils. Alumroot is used with flowering dogwood to stop bleeding and for reducing pain.

Amaranth *(Amaranthus hypochondriacus* and *A. sanguineus)*. Called spring amaranth or blood plant, amaranth was used to relieve profuse menstruation. Mary Chiltoskey mentioned it being used ceremonially in Green Corn Medicine, following the harvesting of corn in September and October. An elder told me that amaranth would be given to the family of young girls during Green Corn Ceremony. The plant was held when the young woman had her first bleeding. Mountain folks called amaranth "lady bleeding." Blood plant is not to be confused with bloodroot *(Sanguinaria canadensis)*.

American hellebore (see Indian poke).

American maidenhair (see Fern, maidenhair).

Angelica *(Angelica archangelica)*. Also known as masterwort, this plant was used as a calming agent by many in the Appalachian mountains. An elder referred to the plant as green bread, or *ga du, a tse he*. The elder could not remember why it was called green bread but also remembered the plant being called prayer plant, or *e me hah*.

Angelica is used for stimulating appetite, especially for women who have been through birthing, and for the elderly for enhancing energy. The earlier Cherokee believed women who were "weakly" could be stimulated to health with a tonic made of angelica and with the help of other blood builders used in traditional sweats. Another elder referred to *Angelica atropurpurea* as "hunting root."

As a member of the Carrot or Parsley family, angelica contains some fifteen anti-arrhythmic compounds, according to James Duke, Ph.D. One of those compounds is the same active ingredient found in the drug Verapamil, a calcium-channel blocker used for treating irregular heartbeat. Angelica is also used for treating indigestion and stomach cramps.

Today angelica is used to relieve postmenopausal symptoms, gynecological disorders, and menstrual discomfort. A cousin plant, dong quai *(A. sinensis)* is a popular Chinese remedy for regulating menstrual disorders and relieving menopausal symptoms. A Chinese delegation to the Cherokee reservation in 1981 was elated to learn that earlier Cherokee also used angelica for similar complaints, as well as for easing the pains of rheumatism or arthritis and as a natural antispasmodic. Men also used it for increased testicular hormone effect.

Chasteberry *(Vitex agnus castus)* is more widely used today as a tonic for normalizing reproductive function and stimulating progesterone production (which normalizes many menopausal symptoms). Earlier Medicine men and women used red clover with angelica for a similar effect.

When considering using phytoprogesterones be sure to consult a physician or a trained herbalist before beginning treatment, for followup concerning your symptoms, and for receiving a preparation with standardized content. Do not use angelica during pregnancy.

Arrowwood shrub *(Viburnum dentatum)*. Also called southern arrowwood, the stems of this shrub were used for making arrows in earlier years. The fruit was gathered to attract birds such as the tanager for its special feathers, used for ceremonial purposes. Arrowwood is a member of the Honeysuckle family.

Ash tree *(Fraxinus americana* or *Sorbus americana)*. American mountain ash, or rowan tree *(S. americana),* was said to be from Roan Mountain in North Carolina. The leaves were crushed for a wash used to cleanse women after childbirth. Ash tree has astringent properties and was used in a tonic formula for "women's needs." It is also used by women as a diuretic, and for bladder complaints.

White ash *(F. americana)* was used to control bleeding due to its tannins and analgesic properties. The inner bark is used for treating fever and as a tonic. Also called Biltmore ash, the tree was used in earlier years for making canoes and oars as well as baseball bats.

Balm, melissa *(Melissa officinalis)*. Lemon balm, bee balm, and balm mint all belong to the Mint family. An elder called the plant "bee," or *wa du li si*. Balm is used to make salves; the leaves are also used to make cold drinks or hot tea. A cold drink popular in earlier years was concocted by letting the crushed leaves sit in water for at least four hours.

An elder said balm is considered an important East Medicine as a helper for women with headaches and anxiety during menstruation. The lemonlike aroma of the plant is most apparent before flowering, which is when the leaves are picked for formulas to ease nervousness and insomnia related to menstruation. Balm is a mild sedative with antiviral and antibacterial value and calming hormonal effects. It is prepared as a tea with two teaspoons of chopped leaves and used as an antispasmodic for stomach upset.

Balm was used in several formulas to calm the spirit of a person who was upset or "acting strange." The remedy for this condition included peppermint and a stronger sedative, such as valerian or skullcap. Lemon balm is used for insomnia related to nervous agitation and for sleep problems, especially of women. It is also used as an antiviral and antibacterial substance. The volatile oils provide antidepressant and sedative value for treating anxiety, insomnia, headaches, and heart palpitations. Balm should only be used for these treatments under the supervision of those trained in the medicinal use of plants.

Balsam apple *(Echinocystis lobata)*. Also known as Indian or wild cucumber, an elder said that the northeastern Indians used this plant for a love potion. The earlier Cherokee used it as a love Medicine and, when combined with dogwood, as a pain reliever to break a fever and the sweats, especially for females during their menstruation.

Banesberry *(Eryngium aquaticum* and *E. yuccifolium)*. This plant is also called button snakeroot, and Oregon grape in the western part of America. Employed as a blood purifier, both *E. aquaticum* and *E. yuccifolium* were used in earlier years to induce vomiting with snakebites. It is also called rattlesnake master.

Eryngium yuccifolium was used to relieve conditions common to children, such as measles, as well as kidney complaints. The plant has thistle-like heads and is a member of the Carrot family.

Barberry shrub *(Berberis vulgaris)*. Barberry, naturalized from Europe, was used in an old formula for "racing hearts, but to be used only by those who were trained." An elder called the plant "yellow eyes," *di ga do li, da lo ni ge i* in Cherokee. The berberine alkaloid in barberry is used as a plant-derived antibiotic in combination with blue cohosh, twin-leaf, and mayapple. Barberry contains several active compounds and is a good source of vitamin C. It was used in earlier years to prevent scurvy. The plant acids act as a mild diuretic while the berberine and other alkaloids reduce blood pressure. Do not use barberry for cardiac conditions without consulting a physician and a trained herbalist.

Basswood tree *(Tilia americana)*. The inner bark of basswood, otherwise known as linden or bee tree, was used in a formula with pine for assisting pregnant women. This use was verified by Hamel and Chiltoskey. Two pieces of basswood were rubbed together to make the "honored fire" in the ceremony honoring the new moon in October, or the Green Corn Ceremony.

The flowers of this impressive twenty-five-foot tree grow in clusters; their coloration changes from yellow to white and they have a strong, sweet fragrance. A preparation of basswood flowers contains flavonoids and tannins, effective for increasing perspiration for sweating out fevers. Carolina basswood *(T. caroliniana)* in South Carolina is used by mountain folks for the same purpose.

An elder who had been writing to me for many years from South Carolina shared many old formulas with me that included inner bark of basswood. When the elder died he left many mixtures of plants and formulas in a side building, which was destroyed by his family. Probably two hundred years of history went up in smoke that night. Thank goodness he had the foresight to preserve this part of our forgotten and unappreciated history of plants and weeds by corresponding with me.

Bay shrub *(Gordonia lasianthus)*. The inner bark of loblolly bay, an evergreen shrub, came to the Cherokee as a trade item from other eastern tribes. An elder said, "It'd take the hide off you. That's what it was used for." He was referring to bay's use in tanning leather, but he was not able to remember how the plant was used in Medicine ways. From the Tea family, bay is known for its large white fragrant flowers, which are a good source for honey found on the Carolina coast.

Bayberry shrub *(Myrica cerifera)*. Bayberry, or southern wax myrtle, another evergreen shrub, is used as an astringent in the Blue Ridge and Appalachian Mountains for uterine hemorrhage and other bleeding problems. The fruit is a source of bayberry wax, which was used in candle making. Bayberry *(M. gale)* is an astringent and aromatic used for digestive disorders and as a cure for itch. Bayberry contains a volatile oil that is potentially toxic. While stimulating the circulation, bayberry affects the body's electrolyte balance and results in potassium deficiency, which can result in high blood pressure and swelling. Bayberry should not be used during pregnancy.

Bear grass *(Yucca filamentosa* and *Y. arborescens)*. *Ga nu la hi, yo nah,* or yucca, was used in Green Corn Ceremony with longleaf pine (*Pinus* and other species), spring amaranth (*Amaranthus hypochondriacus*), Indian tobacco *(Lobelia inflata)*, and tobacco *(Nicotiana rustica)*. (*Yo nah* means "bear" in Cherokee.) Sage *(Salvia officinalis* or *S. lyrata)* was used in the drink for the young dancers, and then sage would be offered with the tobacco to the "sacred fire" in a ceremony. Bear grass was one of the plants used in very old formulas to give strength in competition and in the dancing that was such an important part of the Green Corn Ceremony.

Bear grass, also called Adam's needles, is a member of the Agave family. Indian bear grass *(Xerophyllum tenax)* is used by western tribes for treating liver and gallbladder problems, probably due to the plant's saponin content. The leaves and roots of Indian bear grass were traded in earlier years by tribes.

Bear's foot (see Leafcup).

Bee balm (see Balm, melissa).

Bee tree (see Basswood tree).

Beth root or bethroot (see Trillium).

Birch tree *(Betula lenta).* Birch—sometimes known as sweet birch, black birch, or cherry birch—was called *a ti sa gi* in Cherokee. Birch was used in a formula to "purify the blood of women after birthing," as an elder related to me. Birch oil was used by mountain folks to flavor food, as well as for alleviating pain due to its salicylic acid content. Birch was tapped much like maple trees are for the sap used in birch beer, and birch tea is made by using the sap and the leaves. Birch was also used with bilberry as a blood purifier by mountain folks, according to my grandmother Edna Rogers.

Bird's foot violet *(Viola pedata).* This small violet was used for treating venereal disease in earlier years. The purple and bluish flowers of this small plant are found in bloom from March to June in the Great Smoky Mountains. It is usually found in dry and open areas along the park trails and roads. An elder said it was used in a special formula for women's skin conditions, such as rash that accompanied pregnancy, and was combined with wild pansy and other plants for making the skin soft. There is a rounded-leaved violet *(V. rotundifolia),* smooth yellow violet *(V. pennsylvanica),* and halberd-leaved violet *(V. hastata).* Little is known about their use, but violet *(V. odorata)* has been found to contain volatile oils, saponins, and alkaloids. An elder called several of the violet species "crowfoot," while reminding me that wild geranium was also called crowfoot.

Bittersweet *(Celastrus scandens).* Earlier Cherokee used American bittersweet in a formula to stimulate menstruation and reduce swelling. It contains tannins, which might explain its use with menstrual disorders. It was used in a remedy as an Appalachian ointment for skin cancer, tumors, burns, and swellings. Bittersweet is also a name used for night-shade *(Solanum dulcamara)*.

Black cohosh *(Cimicifuga racemosa* or *C. americana)*. Black cohosh, or black snakeroot, was called *ga na ge* in Cherokee. It was used in a formula for treating reproductive concerns and female problems, especially meno-pause. It was sometimes combined with the root and leaves of Indian root. Black cohosh was used in earlier years to treat fevers, especially in women and children. This plant, part of the Buttercup family, is officially at risk of extinction due to overharvesting from its natural environment. There is much in the herbal literature on black cohosh's estrogenic value and its ability for assisting women with hot flashes and vaginal dryness during menopause. While the estrogen-like effect has been suggested, compounds in the rootstock have an affinity to estrogen receptors in the body.

Black cohosh has a long-standing history of being a helper with meno-pausal ailments. The only side effects mentioned are gastric discomfort and headache. Do not use black cohosh when pregnant or while nursing. Black cohosh should only be used under the supervision of those trained in the medicinal use of plants.

Black-eyed Susan *(Rudbeckia hirta)*. This beautiful plant with its bright yellow flowers and bold black center stands about three feet high and blooms in July and August. It was used as a wash for the "private parts for women," according to Mary Chiltoskey. Another plant called wild golden-glow *(R. laciniata)* is a close relative that was also sometimes used in the formula. Black-eyed Susan was combined with hepatica and fairywand for treating swelling and back pains. It has been said that black-eyed Su-san migrated from the West as the buffalo were disappearing in the East. This flower is good for growing in a wildflower garden, as well as to just enjoy in an open field or woods.

Blackgum tree *(Nyssa sylvatica)*. A wash and tea of black haw shrub or cramp bark was used in a Cherokee formula. Other barks included blackgum, balsam, and sycamore for a "sacred drink for childbirth and cleansing." The blackgum tree is a member of the Dogwood family.

Black haw shrub *(Viburnum prunifolium)*. The bark of black haw (also called sweet haw or cramp bark) was used for "female bleeding and pains," probably due to its astringent properties. An elder called it "black skunk" or *di la, gv na ge i*. This indigenous plant of North America and Canada was used as a sedative and antispasmodic to relax the uterus. Black haw was also used to ease pain and as a tonic in Appalachia for spasms. Some Eastern tribes used it as a relaxant for the heart and as an anti-inflammatory.

Cramp bark *(V. opulus)* is the "cousin plant used for menstrual cramping, as well as for the back and the bladder." Cramp bark should not be used if there is a history of kidney disease.

Both black haw and cramp bark are members of the Honeysuckle family. The Catawba used possumhaw *(V. nudum)* with saltbrush *(Eastern baccharis),* found along the coastal areas of the Carolinas, and magnolia tree bark in a formula for several female-related symptoms. Today black haw is used to ease menstrual pain and to relax the uterus.

Black snakeroot (see Black cohosh).

Blood plant (see Amaranth).

Blue ash tree *(Fraxinus quadrangulata).* The inner bark of blue ash tree was received in trade from our West Virginia Indian brothers to make a blue dye. It was also used in a drink that would represent the North direction in ceremonies. While the elders made mention of the tree and its uses, blue ash is not found in the Smoky Mountains today. Medicinally, blue ash was used as an astringent and a diuretic and was applied for gout and for bladder complaints. It is a member of the Olive family.

Blue cohosh *(Caulophyllum thalictroides).* Blue cohosh, or snakeroot, was called *ga le gi* in Cherokee. The berries are poisonous, and the plant is an irritant to the skin. The Cherokee valued this plant, called "papoose root" or "squaw root" by the mountain folks, for treating female conditons. (Please know that the word *squaw* is offensive to American Indians.)

Blue cohosh was used to stimulate menstruation; it was also used as an antispasmodic. Blue cohosh can bring on contractions and act as an antispasmodic during labor. It is also good for combating dehydration during birth. This was one of those plants that "was used only by those trained on how to prepare and use it," as one elder put it. Another elder said, "You can find *ka na ste te* near the river as a small bush with yellow stems inside and heart-shaped leaves. The root smells like a live snake. It is a good tonic for a sweat." While I agreed to smell the plant, I did not want to get close enough to a live snake to compare the smells.

Blue cohosh is used today for problems related to menstrual flow, to induce labor, and for muscle spasms. This plant is officially at risk for extinction, due to overharvesting in its natural environment.

Borage *(Borago officinalis).* Borage, or bugloss, was mentioned by an elder to be good for "weakly persons to get stronger," especially after a long illness. As a "female" helper it was used for nervous conditions, and the leaves and seeds were used to stimulate the flow of milk in nursing mothers. Borage was an old remedy for "releasing the spirit" after loss, and as an antidote to "feeling down." Borage's tannin content provides an astringent effect. Precautions have been suggested due to borage's hepatotoxic alkaloid content. Today borage is used to treat melancholy and to induce sweating.

Buckeye tree *(Aesculus pavia* and *A. octandra)*. Red and yellow buckeye were used in formulas for female complaints, fainting, and birthing. The largest of the buckeye trees is the yellow buckeye, or sweet buckeye, found in the Smoky Mountains. The seeds and young shoots are poisonous to wild animals. However, earlier Indians washed and roasted the seeds to rid them of the toxic content, and then used the seeds for "fixins in foods." The crushed seeds and small branches of red buckeye *(A. pavia)* were used with devil's shoestring as a "special Medicine" for catching fish.

Buffalo plant (see Alfalfa).

Bull nettle *(Solanum carolinense)*. Also known as Carolina horse nettle, this prickly plant grows to about three feet in open fields and wooded areas. The yellow berries were used to treat nervous stress and as a mild sedative. The Cherokee valued the dried root as a necklace worn by babies who were cutting teeth. Teething pain is still relieved in this way today, with a necklace of dried bull nettle root and colorful plastic beads.

Burdock root *(Arctium lappa* and *A. minus)*. Common burdock is one of the favorite East Medicine plants used in formulas for purifying the blood. It is employed in one formula as a helper for women combating fluid buildup when they are trying to lose weight. The other agents in this formula are catnip and goldenseal. In another old fomula burdock was combined with blackgum and Solomon's seal. Burdock was also used for treating venereal disease. The effects and efficiencies of burdock are little documented in the herbal literature.

Burdock should not be confused with common cocklebur *(Xanthium atrumarium)*, which is said to be poisonous to livestock. Burdock and milk thistle were mentioned by an elder for "the problems of female itching and infection." Burdock and echinacea in combination is still a good mountain remedy for treating vaginal infections.

Burseed *(Hackelia virginiana)*. The plant roots of burseed were used in a special love charm to "endure and ensure love and commitment to that special person." This is an old and sacred formula. An elder also reported that the plant was used for "female problems with kidney problems and itch during pregnancy." While there is very little in the botanical and herbal literature about burseed, it was a plant considered valuable to American Indians in the Southeast. Unfortunately, much of the information about this plant has been lost through the generations.

Butterfly weed *(Asclepias tuberosa)*. Also called pleurisy root or wind root, butterfly weed was used in a heart formula as a diuretic and a cardiotonic. While it is uncertain how it was used, "it was known in earlier days as wind root for its ability to carry a message to the Great One." Butterfly weed enjoys direct sunlight and dry soil, and the orange-yellow flowers make this a good garden flower and a beautiful wildflower for roadside viewers.

Button bush *(Cephalanthus occidentalis)*. The seeds of button bush, or globe flower, were gathered to attract ducks, which were hunted for their tasty meat and for their feathers, which were used in ceremony. Button bush is a member of the Madder family. The white flowers remind me of the sycamore. Button bush is used in sweats to induce perspiration.

Calamus root *(Acorus calamus)*. Also known as sweet flag, this plant is popular in the mountains of North Carolina for "women in labor and with birthing pains"; it is applied both internally and externally. The rhizome is used internally for complaints of gas and gastritis. Calamus root was used as a tonic to stimulate the appetite and digestion following birthing and for those with long-term illness. It was also used with Joe-pye weed and dogwood for treating pain. As an elder said, "You have to know how to gather and prepare the calamus root. You gotta' be trained."

Cardinal flower *(Lobelia cardinalis)*. Cardinal flower was used as a diuretic, and as part of a formula for treating sexually transmitted diseases such as syphilis. Cardinal flower is a beautiful plant that stands about three feet high in the mountains; it has lance-shaped leaves and unique crimson red flowers that appear from July to September. Cardinal flower is no longer used for medicinal purposes.

Another member of the Lobelia family is the great blue lobelia, with its blue to purple flowers. This plant wasn't valued like its cousin *Lobelia inflata* (Indian tobacco); however, the beautiful scarlet red tubular flowers of the cardinal flower appear in early Cherokee stories as red paint. As the story goes, Wolf laid asleep on the riverbank while Racoon packed wet clay on his eyes. The clay dried and Wolf thought he was blind until a little earth bird pecked the clay away so Wolf could see again. In appreciation Wolf led the little bird to "red paint," or cardinal flower, which he used to paint himself red, which is the color of the cardinal today.

Carolina horse nettle (see Bull nettle).

Carolina lily *(Lilium michauxii)*. This lily, also called Michaux's lily, was mentioned by an elder as being a "special gift" from tribes in the eastern portion of the Carolinas. It is related to Turk's cap lily; both were used in "female Medicine, but prepared by those trained." There is reason to be cautious in using and eating the various lilies. As an example, lily-of-the-valley *(Convallaria majalis)* is considered poisonous and not suitable for internal use. However, it was used by earlier Cherokee in a sacred Medicine.

Carolina spring beauty *(Claytonia caroliniana)*. The white spring flower of Carolina spring beauty was a reminder each year of the "special Medicine" that starts the warm season. This plant was one of several early bloomers used in the "spring tonic."

Catawba rhododendron *(Rhododendron catawbiense)*. Rhododendron, or purple laurel, is found in the Great Smoky Mountains. It is an evergreen shrub or small tree that grows to twelve feet and shares its name with the Catawba River in North Carolina. The bark was used in several formulas for pain relief.

The Catawba rhododendron, a member of the Heath family, is often combined with mountain laurel *(Kalmia latifolia)* from the same family. Sometimes mountain folks will refer to rhododendron as "laurel." There is also a dwarf rhododendron *(R. minus)* that grows about four feet tall with short leaves. The dwarf rhododendron was used as a pain reliever in a very old formula, in combination with willow bark and flowering dogwood.

Catawba tree *(Catalpa bignonioides)*. Called Indian bean, this tree with eight-inch-long heart-shaped leaves grows to sixty feet tall. It is sometimes called common catalpa, and a friend once called it "Kentucky tree." The pods are called catalpa. As a member of the Bignonia family, the tree was also sometimes called "cigar tree" or "bean tree" by mountain folks.

An elder said that the flowers are unusual, with two orange stripes and purple spots on each petal. The flowers were used in a formula with willow bark for female complaints. It is unclear how the leaves and bark were used, but I suspect it was for the pains of menstruation.

Catnip *(Nepeta cataria)*. Catnip was used as a mild sedative for women and children, and for babies with colic. Sometimes called "field balm" or "catmint" by mountain folks, catnip was used as a "smoke" for colds and nervous conditions, according to my Uncle Grady and my dad. My grandmother said it was used to delay menstruation. It "drives cats crazy." The active agents in catnip are bitters and tannin used for their value in fighting colic, colds, nervous conditions, and migraines. As a female Medicine, catnip's value was as a sedative and a calming agent, mixed with peppermint tea, which stored easily for use in the winter months. As an elder said, "Catnip and the mint teas were the only way before the black teas could be bought."

Chamomile *(Matricaria chamomilla* or *recutita)*. Chamomile, or wild chamomile, was a gift from the European settlers. It is used for "calming health." It turned out to be a good tonic and essential oil from our English brothers and sisters; chamomile induces perspiration and increases elimination through the skin. It is a helper for circulation and for nervous conditions, as well as for regulating menstrual flow when combined with Indian root.

While there was much conflict between the Indians and the Whites over land, this is a reminder of the many gifts of trading between people, a gift that had much value and benefit for everybody. Chamomile flowers are valued as an antispasmodic and anti-inflammatory. The flowers are also valued as an antibacterial.

The German variety of chamomile on the market today grows upright to three feet, while the Roman variety has creeping stems. Chamomile is used today for alleviating female conditions, in particular menstrual disorders. An old Cherokee name for this herb is yellowroot, or *da lo ni ge i*.

Cherokee bean (see Red cardinal).

Cinquefoil *(Potentilla reptans)*. Also called creeping cinquefoil or five-fingers, this delicate field plant with runners was used as an astringent to stop bleeding, particularly in females and in children with nosebleeds. The entire plant was crushed and applied to the area. This is one of those plants that probably was introduced to American Indians by the White settlers. Erect cinquefoil *(P. erecta)*, which grows about twenty inches high, was also used to stop bleeding. An elder said that common cinquefoil *(P. canadensis)* and wild strawberries were friends who "talk to each other along the side of roads and fields. They are both helpers in the ways of love." The little yellow flower of rough-fruited cinquefoil *(P. recta)*, which reminds me of a tiny dogwood flower, is also common along roadsides, but its use was not mentioned among the elders.

Coltsfoot (see Wild ginger, Bird's foot violet, Geranium, and Alumroot).

Columbine *(Aquilegia canadensis)*. Wild columbine was mentioned by Hamel and Chiltoskey as a tea for heart problems and "bloody flux." It was used with caution, but valued for its narcotic effect. Fox grape was combined with columbine and used by mountain folks for treating varicose veins. An elder said it was used "for the internals of a woman that get out when birthing." Culverwort *(A. vulgaris)* has been researched to identify glycosides and the potential for poisoning agents from the cyanogenic glycosides, but the active amount in the plant is probably too small to measure. The research literature does not include information on *A. canadensis,* but it is likely to be similar in effect to *A. vulgaris,* the glycosides being the reason for the plant's effectiveness in treating female bleeding problems.

Comfrey (*Symphytum officinale*). Common comfrey, or *o se e o se,* was used as a blood purifier in earlier years. It was one of the sacred plants used in a tonic formula for ceremony and for "little wars," or ball playing.

According to an elder, comfrey was used "for women who had bad dreams." Persimmon bark was used with comfrey in earlier years for treating venereal disease. Comfrey contains alkaloids that have been shown to cause cancer when taken internally. I suspect that comfrey has been plagued with suggestions of toxicity by the Food and Drug Administration, possibly too strongly. The carcinogenic constituents are pyrrolizidine alkaloid, an isolated extract, as well as symphytine; however, the amounts of alkaloid found in each plant are very small. Still, confer with a trained herbalist for a safe dosage and use. Do not use comfrey if you are pregnant or while you are nursing.

Corn (*Zea mays*). The shucks of maize, or Indian corn, called *se lu, sha' lou,* or *she lu* in Cherokee, were crushed in earlier years and mixed with water to make "nature's mush," a food for "little ones, old ones, and those who are sickly." There is a very old formula using corn "to tender the heart of a woman." Corn had a mythological and sacred meaning among the Cherokee and other tribes. It was used in ceremonies and for "joining a man and woman together."

Corn would be dried slowly over a fire to preserve it to be eaten in the winter. Cut pieces of wild potato, pumpkins, and squash were preserved the same way.

Corn was also preserved in the husks, which were kept in bins called *u wa da li.* It was also made into cornstarch, which is still used as a powder for babies and to soothe dry feet. Corn silk is still used as a diuretic for women with bloating and water retention problems.

Dandelion (*Taraxacum officinale*). A tea of dandelion, or yellow flower (*hu tsi la ha* in Cherokee), is used as a tonic "to make the woman stronger after childbirth." The entire plant was used in a tea for treating heart problems in earlier years. Dandelion has been used by southwestern Indians for heart trouble. The Cherokee and mountain folks in Appalachia enjoyed dandelion greens in a spring salad. My Uncle Grady and my father called the plant "blowball" when they were children living in the mountains of North Carolina.

Devil's hair (see Virgin's bower).

Devil's walkingstick *(Aralia spinosa)*. Devil's walkingstick was also known as Hercules' club and prickly ash. The formula for using the large compound leaves and bark has been lost, but use of the fruit as an aromatic in other formulas is still in practice today. Devil's walkingstick is not to be confused with true prickly ash *(Zanthoxylum americanum)*.

Dock (see Yellow dock).

Dogwood *(Cornus florida)*. The flowering dogwood's bloom in the early spring triggered the time for "spring ceremony and the early planting season." It is one of the most beautiful and distinctive small trees found in the mountains of North Carolina, Virginia, Tennessee, West Virginia, and Kentucky. The white bracts that look like petals in the summer also carry bright red foliage in the autumn. I always look forward to the flowers in April and May and the fruits in September, and the turning color of the leaves in October.

The hard wood of the dogwood was used for ceremonial purposes, as was hickory. The fresh or dried bark of dogwood is used as a tonic, a stimulant, and an astringent due to its tannins. A bark tea was used for attending to female pain and backaches. Formulas often included dogwood for general pain relief. The flowering dogwood is a member of the Dogwood family and the official North Carolina state flower.

Dwarf sumac *(Rhus copallina)*. The leaves of dwarf, or shining, sumac were used in a tea to increase the flow of milk in females. I was not able to verify any use of this plant today. It should not be confused with poison sumac *(R. vernix)*, which was used in earlier years for treating venereal disease. Dwarf sumac is a member of the Bittersweet family; it makes a nice ornamental shrub.

Eastern wahoo *(Euonymus atropurpureus)*. Also known as Indian arrowroot or Eastern burning bush, the inner bark of Eastern wahoo was used to purge the digestive system. According to Arnold and Connie Krochmal, American Indians used a decoction of the stem's inner bark for uterine problems. It was used as a heart Medicine to slow down irregular beats. The seeds were used as a laxative.

The Eastern wahoo is a shrub that can grow to twenty-five feet, but it's usually about six feet in height. The inner bark would only be used in the fall and early spring for "female problems," as well as in a formula for the "bad disease," or sexually transmitted diseases. An elder said that caution is necessary, "because it affects the heart, and the berries and seeds are poisonous." The Eastern wahoo is a member of the Bittersweet family. It should only be used by those trained in its Medicine.

Echinacea (see Purple coneflower).

Elder shrub *(Sambucus canadensis)*. American elder-root tonic was an American Indian original. The tonic was used to stimulate circulation. The mountain folks used the fermented berries to make a tonic wine for treating fever. A member of the Honeysuckle family, elder was considered a female Medicine and was prepared as an antiseptic and a tonic, like others in the Honeysuckle family. As an elder said, "The bark was used to purge, while the berries were used as a diuretic. The flowers are still used for the lungs [expectorant] and to stimulate the [circulatory] system."

As a youngster I remember the elders making "popguns" and whistles from the American elder by removing the pith from the stem and using a dial-like piece in the pith to make a popping sound.

Elecampane *(Inula helenium)*. Also called wild sunflower in tribute to its daisylike flowers, elecampane is a cure-all plant. It is used as a tonic, a stimulant, an antifungal, anti-inflammatory, antiseptic, and antibacterial. An elder called it *a ga li ha*, "sunshine plant." (This plant should not be confused with sunflower, *Helianthus strumosus*. Elecampane plant grows three to six feet high, with alternate and serrate leaves with white veins and large yellow flowers in clusters. It is a member of the Aster or Composite family.

Elecampane is often overlooked for medicinal uses, but the Cherokee used it for the female problems of weak bowels and "fallen wombs." An old formula combined it with cowslip and Indian pink for treating menstrual problems. Elecampane is sometimes called "horseheal" by mountain folks, as it was used to treat respiratory and digestive problems in horses and dogs. The plant has a fibrous rootstock that is used in Medicine. It is listed in the East Medicine because of its value for women and children. Honey or horehound was added to a formula using elecampane due to its bitter taste. An elder warned of the importance of learning how to use the plant from someone trained, "because too much will make you sick and vomit." Although elecampane can be irritating to the mucous membranes, it is used to treat bronchitis and coughs as well as menstrual complaints.

Elm tree *(Ulmus americana)*. The inner bark and roots of American or white elm was called *ha wa tsi la, tlu gah i*. It was used for treating skin infections, colds, and chronic bowel problems. The Cherokee used it for "the tender breasts of women, and young men in their change." Interestingly, it was used as a "chew" to spit on the baseball glove so the ball would stick to the glove, according to Mary Chiltoskey. An elder called the elm a "flyer" because the fruit has winglike seeds that "fly in the wind, carrying the tree to other places to grow."

Evening primrose *(Oenothera biennis)*. *Sa no yi*, "falling sun rose," was used in earlier years for women's health. This is a very old formula. Uses included weight stabilization, easing premenstrual pain, and soothing tender breasts. Evening primrose was used with rose pink *(Sabatia angularis)* for addressing menstrual cycle pains. Evening primrose is still used today for lowering blood pressure and for treating rheumatoid arthritis.

Evening primrose seeds have been found to contain gamma linolenic acid, or GLA, used for treating inflammation. This fatty acid is necessary for cellular metabolism and is a helper to women, especially during the monthly menstrual cycle. An elder showed me the four yellow petals of the evening primrose flower and said it was referred to as a sacred plant for female Medicine that someday we would know more about. Sundrops *(O. fruticosa)*, a plant cousin, was used by earlier Cherokee for the same purpose, but it has not been studied for chemical content. Today GLA is used to treat high blood pressure and high cholesterol, as well as premenstrual syndrome.

Fennel *(Foeniculum vulgare)*. The entire fennel plant was used in a tonic for colic and for women in labor. It was mixed with bracken fern *(Pteridium aquilinum)* and used for children with colds and as a tonic for females with nursing and bladder problems. Fennel is combined with partridgeberry for treating sore nipples. Fennel also helps promote milk flow in nursing mothers. Fennel was combined with American chestnut for treating heart problems.

One elder Medicine person said it was "a children's Medicine for colic." Fennel is also used as an expectorant and as a diuretic in several formulas. Today fennel is used for treating menstrual problems, to increase lactation, to enhance sexual drive, and for easing childbirth. An elder said that fennel should not be used without the input of "someone trained, because it can be toxic and even cause a miscarriage if pregnant," in the quantities used for female problems.

Fern, maidenhair *(Adiantum pedatum)*. The maidenhair fern was considered a "powerful Medicine for the heart," but few today know the sacred formula, which included hawthorn and Indian root. This Cherokee use was verified by Paul Hamel and Mary Chiltoskey. I believe it was used particularly for female irregular heartbeats, "only by those who were trained in the sacred preparation of the entire plant."

Feverfew *(Chrysanthemum parthenium)*. The word *parthenos* is derived from the Greek word for "virgin." While used by earlier Cherokee for assisting with young women's menstrual cycles, it is not clear how that use originated. The general use of feverfew for pain relief and to reduce fever is still popular in the culture of mountain folks today. Feverfew contains a compound called parthenolide, which helps protect blood vessels and muscle tissue; this might explain why it was used for easing menstrual pains and for childbirth in combination with four-o'clock plant. Feverfew is used today for treating migraines, arthritis, rheumatic disease, and allergies.

Feverfew is a great daisylike plant to grow indoors. It grows about two feet tall. This plant has its place in my Medicine bag as nature's vasodilator and an anti-inflammatory, as well as for its use in treating arthritis. An elder reminded me that in earlier years feverfew was used as a "bugbane" to repel insects. The leaf would be placed in bean bread dough as a way to take it without upsetting the intestines. Feverfew affects the smooth muscles of the digestive system, which could cause contraction problems if used too frequently. This plant should not be taken during pregnancy.

Five-finger (see Cinquefoil and Ginseng).

Flax *(Linum usitatissimum)*. Flax seeds are a source of omega-3 fatty acids, which benefit women with ovarian and breast problems who also are at risk of cancer. Earlier use of flax was as a laxative in "cleansing" the system. It was also used for cleansing following childbirth. Flax oil is still very popular for "keeping a strong system for working the fields."

The simple name *flax* is a much longer word in Cherokee; it is *u do la nv s di*. As a member of the Milkwort family, flax is a good healing oil for just about everything. Today it is used for protection against cancer, heart disease, and gallstones and is used to treat inflammation with gout. It is still very popular as an East and West Medicine. The alpha-linolenic acid is also protective for the heart.

Foxglove *(Digitalis purpurea)*. Cherokee Indians knew of this plant's ability to be a helper in regulating heartbeat and swelling. The discovery of foxglove has been attributed to an English physician in 1775, who recognized its properties as a cardiac agent and made the first digitalis medicine.

Due to its poisonous nature foxglove is not recommended for use today, but it has been a key element in the past for treating swelling or edema associated with congestive heart failure. It can cause a rash in some people and can be poisonous due to the glycosides digitalin and digitoxin. An elder said foxglove was used for "weakly females who passed out a lot," and "for men who had weak hearts." The plant's effect in the latter instance was possibly to stabilize the pulse and the blood pressure.

Take foxglove only under the supervision of a trained herbalist or Medicine man or woman with expertise in preparing the dosage. The beautiful, tall stems of white or purple flower clusters are very showy in home flower gardens.

Fox grape *(Vitis labrusca)*. Fox grape, called *tsa la* or *soc lol,* was used to treat soreness of the breasts after childbirth. It was called "frost grape" and "summer grape" by Paul Hamel and Mary Chiltoskey. They also mention its use with geranium to relieve breast soreness.

Fraser fir tree *(Abies fraseri)*. This fir tree, called big tree, or *tlu ga i, e qu a* in Cherokee, was sometimes known as she-balm or balsam-in-the-mountains. The inner bark was used for "weakness with women, especially with cleansing and healing after the birth of a child." The resin was used by some Indians by rubbing it on the chest and back for pain relief. In traditional sweats the needles were used as a clearing-way when placed on the hot rocks. Fraser fir is a member of the Pine family.

Garlic *(Allium sativum)*. The cloves of garlic were used in earlier years for purifying the blood, along with Indian root. Today garlic is used to stimulate the circulatory system and to reduce blood cholesterol level. I suspect that every culture of people on Mother Earth has valued garlic for a special medicinal purpose and for its abilities as an antibiotic.

An elder shared a story about the Great One giving garlic the assignment to taste like the wet ground that gives it life and to be a helper from the bacteria, fungi, and yeasts that come from the ground. In the story garlic is called ground bulb. The volatile oil and sulfur compounds in garlic together have an antibiotic action. Garlic is a helper with blood pressure, cholesterol, and blood sugar. American Indians recognized "this gift from another world" as an antihistamine and its ability to rid the intestines of parasites. Today it is used to fight infections, reduce high cholesterol, and for diabetes.

Ginseng *(Panax quinquefolius)*. American ginseng, or five-finger, was a cure-all plant; it is called "sang" by mountain folks. Earlier Cherokee considered it to be one of the sacred plants, and it was included in several formulas as a stimulant and tonic. Ginseng was used with elders to improve appetite and for "just feeling good," and with children who were "too anxious to play." Today ginseng is considered an adaptogen herb for its power to enhance the body's ability to deal with stress. Ginseng was particularly used with elders and for treating female disorders. As an elder said, "The sang is for the female weakness and feeling good after childbirth and illness of any kind." It was also used in a general spring tonic with sassafras, Indian root, and other plants.

James Mooney recorded ginseng as *a tali kuli* in Cherokee, meaning "it climbs the mountain." It has been my experience that ginseng seems to like living in patches of poison ivy. My friends from China use it in a similar way as the earlier Cherokee for balancing and to bring harmony to the entire system, especially for elders.

It seems fitting that the Greek word *panax* means "panacea." My friend refers to American ginseng as an herb "for cooling down the body, and for balance." Panax ginseng seems to have a positive effect on athletic performance, increasing oxygen absorption for quick recovery, with less serum lactate and muscle fatigue. This means less effort is expended and energy is conserved. Because of these properties ginseng was used in earlier years in Indian ball competition and by "deer-riders," or runners.

Today it is used for exercise tolerance, to stimulate the immune system, to increase stamina, to improve the circulation, and for mental conditions in the elderly. In its natural environment ginseng is officially now considered to be at risk for extinction.

Globe flower (see Button bush).

Goat dandelion *(Pyrrhopappus carolinianus)*. Goat dandelion was made into a drink to purify the blood. An elder said it was used as a spring tonic, but little is known about how it was decocted. It was used with Indian root by several elders as a stimulant and "to get the blood going after a cold winter." Goat dandelion is not a plant that is referred to by Cherokee Medicine men and women today.

Goat's beard *(Aruncus dioicus)*. Called *tsu s qua ne gi dah,* goat's beard was used with other plants to control the loss of blood in childbirth. It was also popular in earlier years as a bath for swollen feet. The unusual cream-white flowers appear in plumes that remind me of strings blowing in the wind. Goat's beard is not to be confused with goat's rue *(Tephrosia virginiana)*, a plant with white petals mixed with purple color found along roadsides.

Goldenclub *(Orontium aquaticum)*. An elder told me that earlier Cherokee believed bathing a baby in a formula made with goldenclub during a new moon for the first seven months "would give the baby the spirit strength necessary for survival. You gotta' remember that in those days it was difficult for babies and mothers to survive the ordeal of birthing in that rugged environment." This ritual bathing was also seen as a way to give thanks to the Great One for the gift of life.

Goldenrod *(Solidago erecta* and *S. odora)*. As "special Medicine," in October of each year the sacred fire was rekindled at the fall ceremony, called *A tsi la, ga lun ka we tsi ye.* Dried goldenrod, or *sa ni ti,* was used in this ceremony, along with a prayer-chant giving thanks in the Four Directions. Sacred tobacco was offered to the fire. An elder said, "The small clusters of yellow flowers reach out to let you know they are there to help you or make you sneeze. You cannot miss them in the field. Goldenrod was always a special plant to the Cherokee." It was used externally as an astringent after birth, and for treating fungal conditions, such as *Candida albicans,* common to women.

Goldenseal *(Hydrastis canadensis).* Goldenseal was also known as yellowroot or Indian paint (*da lo ni ge i* in Cherokee). A member of the Buttercup family, it should not be confused with butterfly weed *(Asclepias tubersoa),* pleurisy root, and other plants called yellowroot. Goldenseal has a hairy stem six to eighteen inches high; the white flowers bloom in April and May. The plant's fruit looks like a raspberry.

To the Cherokee goldenseal was an important female medicinal herb; it was used as both an antiseptic and a hemostatic. Goldenseal douche treated vaginal inflammations. Goldenseal was also used before sweats and ceremonies as a natural antimicrobial. Also known as Indian dye, Indian plant, and Indian turmeric, goldenseal was used as a laxative and to raise blood pressure.

Today goldenseal is used as an astringent to control bleeding after childbirth; as well, the berberine in the plant makes it useful for treating vaginitis. Goldenseal is officially at risk of extinction due to overharvesting from its natural environment.

Gourd *(Lagenaria vulgaris).* According to Mary Chiltoskey, the seeds of gourd, or *ga na tse ti,* were used as a poultice for treating boils. The dried gourd was used for ceremonial rattles and as dippers for water. The Gourd family includes pumpkin, squash, gourds, melons, and cucumbers. In earlier years gourds also made very nice decorated purses, carriers, and keepers for special things.

Greenbrier *(Smilax rotundifolia).* A formula of greenbrier, or bullgrip, was mixed with equal amounts of sycamore and Carolina hemlock *(Tsuga canadensis)* or Eastern hemlock to expel afterbirth, according to Mary Chiltoskey. A formula for treating sexually transmitted diseases contained greenbrier, hearts-a-bustin' (or strawberry bush), sweetgum, fox grape, beech, and blackgum.

Hawthorn shrub (*Crataegus intricata* and other species). The primary use of hawthorn with the Cherokee was as a relaxant, but mountain folks used it for the treatment of kidney and bladder problems. The leaves of Biltmore hawthorn were used to treat heart ailments and circulatory disorders, as well as in a tonic for the heart. Hawthorn dilates the blood vessels to lower blood pressure. An elder called it "white speckled," or *u nv tsa dv, u ne ga.* There is also an English hawthorn *(C. laevigata).* Hawthorn is not to be confused with black haw *(Viburnum prunifolium)* or cramp bark *(Viburnum opulus).*

Hawthorn should not be used without medical direction if you have a heart condition. Earlier use was to steady the heartbeat and to dilate the arteries for increased oxygen and blood. Hawthorn has a mild sedative function; a formula mixed for this purpose included lemon balm, lavender, or another mild relaxant. There is much good research and testimony in the literature about the benefits of hawthorn. A drink for the Cherokee ballplayers that would be given to them by the Medicine man or woman included hawthorn for "good circulation, and to keep the defense from being caught while running with the ball." The Biltmore Estates in Asheville, North Carolina, is home to several of the hawthorn species that were studied in earlier years.

Today hawthorn berries are used for their flavonoids, compounds that are beneficial to the blood vessels and the heart and help to alleviate high blood pressure. Hawthorn is used for cardiac insufficiency where there is a feeling of tightness or pressure in the heart. Use hawthorn only as instructed by a physician for cardiac and arrhythmia problems. Hawthorn is a member of the Rose family.

Heal-all *(Prunella vulgaris)*. Called self-heal or wild sage, heal-all was used as an astringent and in ceremonies. An elder called it "spoon," or *di do di* in Cherokee. Heal-all was recognized as a "special Medicine" for females, and was used in ceremonies. A carminative, it was also used in treating hemorrhage. As a member of the Mint family heal-all is an aromatic; it grows up to twenty-eight inches tall, with several stems arising from the root base. Leaves grow in opposite pairs; the plant bears purple flowers that bloom from April to November as spikes at the tops of the stems. Heal-all is used in the mountains today as a gargle for sore throats more than anything else.

The name heal-all is also given to stone root *(Collinsonia canadensis)*, a member of the Mint family, and to figwort *(Scrophularia nodosa)* in the Figwort family. Both were used primarily as an ointment for bruises and scratches.

Hearts-a-bustin' *(Euonymus americanus)*. Also called strawberry bush, this plant was used as a tonic in earlier years, as well as for treating breast complaints. It is used as an antiseptic and for urinary problems. Hearts-a-bustin' is a beautiful plant with bright green leaves and unusual crimson red flowers with red pods that burst open in the early fall with orange seeds. Hearts-a-bustin' is found in many home gardens and landscapes.

An elder said that the common bleeding heart *(Dicentra spectabilis)*, a plant with many heart-shaped flowers, grew from each heart-filled tear from the young Cherokee who hid behind the strawberry bush to watch his love at a distance. (See the story in chapter 3.) This love brought a smile from the young Cherokee girl, which became what we call the new moon in the sky today.

Hickory tree *(Carya tomentosa)*. Mockernut hickory was used as an anti-septic in combination with other tree barks. It was also used in several formulas for ballplayers and for addressing "female problems." Hickory is still used for making blowgun darts and arrow shafts and in basket weaving.

Hickory appears to be an astringent; it was considered to have "special power" by earlier Cherokee. Hickory ashes were used in tanning hides. Sometimes called white hickory, it is a member of the Walnut family "with a nut that squirrels and humans will gather as soon as they fall."

Holly *(Ilex opaca)*. American holly was used for "weak blood or for circulation in elders." While stories of holly's Medicine power tell that it was very popular in earlier years, and even though it is mentioned often in descriptions of "the old formulas," holly is mostly used today for decoration. The leaves (not the berries) have been used to treat fever, bronchitis, gout, and rheumatism.

Hops *(Humulus lupulus)*. A drink from common hops or hops vine was used for treating "female problems," and hops is mentioned by Paul Hamel and Mary Chiltoskey as being useful for womb problems. Hops are thought to have an estrogenic effect for females. In addition to being used for insomnia, the hops' bitter acids are also antibacterial. Its primary use today is as a sedative.

Horse balm *(Collinsonia canadensis)*. The roots of horse balm, also called stone root or richweed, were prepared as an antispasmodic tea for treating menstruation as well as pain and nausea. Horse balm was used as an astringent and tonic for children with colic, indigestion, and bronchitis. As an elder said, "When the child didn't want to go to school, pull out the horse balm and castor oil." Another elder said that "before we knew how to use horse chestnut, chamomile was added with stone root for the problems and pains of varicose veins." Today horse balm is used for treating fluid retention, swelling, headaches, menstrual discomfort, and varicose veins.

Horseweed *(Erigeron canadensis)*. Called bittersweet or fleabane, *so qui li* was used by the Cherokee and mountain folks to stop bleeding. The plant was probably originally from Europe. An elder said, "You see, we [Indians] did learn something from the White people that came here. We enjoyed the sharing of Medicine, music, and food. We should remember those things too." Horseweed was used to stop the flow of blood externally. It is used as a hemostatic due to tannin in the leaves. It is also used as a natural diuretic for bladder conditions. The erect stem can grow to seven feet tall, crowned with a tuft of basal leaves similar to mullein's.

Horseweed is also another name for scabious *(Scabiosa succisa),* commonly used for treating scabies and other skin itches.

Indian apple (see Mayapple).

Indian balm (see Trillium).

Indian bean (see Catawba tree).

Indian cucumber (see Balsam apple).

Indian hemp *(Apocynum cannabinum).* Indian hemp should not be confused with *Cannabis sativa,* or what mountain folks called "loco weed" (marijuana). The roots of Indian hemp, also called bowman's root, were used to treat uterine problems. The plant was used for treating female depression and nervousness, "but only by those who were trained." The glycosides in Indian hemp can lower blood pressure precipitously, causing bradycardia. This plant should not be confused with *Cannabis indica,* which is used for making latex and fiber but is not taken internally.

Indian hyssop (see Vervain).

Indian paintbrush *(Castilleja coccinea).* Earlier Cherokee used this plant in a sacred and mythical way to "do combat with the enemy." This use was mentioned by several elders, as well as by Paul Hamel and Mary Chiltoskey. The mountain folks called the plant scarlet "paint-cup" or "painted-cup."

Indian paintbrush grows to fifteen inches in height; it bears clusters of flowers with the reddish bracts that are green where it connects to the stem. The beautiful red stands out in the mountains, along with hearts-a-bustin', crimson bee balm *(Monarda didyma),* trumpet honeysuckle *(Lonicera sempervirens),* Indian pink, purple wake-robin (trillium), and fire pink *(Silene virginica)* that add to the East Medicine color of the Great Smoky Mountains National Park and the Appalachian Trail. A similar plant for home gardens is blanket flower *(Gaillardia grandiflora),* which has yellowish tips on its daisylike flowers. Blanket flower is great in pond or rock gardens. Another plant with scarlet flowers reminiscent of Indian paintbrush is fire pink, or red catchfly.

Indian poke *(Veratrum viride).* Indian poke, also known as American hellebore, pokeweed, or devil's bite, was used as a mild sedative for "control of the heart and vessels." The plant was mentioned by several elders, but they could not remember how or in what quantities it was used. This plant should not be confused with poke *(Phytolacca americana),* the green eaten as a salad. My father and Uncle Grady called Indian poke "earth gall"; my grandmother used it as an antispasmodic and for treating fevers. It was also used as a diuretic and sedative. White hellebore *(V. al-*

bum) is listed in the herbal literature as helpful for blood circulation, digestive problems, cold sweats, vomiting, and cramps. The dosage of white hellebore can be difficult to determine due to toxicity and other side effects from plant alkaloids, which irritate the mucous membranes. As an elder cautioned, "Only seek those trained in the use of this plant."

Indian root (*Aralia racemosa*). Also called American spikenard, or *yo na tsu ne ste,* this plant was used by the Cherokee and other southeastern tribes to treat blood poisoning. A "cure-all" plant, the rhizome was used in the Medicine of each of the Four Directions. Indian root grows to ten feet high with a single leaf stalk; the leaves are divided into three parts, each carrying five leaflets. The yellowish green flowers grow in clusters with a purple berry. Only the roots of Indian root were used medicinally.

As a boy I remember this plant being called bearberry bush. Do not use Indian root during pregnancy.

Indian tobacco (*Lobelia inflata*). The leaves of Indian tobacco, or pukeweed, are called *tso la* or *sah lol* in Cherokee. They were used by earlier Cherokee and other American Indians. Indian tobacco was classified as poisonous by the U.S. Food and Drug Administration in recent years; however, Indian tobacco was used in earlier years as a smoke for treating asthma and other lung ailments.

Also known as Hercules' club, Indian tobacco was thought to be a "cure-all" in the early nineteenth century. The plant contains an alkaloid called lobeline, which relaxes muscles. It is used to help smokers to quit smoking; however, too much lobelia can produce nausea and vomiting.

The Cherokee used Indian tobacco as a sacred tobacco for ceremonies. The buds were used as an ointment to treat burns and inflammation. Crushed leaves were placed on and around the head to treat headaches. The Cherokee used Indian tobacco in a smudge, and "gifted it to the fire to send a message to the Great One." Indian tobacco was considered a sacred power plant that would carry our messages and prayers as the smoke rose into the sky. While used in several formulas, it was best known for treating "female problems." The alkaloids in Indian tobacco are potent compounds that can be deadly poisonous; they are not to be used in teas.

Juniper bush (*Juniperus communis*). The oil from the juniper or dwarf juniper berry cones were used for "the flitters and hot feeling of the head with giddiness." Juniper was used to lower blood pressure and as a diuretic. It was also given to elderly who had been sick and experienced "lacking appetites" and those with blood sugar problems, such as diabetics. Juniper is a member of the Cypress family.

Ladies' tresses (*Spiranthes cernua, S. lucida,* and *S. vernalis*). This plant was used to treat urinary problems associated with pregnancy, along with twayblade. In earlier years it was also used in a bath for an infant to grow healthy and strong. A member of the Orchid family, the tiny flowers grow out from the spiraling stem. The plants grow nearly a foot high with the nodding and slender ladies' tresses "reminding us of a young Cherokee woman's braided hair." My grandmother called this plant "pearl twist" or "spiral flower."

Lady's slipper (*Cypripedium calceolus*). *U tsu wodi,* or moccasin flower, was one of the oldest plants in a Cherokee formula for nerve conditions, particularly for females who are "weak from the rigors of childbirth." An elder called the plant *oo ka ou la su lo,* or "nerve root." It was used in a formula for sexually transmitted diseases but was prepared, with Indian root, only by those trained in its use.

Lady's slipper was one of the plants that John Bartram noted in his travels; it was also mentioned by Vogel as a plant used by the Iroquois. A member of the Orchid family, the dried rhizome and roots were used to reduce bleeding during birthing. Lady's slipper is a sedative and antispasmodic. The plant is protected by federal and state laws. Today it is used for hysteria, headaches, and nervous conditions.

Larkspur (*Delphinium ajacis* and *D. tricorne*). Larkspur, or field larkspur, was used in a formula for treating heart problems. An elder remembered the formula as one for "settling the heart down with ginger and sometimes hawthorn." An elder said, "This plant is poisonous and should be prepared only by those trained." An active agent, delphine, has a paralyzing effect on the central nervous system.

A substitute for larkspur used for herbal medicinal purposes in recent years is ginkgo (*Ginkgo biloba*), a native tree of China and one of the oldest trees in the world. It is used today in the way that elder, hawthorn, juniper, lily-of-the-valley, and others were used in earlier years: to improve circulation. Ginkgo can replace those plants for treating elders with "fuzzy feelings, or those with weakly conditions due to their heart." The use of gingko is a good example of the way in which Indian Medicine men and women are willing to learn new applications from plant uses of other cultures. Ginkgo is cultivated in the Carolinas today.

Lavender (*Lavandula vera* or *L. officinalis*). While it is uncertain how or when American Indians learned about the value of this aromatic plant, it is without a doubt true that lavender was a favorite among many Indian women, according to an elder. She said that "the entire plant was crushed for the juice [oil] and used on the skin. A little could be mixed with other plants for women who had the itching and irritation [vaginitis]." The essential oil from the lavender flowers is a mild sedative, as well as a helper with internal gas. It is used today to stimulate appetite and to treat nervousness and insomnia. *Lavandula angustifolia* is the variety most often found in home gardens.

Leafcup *(Polymnia uvedalia)*. Leafcup, or bear's foot, was used in a formula for expelling afterbirth. Little is known about its use today, but an elder remembered that "the bear used it for pain in the paw."

Lemon balm (see Balm, melissa).

Licorice *(Glycyrrhiza lepidota)*. Licorice, also called American licorice, and *u ga na s da* or *oo gah nah see doh* in Cherokee, was used with horehound in a formula intended only for females. Its use was restricted to young women with digestive upsets during the "changing to womanhood," which is different from its use for balancing estrogen levels in premenstrual and menopausal periods of life. Licorice was also used as a natural anti-inflammatory.

Licorice was used by southeastern Indians in many remedies or formulas in each of the Medicine directions. It was and still is a favorite for viral and yeast infections affecting males and females. Caution with using licorice root is recommended due to possible loss of potassium and retention of sodium in the body.

Lily, Easter *(Zepbyranthes atamasca)*. The Easter lily, or an older variety not identifiable today, was considered a sacred plant of the Cherokee. It was referred to as "west wind flower." It is mentioned here rather than under West Medicine because the teaching was about using the lily "to open the West door from the East." The formula for that use has been lost; it was a "clearing" formula, used with a prayer-chant to seek healing for the family and clan. It is unclear when this plant started being used in ceremony, but European and Christian traditions have certainly influenced Indian use of certain plants, including the Easter lily.

Lily-of-the-valley *(Convallaria majalis)*. As a member of the Lily family, *ka la wi yi* was used in the North Carolina mountains for the heart. It contains a substance that acts like digitalis (foxglove); like foxglove, lily-of-the-valley can be poisonous. *Cullowhee,* a Cherokee word meaning "lily of the valley," is the name of a place in North Carolina and the home of Western Carolina University. It is also where I did my undergraduate work in biology, botany, and Appalachian studies.

Lily-of-the-valley contains a cardioactive steroid glycoside. Earlier use of lily-of-the-valley for treating arrhythmia has been demonstrated. It was also found to elevate diastolic pressure and was used for mild cardiac insufficiency or changes of the heart due to age or chronic condition. Today lily-of-the-valley is used as a heart tonic and for heart valve problems and seizures. It is also still used in the eastern mountains for treating kidney and bladder stones. *Caution:* Use lily-of-the-valley only under the supervision of one who is trained in its therapeutic dosages.

Life root (see Ragwort).

Linden (see Basswood).

Lizard's tail (see Swamp lily).

Lobelia (see Indian tobacco).

Loblolly bay (see Bay).

Locust tree *(Robinia pseudoacacia).* An elder told me that "a chew of the [locust tree] bark was used in ceremonies, and for women who wanted to just clear the sick feeling." Black locust was used for making blowgun darts, fence posts, and log cabins. According to my Uncle Grady, the first settlers to Swain County, North Carolina—a group that included my forefathers—used the wood of the strong black locust tree as corner posts in building their new cabins.

Loosestrife *(Lysimachia vulgaris* and *L. quadrifolia).* Loosestrife and whorled loosestrife was used for addressing female problems. An elder recalled a formula with sage or rue "to settle the nerves during that time of the month." An active agent in loosestrife is rutin, an astringent.

Another plant, called rough-leaved loosestrife *(L. asperulifolia),* is very rare in North Carolina. With the help of an elder I was able to locate one rough-leaved loosestrife, which the elder said was a gift from another eastern tribe, from a place where they are plentiful. Other species of loosestrife *(L. vulgaris* and *L. salicarici)* are used as astringents, anti-inflammatories, and antibiotics. These are natural helpers for diarrhea, intestinal complaints, varicose veins, bleeding of the gums, and hemorrhoids.

Love plant *(Alertris farinosa).* Love plant, also known as blazing star and colic root, was used to treat female problems such as painful menstruation, the threat of miscarriage, and spasms of the uterus. An elder referred to the plant as *oo wa sa ou e,* a word related to the female that defined this plant as a helper for strengthening a woman for birthing and to prevent abortion.

The plant is called "devil's bit" by mountain folks. My Uncle Grady said that folks in Appalachia used it with "homebrew" for treating rheumatism. My uncle knew a lot about the years when the White man settled in the Smoky Mountains. He and my father grew up in what is now the Great Smoky Mountains National Park. They knew this plant as "true unicorn root," used by my grandmother for "female complaints" as well as for chronic bronchitis. An elder called the plant "stargrass" or "agueroot."

Magnolia vine *(Schisandra chinensis).* According to an elder, the fruit of the magnolia was a gift from a southern tribe of Indians, who used it as a tonic for the liver. Little is known about how it was prepared or used, but it was combined with Indian root in one of the old formulas.

Maidenhair *(Adiantum capillus-veneris).* The Cherokee and the Creek Indians used southern maidenhair fern in a tea made from the roots and leaves for easing menstrual discomfort. This plant is not to be confused with the maidenhair tree *(Ginkgo biloba),* which is a plant used to relax the vessels and to stimulate circulation. The maidenhair fern has small, fanlike leaves on brown stems. An elder called this plant "five-finger fern," and mountain folks knew it as "Venus hair." Do not use maidenhair during pregnancy.

Maple tree *(Acer rubrum* and *A. saccharinum).* The barks of both red and silver maple are used with white and black oak and chestnut for female concerns. An elder said that maple was used for cramps and other menstrual problems. Today maple bark is used for treating sore eyes and as an astringent in several remedies. The bark strips are used for making baskets and the inner bark for making red dye. Striped maple or goosefoot *(A. pensylvanicum)* and mountain maple *(A. spicatum)* are used by Cherokee and mountain folks from Indian Gap in the Smoky Mountains to Indian Creek in West Virginia.

Marigold *(Calendula officinalis).* Sometimes called "pot marigold" by mountain folks, this plant was used as an astringent for treating menstrual problems. Marigold is used to treat yeast infections due to its antifungal value. Its anti-inflammatory properties also made it good for healing wounds, particularly following birthing. Today marigold is popular for treating inflamed wounds, burns, and mouth sores and as a facial wash and eyewash.

Marigold flowers are antimicrobial, antifungal, antibacterial, and antiviral and tend to stimulate the immune system. It is no wonder that it was considered by mountain folks to be "a European heal-all." The Cherokee preferred it as female medicine, for treating what we now know as vaginitis, and for treating young children and babies with colic, fever, and unspecified pains. Earlier Cherokee women used it as a bear salve (bear grease) for treating baby rash. Marigold was used with bloodroot *(Sanguinaria canadensis)* for treating venereal disease and to kill bacteria and fungus. For a home garden with moist soil, marsh marigold *(Caltha palustris)* provides beautiful buttery yellow flowers.

Marshpepper smartweed *(Polygonum hydropiper).* The juice from a leaf of marshpepper smartweed was put on a child's thumb to stop her from sucking the thumb. Other purported uses were for inflammation and swelling, but I was unable to verify this with the elders. One elder did say that marshpepper smartweed "helped to catch fish." He did not expound on how to use it for this purpose.

Mayapple *(Podophyllum peltatum).* This plant was called Indian apple or mandrake, and it was used as a "special Medicine." Like sunflower and evening primrose, Cherokee myths hold mayapple as sacred. Mayapple is a member of the Barberry family, along with twinleaf in the West Medicine and blue cohosh in the East. Mountain folks used it to treat cancer and as a liver tonic. Mayapple contains agents that are irritating to the skin. Do not use mayapple without the guidance of a person trained in its handling and use. This member of the Barberry family should not be used during pregnancy.

Milkweed *(Asclepias syriaca).* Earlier southeastern Indians used *u na di* for treating sore breasts. Common milkweed was called "elder plant" for its use in "strengthening and purifying the blood of weak elders." Sassafras was used with it in the formula, along with ginseng "to improve the elder's appetite and spirit." It was also used for "the backaches of pregnant women and for the bad disease [venereal disease]." This use was verified by Paul Hamel and Mary Chiltoskey. Swamp milkweed was also used for treating digestive disorders. Close cousins to milkweed are pleurisy root *(A. tuberosa)* and swamp milkweed *(A. incarnata)*, but these plants are used for different conditions.

Mistletoe *(Viscum album* and *V. abietis).* Called *oo ta le,* mistletoe was used to treat heart conditions, headaches, and "the nervous condition of some women." It was used in earlier years as a stimulant or tonic. One elder said that it was the "best Medicine, if grown on an oak tree." It was used in a special formula for those with epilepsy, as well as in a love charm to take care of love sickness. An elder said, "You were given two leaves to carry in your Medicine bag for twenty-eight days by the Medicine man for love sickness." Today mistletoe is used to treat depression, as a helper with cancer, for high blood pressure and irregular heartbeat, and for easing tension. It strengthens capillary walls and reduces inflammation while slowing the heart rate. It was also used in Green Corn Medicine, considered sacred.

Mistletoe was used in the Friends-making Ceremony as a clearing-way, along with greenbrier, heartleaf, and ginseng. It was considered a "male Medicine" for strength and love, and a "female Medicine" for imparting protection. In addition to regulating blood pressure, mistletoe was also used for treating gout and rheumatism and as a blood purifier in earlier years. Always consult with someone trained in the use of mistletoe.

Moonseed *(Menispermum canadense)*. *Udo sa no e hi,* or "moon root" as it is called by some American Indians, was used as a diuretic and for "females that are weak, especially before or after childbirth." Mary Chiltoskey reported it as being used for sickly or weak stomach.

Mother of corn *(Coix lacryma-jobi)*. Sometimes referred to by mountain folks as "Job's tears," mother of corn was called *se lu oo sti* by the Cherokee. The seeds were used for cooking and were strung in a necklace to put around the baby's neck so he could chew on it when teething. Bull nettle was used for the same purpose by the Cherokee.

Motherwort *(Leonurus cardiaca)*. The common name of this plant tells its use—to help the mother. The Latin species name, *cardiaca*, tells of its other use—a helpmate for the heart. It was used with evening primrose and bilberry for blood pressure problems and blood clotting.

In earlier years motherwort was used as a stimulant and a tonic. The plant was referred to as "mother," or *e tsi*. One elder said motherwort was a gift from the Iroquois for treating "the cramp and weak hearts of women." One had to be trained in the proper use of the plant. Motherwort should not be used when taking blood-thinning drugs, or when a woman is pregnant. It is used as a stimulant for "weakly females with nervous conditions, and works where others don't." My father called it "lion's ear." Today motherwort is used for treating menstrual cramps and for easing childbirth. A sedative, it is also used in treating heart palpitations.

Mountain dittany *(Cunila origanoides)*. This plant was included in a snakebite formula in earlier years. As a tea it was used for "female pains, and with the gift of birth." Mary Chiltoskey mentioned this same use. Another elder said it was "used with the 'five-finger plant' [ginseng] to help women in labor and with the pains of childbirth."

Mountain mint *(Pycnanthemum flexuosum* and *P. virginianum)*. Mountain mint was mentioned by Paul Hamel and Mary Chiltoskey as a leaf poultice for treating female headaches and for treating heart problems. The plant was used to settle the nerves, usually with rue and willow, among others. Other plants called mountain mint include calamint *(Calamintha nepeta)*, oregano *(Origanum vulgare)*, and Oswego tea or bee balm *(Monarda didyma)*.

Mullein *(Verbascum thapsus)*. Common mullein, *ga lah la di, i ga di* in Cherokee, is probably best known for its furlike leaves, which were smoked to ease throat and lung problems. French traders who lived among the Cherokee probably shared mullein's use for treating irregular heartbeat, palpitations, and other heart problems.

A handful of cut leaves would be boiled until reduced to about a pint. This infusion would be strained and mixed with a popular tea, one teaspoon twice a day, just to preserve the formula. I do not recommend using mullein without consulting with a trained herbalist who knows about dosage control. Mullein's most common use is for treating cough and bronchitis.

Nettle, stinging (*Urtica dioica*). This plant was used to promote the flow of milk in new mothers. It was also used for "poor blood," or anemic conditions with low hemoglobin levels, especially in women who experienced heavy menstruation. Today nettle is used for complaints of uterine bleeding and for treating inflammation. It is an effective diuretic and is used in a formula as a sedative for female anxiety and uterine pain, but its effectiveness in promoting milk flow is in question.

The tiny hairs, or stingers, on the nettle plant contain formic acid and histamines, which protect the plant from animals and unwanted insects. When the hair tips are touched they leave the acid and histamines on the intruder's skin. These substances are so toxic to insects that some can actually experience genetic damage to the larvae.

Nettle has been used for male prostate complaints and for everything from respiratory ailments to arthritis. The tops of young plants are carefully removed with gloves, then crushed with the leaves of dock *(Rumex crispus)*. An earlier formula combined nettle with plantain and milkweed "for difficulty of men urinating" (benign prostate hyperplasia). This formula is not in use today. Some tribes considered stinging nettle a sacred plant that could only be used by those specially trained in the ways of this Medicine. There are good references today for the specific uses of nettle.

Nightshade, black (*Solanum nigrum*). The stem and leaves of black nightshade were used as a tea for "grieving persons after the death of a family member." An elder reported that "it was mixed with the Moon Medicine to calm the spirit." In earlier years the Moon was always associated with someone passing to the "darkening land." A sacred formula for grieving included a sedative as well as a stimulant to ward off depression. Black nightshade should not be confused with bittersweet nightshade *(S. dulcamara)*, which was used with yellow dock for sores and swelling.

Black nightshade was used for treating heart rhythm problems and a "nervous heart," as well as for treating digestive problems in earlier years. Caution is recommended if black nightshade is used internally, because it can be slightly poisonous. This plant should also not be confused with deadly nightshade *(Atropa belladonna)*, sometimes called poison black cherry.

Oak tree (*Quercus alba* and other species). The inner bark of *ge ga a ta u* (or *e qua, gu le,* for "acorn") was used in a formula with other tree barks as a wash for sores and itching skin. It is also used as an astringent, due to its tannin content, and as a natural antiseptic, antifungal, and antibacterial. Oak was used along with locust, redbud, and plum to make the sacred fire. The inner bark on the east side of the tree was used for ceremonial purposes, along with white oak, black oak, basswood, and chestnut. The inner bark of black oak and yellowroot were used to make a dye. Black or yellow oak *(Q. velutina)* was used as an East Medicine for birthing, with chestnut or rock chestnut oak *(Q. prinus)*. The latter was also used to tan leather.

As members of the Beech family, other oaks were used not for their medicinal value but for making sacred fires. These included post oak *(Q. stellata)*, red oak *(Q. rubra)*, Black Jack oak *(Q. marilandica)*, red or black oak *(Q. coccinea)*, and chinkapin or chestnut oak *(Q. mueblenbergii)*. Today oak is used for treating vaginal problems, to harden nipples for breastfeeding, and for treating bacterial and viral infections.

Partridgeberry *(Mitchella repens)*. Sometimes called twinberry, foxberry, or squaw vine, partridgeberry was used on breasts before breastfeeding; it was also used to ease the pain of sore breasts. Earlier Cherokee called it *gu qua,* or deer plant, and *a wi* for its use in soothing abdominal pain and menstruation. Partridgeberry was used as a uterine stimulant and an astringent for the nervous system in a formula that would include raspberry leaves. It is a member of the Madder, or Bedstraw, family.

Partridge pea *(Clitoria mariana)*. Called "butterfly pea" by mountain folks, "it was said to be a good love Medicine to give to a woman. Just don't tell her it's called 'clitoria,' and was used by the Old Ones in other countries to enhance fertility."

Passionflower *(Passiflora incarnata)*. The flowers and roots of passionflower were used as a sedative for painful menstruation. It was also used in a tea for nervous conditions and "pains of the heart," along with flaming azalea roots and twigs. The formula also mentioned the use of hawthorn and hazel alder *(Alnus rugosa)*.

Passionflower was known as "old field apricot" or "maypop" by earlier Indians and mountain folks, who used it "to draw out inflammation." It was used for babies who had a difficult time weaning, and with chamomile for young mothers, to "calm the spirit."

There is much to be said about this sacred plant, used earlier in "love Medicine" and in ceremonies. A beloved elder said that passionflower was "a gift from our Mexican brothers and sisters to calm the heart and spirit." It was also used in sacred ceremonies for those who had passed on. Today passionflower is used for its calming effects. It is a member of the Passionflower family.

Pepper *(Capsicum annum)*. Red pepper is a systemic stimulant that was not used much by earlier Cherokee, but it was traded as a stimulant. However, pepper has become more popular in modern days and is included in several formulas as a tonic and stimulant for the digestive and circulatory systems of "sickly females" and the elderly during cold weather. Pepper has antiseptic and antibacterial qualities. Earlier Cherokee give credit to our Mexican Indian brothers and sisters for introducing capsicum through trade.

Pepper grass *(Lepidium virginicum)*. Pepper grass was a gift from the southeastern Indians, who used the native plant with ginseng, or "five-finger," root. Knowledge of its use in earlier years seems to have been lost.

Periwinkle *(Vinca minor)*. Common periwinkle, sometimes called myrtle or lesser periwinkle, is identified by its runners and shiny leaves, with violet or sometimes whitish flowers that bloom in May and June.Common periwinkle was used as a hemostatic, an agent that stops the flow of blood. While that application was mentioned in earlier Cherokee Medicine teachings, it was not clear what part of the plant was used. We do know that the entire plant was used for treating circulatory complaints. Periwinkle was only used by those "trained in plant Medicine."

Persimmon tree *(Diospyros virginiana)*. In earlier years persimmon fruit was dried for traveling food and to use as a lure when hunting animals. The bark was used in a formula for treating venereal disease. According to an elder, sweetgum was used in that formula. Persimmon is a member of the Ebony family.

Peruvian bark tree *(Cinchona ledgeriana)*. It was a little surprising to me when use of this bark was mentioned in Cherokee Medicine. Peruvian bark tree was valued as an astringent, a tonic, and a stimulant for the uterus. The bark was used for its quinine content in treating malarial infections in earlier years. The tree is native to Peru and Ecuador.

Phlox (see Sweet William).

Pine tree *(Pinus virginiana* and other species). All species of pine were considered sacred among the earlier Cherokee. Pine was used in many earlier formulas. The bark was used for treating swollen testicles and sexually transmitted diseases. The primary use as an East Medicine was for ceremonial purposes and for treating swelling of the breasts. According to Mary Chiltoskey, a pine branch or bundle of needles was placed on the hearth and would be used to rekindle the hearth fire after a death in a Cherokee family.

The inner bark of white pine taken from the east-facing side of the tree was used in the sacred fire on the seventh day of the Green Corn

Ceremony. Other woods included in the ceremonial fire were Black Jack pine and chestnut; the ashes would be used for ceremonial purposes. White pine was also used in a Friends-making Ceremony that was held each year, along with cedar and hemlock. Other tree bark and roots were used for the fire, including mountain birch, willow, dogwood, and spruce. The new fire would be carried to each clan and family home as a symbol of beginning-again. As an elder said, "The Great One gifted us with the pine that is used for everything in the physical circle, including the Universal Circle."

Piney weed *(Hypericum hypericoides* and *H. gentanoides).* Earlier use of this plant included a formula for promoting menstruation. The formula included skullcap, partridgeberry, and several other plants for "fixing a female problem." It was also used in a formula for venereal disease, in which it was referred to as St. Andrew's cross. In earlier years other plants were used with piney weed for treating sexually transmitted diseases. Those plants include burdock, comfrey, devil's walkingstick, lady's slipper, pine, and prickly ash. Mountain folks added balsam, persimmon, Eastern wahoo, greenbrier, milkweed, dogbane, figwort, and cardinal flower.

Pipsissewa *(Chimaphila umbellata).* Also called pip, this plant was used for treating menstrual difficulties and was part of an old formula for controling menstrual flow. While little was said about pip, a Cherokee elder felt that it was very effective, especially when used with goldenseal.

Pitcher plant *(Sarracenia flava).* While this plant was known by several common names, such as flycatcher or trumpets, it was known by earlier Cherokee as *ta lu tsi,* "cup plant" or "basket plant." Pitcher plant was considered to be special Medicine; the formula for its use was kept secret. An elder said, "Only a few knew the formula of the pitcher plant, and they have passed into the otherworld." An elder said the plant was "a gift from the Catawbas and other eastern tribes who live in the east of North Carolina and south, down in South Carolina, where this plant is commonly found." An elder referred to the plant as "trumpets calling to insects and little flyers to catch them on a stick death." It is a carnivorous plant found in the damp soils of bogs and swamps.

Plantain, broadleaf *(Plantago lanceolata* and *P. major).* Broadleaf, or lance leaf, plantain was also called English plantain. American Indians referred to this common weed as "White man's foot." Common, or great, plantain *(P. major)* was a popular remedy for children, especially in treating insect bites and stings. Earlier Cherokee believed that an infusion of the leaves would strengthen the child for learning to crawl or walk. According to Mary Chiltoskey, plantain was used as a wash for babies and as a tea for cleansing the bowels of a baby with complaints. A combination of broadleaf and rattlesnake plantain (*Goodyera pubescens* or *repens*) was used with alder, wild cherry, wild ginger, and yellowroot (*Xanthorhiza simplicissima*) as a tonic to "build the blood and give spirit to the body." Rattlesnake plantain was mentioned in the formulas as useful for treating swelling. Today plantain is used to treat urinary tract infections and skin inflammation resulting from poison ivy and as a helper in treating cancer.

Poke or pokeweed (*Phytolacca americana*). While primarily known for its use in "poke salad," pokeweed was used as an East Medicine to stimulate the metabolism. It was also used to treat what we now know of as breast cancer and for swelling and related pains of the breast following childbirth. The formula has been lost, but I believe it included wild ginger, ginseng, and *ga na s da tsi,* or sassafras.

Today poke is used for treating inflammation and swollen lymph nodes. Poke has many side effects and can be extremely toxic. An elder reported that "only those trained would be allowed to work with this plant in earlier years." It is also a persistent plant and can be difficult to get rid of in the yard or garden.

Prickly ash tree (*Zanthoxylum americanum*). Prickly ash was used in several formulas to "purify the blood" and was combined with Indian root for treating sexually transmitted diseases. Also known as toothache tree, it is an astringent and is used to stimulate the circulation. An elder said it was also used to lower blood pressure and reduce fevers and inflammation. An elder said, "Prickly ash was used to stimulate the circulatory system and for fever that comes with being sickly and having no energy." See also Devil's walkingstick.

Puffball (*Geastrum hygrometricus*). Earlier Cherokee put some of the "dust snuff" from puffball, or earth star, on a baby's navel after birth to help the umbilical junction to heal. Puffball is a natural antibiotic and an astringent. It has also been used for "earaches and infections with children." It was mentioned by Mary Chiltoskey as being called "earth star."

Puffball is a fungus not to be confused with dandelion, which is also called puffball or blowball because the dried flower is a globular cluster of achenes that can fly through the air. Puffball has a shell-like ball that is brown. When stepped upon it releases a light, airborne substance that looks like snuff.

Purple coneflower (*Echinacea purpurea*). Purple coneflower was used for treating snakebites in earlier years. The Cherokee recognize echinacea's value as an antibacterial and an anti-inflammatory. It was used in several formulas, including formulas to support birthing. Please encourage others to leave this beautiful gift of Mother Earth unharvested in its natural environment. Like goldenseal and ginseng, echinacea is popular and it is very rapidly being stripped from the mountains. This plant is easily grown in a home garden where the soil is moist but well drained and sunshine is abundant.

Rabbit tobacco *(Antennaria plantaginifolia)*. An old formula included rabbit tobacco, or sweet everlasting, for reducing menstruation for "women with profuse bleeding." A story in Cherokee mythology tells about how Rabbit got caught in the briers and laurel roots, and in the process of freeing himself discovered this plant's gift for stopping the bleeding at a cut or wound. There are many stories about how the plants got their names, and in earlier days stories were a means for remembering a plant's use.

Mountain folks called rabbit tobacco "pearly everlasting." Another plant called rabbit tobacco by early Cherokee is *Gnaphalium obrusifolium,* which is also known as cudweed or sweet everlasting.

Ragweed *(Ambrosia artemisiifolia)*. Common ragweed and great ragweed were used in the Green Corn Ceremony to celebrate the beginning of the health of the corn crop. This was a special occasion in earlier years, for the survival of the families, clans, and the Cherokee tribe was determined in part by the corn crop. As an elder said, "Full corn bins meant a good winter, but empty bins meant slim or no survival in the harsh mountain winters."

Ragweed pollen is recognized as a common cause of hay fever.

Ragwort *(Senecio aureus)*. The Cherokee called ragwort *da lo ni ge i,* or "gold"; mountain folks called the plant "squaw weed" or "golden ragwort." An elder said that ragwort was used in a formula to prevent pregnancy. It was also used in a heart formula, probably as a diuretic. It was used to suppress menstruation and was even used by some American Indians to induce abortion. The toxic alkaloids in ragwort make it a plant to use with caution.

Mountain folks considered ragwort a good heart remedy because it has heart-shaped leaves. Sometimes it was called "old man," "squaw weed," or "wild valerian." (Please keep in mind that the term *squaw* has negative connotations for American Indians.) Today ragwort is used for treating menstrual concerns.

Ramps *(Allium tricoccum)*. This species of wild onion, *was di* in Cherokee, is an important ingredient in the Cherokee "spring tonic" for vigor, and for "purifying the blood." Today ramp festivals are popular events in the Southeast. An elder said, "You gotta' cultivate a taste for cooked ramps or get out of town when they are being prepared, 'cause they smell something awful."

Raspberry (*Rubus idaeus, R. occidentalis,* and *R. strigosus*). Raspberry root was used as a uterine tonic for easing labor. It was also used to ease the pains of childbirth and for addressing menstrual problems. While useful during pregnancy, an experienced midwife recommended not using raspberry root during the first trimester because of its ability to stimulate bleeding. It is a mild astringent with tannins.

In earlier years raspberry root was thought to be a way of relieving rheumatism. The painful or inflamed area would be scratched by the prickly stem of the raspberry, and then the root wash would be applied to the scratch. Raspberry was also used to prevent miscarriage and increase milk, and for addressing cardiovascular problems. The active agents are tannins, flavonoids, and vitamin C. If harvesting the plant for personal use, be sure it is raspberry rather than blackberry.

Red cardinal (*Erythrina herbacea*). An elder referred to this plant as "Cherokee bean." The seeds were used in the winter as a special Medicine for fishing; it was also used as a natural poison for rats, along with horse chestnut seeds. Red cardinal was considered a sacred plant for "moon Medicine," referring to female issues. It was usually used as part of a formula or a remedy that a grandmother would have that would be kept secret until needed for starting a period or avoiding pregnancy, or for treating a disease "that was not to be mentioned for open ears."

Red clover (*Trifolium pratense*). Red clover, also called broad-leaved clover, is a plant naturalized from Europe. Earlier Cherokee and other tribes used it along with Indian root as a blood purifier and for menstrual problems, as well as for menopause. An elder called it "red horse" or *o li ga*. Red clover is an excellent source of what we know today to be phytoestrogen isoflavones, which help prevent cancer. An elder said, "Clover is like ginseng and evening primrose—there are some special things the Great One put in them to make them special Medicine, and it is up to us to figure that out." Red clover is a member of the Pea or Bean family. Today it is used as an estrogen replacement after menopause. Do not use red clover during pregnancy.

Redroot (*Amaranthus retroflexus*). Redroot is sometimes referred to as "pigweed" by mountain folks. Due to their saponin content the leaves of redroot were used by some Indian tribes for washing clothes. Redroot was used in earlier years to stop bleeding from diarrhea and in the event of profuse menstruation. An elder remembered that there used to be a story about the red bark of this plant, which grows about two feet high and has white flowers, and its strong friendship with the hickory and pine trees. While the story has been forgotten, the relationship of plants and trees were very important in learning about which ones to choose and from which direction on the Medicine Wheel to harvest the plants. Stories were also a way to remind us of our harmony and balance with all things in nature "for the Medicine to work as a helper for us."

The roots of redroot were used to treat internal bleeding, difficult sores, and venereal disease in earlier years. Amaranth pigweed (*A. hybridus*) was also used as an astringent for reducing menstrual flow.

Red root (*Ceanothus americanus*). This plant, also known as New Jersey tea, was used in a spring tonic with sassafras, sarsaparilla, Indian root, and ginseng in earlier years. An elder said, "It would set your heart and spirit straight." Red root was used in a formula in earlier years for treating venereal disease as well.

Rhododendron (*Rhododendron maximum* and *R. catawbiense*). A tea was made for the heart in a formula using the bark of rhododendron and several other plants. Rhodendron leaf was used in a poultice for treating pain. Rhodendron-leaf fans were used in the Friends-making Ceremony as a traditional way to "call upon the spirit of the winter to be kind, to clean the air, and to call for an early spring." This plant is sometimes called Catawba rhodendron, the name coming from the Catawba River in North Carolina. According to an elder rhodendron was also called "purple laurel" or "mountain rhododendron."

Rosemary (*Rosmarinus officinalis*). Rosemary is an antiseptic, diuretic, and antispasmodic used in earlier years for relieving pain, stress, and cramping. The essential oil in the rosemary plant has been identified as stimulating menstrual flow and treating circulatory problems. It is unclear how it was prepared. This small evergreen herb with aromatic leaves continues to be grown in kitchens and used in cooking. In earlier years, as one elder put it, "This little plant represented the liberation of women, long before these young girls thought of the idea." Rosemary was also used with walking fern (*Asplenium rhizophyllum*) for treating swollen breasts. The essential oil was considered a "gift to females" and was added to shampoo.

Rose pink (*Sabatia angularis*). Rose pink was one of the plants that Bartram took back to Philadelphia from his trip to the Carolinas in the 1790s. It was used as a tea for yellow fever at that time. The Cherokee also made a tea from rose pink for treating menstrual pains. This use was verified by Paul Hamel and Mary Chiltoskey. Also called meadow beauty, rose pink has beautiful pinkish to purple flowers; it grows in the open areas of the mountains and along roadsides.

Rosin weed *(Silphium compositum* or *S. laciniatum).* Rosin weed was mentioned by Paul Hamel and Mary Chiltoskey as being used for treating weak females. Mountain folks used it in a "sang [ginseng] tea" for stimulating the body and building strength. The plant is a cousin to Indian cup *(S. perfoliatum)*, which was used by several midwestern tribes to treat rheumatism and for "strength for hunting." An elder called it the "plant pilot weed"; it was used in sweats to increase perspiration and to rid the body of toxins each spring.

Rue *(Ruta graveolens).* Common rue was called *u ne ga, u s di,* "little white," by earlier Cherokee. It was used to treat nervousness during menopause, as well as heart palpitations. It was also combined with alumroot, or wild geranium, to reduce menstrual flow and for vaginal discharge.

There may be some confusion about this plant as recorded by Mooney, who identified meadow rue *(Thalictrum anemonoides)* as being used by the Cherokee for diarrhea. The purple meadow rue *(Thalictrum revolutum)* was used for stomach cramps, but the rue mentioned in the old formula for avoiding pregnancy and treating menstrual concerns and cramping is *Ruta,* or *u tsa ti* in Cherokee.

Rush, common *(Juncus effusus* or *J. tenuis).* In earlier years this plant, which was used with babies and children, had a mythical quality. An elder said it "was given by the Medicine man for strength of the little ones, for them to grow to be good hunters and ballplayers." It was used with plantain to prevent infant walking problems.

Sage *(Salvia officinalis).* Sage, or purple sage, is used in ceremonies and traditional sweats as a "clearing-way" formula. It is used for nervous conditions, especially during menopause. An elder said that "a tea with honey would be given to weakly females for strength before birthing." Sage was used to stop the flow of milk, but the elders could not remember the formula. It was combined with shepherd's purse to raise the blood pressure. One Medicine woman combined sage with sarsaparilla and red clover "to stimulate the female," or provide an estrogen-like action. Sage was also combined with rosemary for improving circulation, and with raspberry for treating "the pain of menstruation."

Sage was used as an antispasmodic, an astringent, and an antiseptic, and for reducing blood sugar levels. Today it is used for treating menstrual pain, muscle spasms, and excessive flow of milk.

Scarlet sage *(Salvia splendens)* makes an interesting variety for East ceremonies. The flowers are also white and purple, which can be used for South and North Medicine ceremonies to burn or offer to a fire for a "clearing-way" and to give thanks to the Great One for healing or going on a long trip or journey. There is also a blue or azure sage *(Salvia azurea)* that was gifted to the Cherokee by eastern tribes, but its use is uncertain now.

Sassafras tree *(Sassafras albidum)*. The bark and roots of sassafras, *ka na sti* in Cherokee, were mentioned by an elder as being used for treating venereal disease and as a blood purifier. The inner bark was considered a cure-all by American Indians in the Southeast. The Cherokee used sassafras as a diuretic, and the oil was extracted and used as an antiseptic. It is used as a tonic with calamus root or blue flag to "settle the spirit and body." It was also used for "people with weak hearts."

Earlier use of sassafras by American Indians and mountain folks was as a spring tonic. An elder called it *ga na s da tsi,* a word relating to sassafras's clearing actions, a testimony to its use in treating bowel and stomach problems. It was also used as a cough medicine and a blood tonic. The roots were used for making yellow dye. Today sassafras is used as a tonic for addressing ill health and malnutrition, fluid retention, and sex-related diseases, and to enhance physical performance. Sassafras was banned for use by the U.S. Food and Drug Administration due to safrole, a poisonous constituent of the plant. It is mentioned here only for educational purposes.

Saw palmetto *(Serenoa serrulata)*. The berries of *ga na do gi,* "leaf saw," were crushed for their juice and applied to sore nipples. Today saw palmetto is a popular remedy for genital and urinary problems, as well as for treating sexual dysfunction. It is a member of the Palm family.

Scurvy grass *(Cochlearia officinalis)*. Scurvy grass was used as a blood purifier and in a formula as a spring tonic, along with other plants, including sassafras. Scurvy grass is known as "spoonwort" by my herbalist friends in England, who grow it as a garden plant.

Senna, wild *(Cassia marilandica)*. Also called sensitive plant, senna was used as a root tea for "weak hearts, and those who have fainting spells." It was favored as a mild tea for treating children with fever, and for women "during the time of cramps." Mooney mentioned the Cherokee calling this plant *u nagei* or *u neg,* "black plant," for use when there was darkness around the eyes. Partridge pea is combined with senna to alleviate fatigue and syncope, as verified by Paul Hamel and Mary Chiltoskey. Do not use senna during pregnancy or while nursing.

Serviceberry tree *(Amelanchier arborea)*. Serviceberry was included in the spring tonic. It is sometimes called downy serviceberry; my father called it "shadbush," and his grandfather called it "sarvis." It is popular for its beautiful white flowers, which bloom in the early spring. The Cherokee called serviceberry "little apple" for the sweet and edible fruit. Serviceberry is a member of the Rose family.

Seven-bark shrub *(Hydrangea arborescens)*. Also known as wild hydrangea or seven-bark shrub, *te ta na we ski* was used in a tea for assisting with a woman's menstrual cycle. It was also used for high blood pressure, and the bark and leaf were made into a diuretic for women's Medicine. Seven-bark shrub was mentioned for women who had "bad dreams during their periods." Other female Medicine uses included treating weak bladders, edema, and gout. Seven-bark shrub was also used to treat prostate problems in men. Seven-bark shrub has tiny clusters of light yellow to cream-colored flowers that rest among the large and broad leaves of the shrub.

Shepherd's purse *(Capsella bursa-pastoris)*. Called *de ga lo di, yv wi ya hi,* "Indian bag" in Cherokee, shepherd's purse was used along with alumroot or wild geranium to stop bleeding, or as a mild hemostatic. An elder referred to it as "a bristle plant that hooks on whatever goes by to catch a ride to higher ground." The name shepherd's purse is said to have come from the shape of the seedpod, which looks like a purse. Some mountain folks called it "mother's heart."

Shepherd's purse is a member of the Mustard family. Shepherd's purse acts to constrict blood vessels; it regulates the heart as well as the menstrual cycle. As an astringent it reduces blood pressure and bleeding; it is also used as a urinary antiseptic. Today it is used for treating bleeding disorders, blood in the urine, and heavy menstrual bleeding. It is not recommended for use during pregnancy as it brings on uterine contractions.

Skullcap *(Scutellaria lateriflora)*. The Cherokee used skullcap as a sedative and to relieve breast pains, a use which was verified by Mary Chiltoskey. I could not verify its reported use for expelling afterbirth. The Cherokee called skullcap *ga ni qui li ski*.

Slippery elm *(Ulmus rubra)*. The inner bark of slippery elm was used in earlier years for addressing breast complaints, and for treating children "who complained of pain in the stomach as a way to get out of going to school." It was combined with chamomile for a vaginal douche. Eastern tribes called it "Indian elm."

Snakeroot (see Blue cohosh and Wild ginger).

Snakeroot, black *(Aristolochia serpentaria)*. The root of black snakeroot is used for treating "female weakness, headaches, and other pains." Also called Virginia snakeroot, this plant was mentioned by John Lust as one that stimulates bloodflow. Mooney recorded the Cherokee name as *tstiyu,* or "very small root." The plant is probably best known as black snakeroot; it is still used for treating fevers and "to strengthen weak males for endurance." It was also used to treat syncope, vertigo, and chest pains.

Snakeroot, sampson *(Psoralea psoralioides)*. This plant was used in earlier years for treating menstrual problems. It was considered an East Medicine "cure-all" for female problems. Indian snakeroot *(Rauwolfia serpentina)* has a chemical called reserpine, which dilates the blood vessels.

Snakeroot, white *(Eupatorium rugosum)*. White snakeroot was used as a diuretic, in particular for women during and following pregnancy. It was also used in a tonic formula and to help reduce fever in "weakly females."

Sneezeweed *(Helenium autumnale)*. The common name of sneezeweed probably came as a result of the crushed dried leaves being used in earlier years to induce sneezing. It was mentioned by an elder as being used with ironweed *(Vernonia fasciculata)* roots to prevent menstruation, according to Mary Chiltoskey. Other plants, including sorrel, were part of this formula. The formula is thought to be lost now; it was a very old remedy. This plant is a good choice for a home garden with moist soil. The daisylike yellow to orange flowers have the shape of purple coneflower.

Solomon's seal *(Polygonatum biflorum or P. officinale)*. While used as an astringent and to evoke "throw-up and for a clearing," Solomon's seal was most commonly used "for those with too much bleeding [female menstruation]." Mary Chiltoskey verified Solomon's seal's use for the same purposes. Solomon's seal was collected for making a "wild salad," along with watercress and dandelion. An elder referred to it as *oo te ste ski,* used as a female tonic.

Solomon's seal is a member of the Lily family. The drooping stem has greenish white bell-shaped flowers that hang down, which is a way to differentiate it from false Solomon's seal.

Souchan *(Rudbeckia laciniata)*. While these natural greens are gathered in the spring for cooking, they are also used as a "spring tonic and good Medicine for women and children, to give them strength." It is called wild golden glow or green-headed coneflower in the herbal literature, but it has always been known to the Cherokee as souchan.

Southern lady fern *(Athyrium asplenioides)*. Southern lady fern was a "special headache Medicine for females." There was no mention of how this remedy was prepared, but it was included in a formula that also used white willow and other plants for calming female anxiety.

Southern wax myrtle (see Bayberry).

Spicebush *(Lindera benzoin)*. Spicebush was valued for all disorders of the blood and was particularly valued as a "female Medicine." An old remedy using spicebush eased "the itching of a female [vaginitis]." The plant has a microbial effect and is therefore effective in treating *Candida albicans* and yeast infections.

Spiderwort *(Tradescantia virginiana)*. Some referred to this plant as day-flower. It was used for females experiencing kidney problems associated with pregnancy.

Spikenard, American (see Indian root).

Spleenwort *(Asplenium platyneuron)*. This evergreen fern was used to improve the flow of milk in nursing mothers. Little else is known about the earlier use of spleenwort as an East Medicine.

Spotted cowbane (see Water hemlock).

Spotted spurge *(Euphorbia hypericifolia* and *E. maculata)*. Both varieties of spotted spurge were used in an earlier cancer formula, especially for women. This formula is known by only a very few Medicine men and women alive today. As is common with "special Medicine," the formula is passed down through the family to preserve the mixture and its use. Spotted spurge is thought to be a helper to the immune system. It is considered poisonous and should be handled only by those specially trained in this Medicine.

Spreading dogbane *(Apocynum androsaemifolium)*. Some Indians believed that eating the boiled root of this plant would confer sterility. The root was used as a stimulant and tonic during pregnancy. The fruit was used for heart and kidney function, and a root tea was made for "flushing." Spreading dogbane was also known as "colic root" and "rheumatism root" by mountain folks.

Spring crocus *(Pulsatilla patens)*. Spring crocus was called pasqueflower. It was gathered in the early spring or April. An elder said, "It reminds us of spring, romance, and ceremonial time a-comin'." Spring crocus was used in an old ceremonial drink. There was also a pasqueflower *(P. vulgaris)* used in assisting women "in the change of life."

St. John's wort *(Hypericum perforatum)*. Earlier use of St. John's wort was "to calm the nerve pain of wounds." It was used for treating menopausal conditions, especially those associated with anxiety and irritability. Infants would be bathed in "root water" for strength. St. John's wort is an astringent and an anti-inflammatory and was used to relieve pain. An elder said this plant was a gift from the Catawba and other eastern tribes. Mountain St. John's wort varieties *(H. graveolens* and *H. mitchellianum)* are used for the same purposes. The five yellow petals have an extended pistil of what an elder calls "golden yellow sparklers that get your attention if you are a bee or a bird."

Strawberry *(Fragaria vesca* and *F. virginiana)*. Wild strawberry and Virginia strawberry were used for women "for strength and clearing during pregnancy." The families would look forward to spring "berry huntin'" in the mountains of North Carolina. Strawberries, like blackberries, were given to children for minor inflammations.

There is a Cherokee story about a woman and man having a conflict. She leaves and he follows, but he is not able to find her. He sees the strawberries that she leaves, and they come back together to enjoy strawberry eating and "clearing-way" discussions. Strawberry-leaf tea was made to calm the nerves. It is used in an old formula with yarrow or raspberry for relieving cramps.

Strawberry bush (see Hearts-a-bustin').

Sunflower, common *(Helianthus annuus)*. Common sunflower, or *a ga li ha*, is a sacred plant that appears in many Indian myths and stories. Sunflower has a special place in Indian Medicine. The seeds were used for treating the pain that females experience with the menstrual cycle; it was thought to help due to the Sun having a daily cycle, which keeps us warm and helps to grow food and medicinal plants. Men ate the seeds for "strength in love," said an elder; sunflower seeds are a good source of arginine, which helps boost sperm count.

The plant contains one of the best sources of phenylalamine, helpful in the control of pain, and is a rich source of vitamin E. An earlier formula combined it with peppermint and thyme for "soothing relief of the druthers and life's daily pain." Sunflower oil is used in cooking and as a dietary supplement, as well as an oil for smooth skin and massage. Sunflower is a member of the Aster or Composite family.

Swamp lily *(Saururus cernuus)*. An elder said swamp lily was a gift from the Catawba people, "who used it for female pains of the heart and labor." It is a member of the Lizard's Tail, or Water Dragon, family. Sometimes called by those names, it is one of the remedies that seems to have been lost with time. John Bartram reported on swamp lily in 1751 in his travels that took him through the swamp areas of South Carolina and Georgia.

Sweet flag (see Calamus root).

Sweet violet *(Viola odorata)*. The entire sweet violet plant is used in a tea for "female nerves," as a cousin to wild pansy. This is "nature's little beauty," with an essential oil being made from the leaves and flowers. In earlier years sweet violet was used in several formulas for treating skin problems, "nervous conditions of females," and sore throats.

Sweet William *(Phlox maculata* and *P. divaricata)*. A bath of sweet William or wild blue phlox was used ceremonially to protect and help young babies and children to grow strong and healthy. Mary Chiltoskey also mentioned mountain folks using the root infusion to make children grow. The blue flowers of the wild variety provide fragrance and a nice speckle of color to a rock garden. Creeping phlox *(P. stolonifer),* a pink- to mauve-flowered variety, is found in shaded areas.

Sycamore tree *(Platanus occidentalis).* In earlier years this member of the Sycamore family was used in birthing with Carolina hemlock *(Tsuga caroliniana)* and golden ragwort *(Secenio aureus).* The bark was used in several formulas for female problems. It was also used in a formula for the "bad disease" (venereal or sexually transmitted disease); that formula included sweetgum, blackgum, beech, mountain laurel, dogwood, and Virginia creeper. Traditional sweats included sycamore bark, tulip or cucumber, and wild parsnips for healing. The sacred and ceremonial fire was made from this tree, as well as Black Jack pine, post pine, and red oak.

Tansy *(Tanacetum vulgare).* Tansy was used primarily for treating bruises and sprains; however, it was also used as a tea "for those who are slow to menstruation." The plant has fernlike leaves with cluster flower tops bearing golden yellow flowers. It was used in a "tonic water." An elder said that in earlier years the leaves were placed in the moccasins of pregnant women to prevent miscarriages. The plant has also been called daisy, or buttons, and the bright yellow flowers were called "nature's eyes" by earlier Cherokee. An elder said the plant was used to "rid children of those pesky parasites." Today tansy is used to stimulate menstruation and for treating muscle spasms and swelling. Do not use tansy internally during pregnancy.

Thyme *(Thymus vulgaris).* A member of the Mint family, this plant gift originally from Spain was included in the Cherokee Medicine bag for painful menstruation. An elder called it "snake," or *u nu tsi.* It has value as an antiseptic, an astringent, and an antispasmodic. Thyme is used today for treating female menstrual problems and for headaches and tensions of males and females.

Tobacco *(Nicotiana rustica).* The leaves of *tsa lu,* or wild tobacco, were smoked and used to gift the sacred fire during ceremonies. Sacred tobacco is offered to the fire for sending a message of thanks to the Great One. The ashes were offered to each family to keep sacred for the entire year, until the next clearing and rekindling of the sacred fire.

Tobacco leaves are poisonous; nicotine, a toxin, is an alkaloid that can be absorbed through the skin. Tobacco is used today primarily as a ceremonial plant and for gifting. A variety of flowering tobacco *(N. alata)* with red flowers is a great plant for home gardens.

Wild tobacco is different from Indian tobacco *(Lobelia inflata)*, or puke-weed, used by American Indians in ceremonies. Another plant, called rabbit tobacco *(Antennaria plantaquinfolia)*, sometimes called sweet ever-lasting, is also used as a "smoke, particularly by women in earlier years." Mullein *(Verbascum thapsus)* was also called Indian tobacco in the mountains of Appalachia.

Trillium *(Trillium erectum)*. Trillium—also known as Indian balm, Beth root, purple wake-robin, or stinking benjamin—was used as a helper for women in childbirth to stop bleeding, and as an astringent. An elder called it "three wolf" or *tso i, wa ya*. A formula containing trillium was used to help slow heart palpitations, but little was said about how it was prepared by earlier Medicine men and women. The use of yellow trillium *(T. luteum)*, large-flowered trillium *(T. grandiflorum),* and white wake-robin *(T. erectum)* were different in earlier Cherokee Medicine. Only the white wake-robin is still used; the other two species are not used in Indian Medicine today, to the best of my knowledge.

Trillium's best-known use is probably as an antispasmodic and a uterine astringent. There were tales of a piece of the root being placed in food to create a "love Medicine." It is considered a sacred plant for "keeping the family together." Do not use during pregnancy.

Trillium is at risk of extinction in its natural environment today. A good choice of trillium for the home garden is large-flowered trillium *(T. grandiflorum)*, which has large and showy white flowers.

Twinberry or twin berry (see Partridgeberry).

Venus flytrap *(Dionaea muscipula)*. Venus flytrap was one of those "special Medicines" that was "just not talked about to anyone." It was considered as having special powers in fishing. Mary Chiltoskey and I confirmed that a small piece of the root would be chewed and spit on the worm or bait. An elder said this plant was a gift from the eastern tribes, who considered it "special Medicine." Venus flytrap is at risk of extinction in its natural environment. Sundew *(Drosera rotundiflora)* is another plant used in female Medicine and is also at risk.

Venus looking glass *(Specularia perfoliata)*. Venus looking glass was used to help control eating, especially for women "who were in waiting for birthing," and afterward. It was considered a sacred plant in earlier years; little more is known about this plant and its use today. It is a carnivorous plant that traps insects. The entire plant is used today to stimulate the immune system.

Vervain *(Verbena officinalis)*. Vervain, or Indian hyssop, was used for treating vaginal itching and yeast infections. It is a weed that has opposite, three-lobed leaves and small stalks of light purplish flowers. As an elder said, "Everybody has seen it, but few know its power. I guess the Great One calls this plant 'the humble one' as it gives thanks each day from the roadside." It is a member of the Vervain family. Do not use vervain during pregnancy. There is also a plant called Indian carrot (V. edulis) in Appalachia that was used as food by earlier American Indians.

Virgin's bower (Clematis virginiana). Also called little vine, virgin's bower was used to treat female problems associated with kidneys and backaches. An elder said, "A tea was used for the nerves women have at that time of the month." It was mixed with dogwood and black haw. The plant was used in a sacred formula in earlier years for Green Corn Medicine, in ceremony for young females. Common clematis (C. recta) is also called virgin's bower. The plant is considered poisonous and should be prepared only by a trained herbalist.

Walking fern (Asplenium rhizophyllum). Also called walking leaf, walking fern was used in a formula for treating swollen breasts and pain following birth. I could not verify the other plants or barks in that formula except for pine and willow bark. I do know that an astringent was used in the mixture.

Wallflower (Cheiranthus cheiri). As an East Medicine, this plant from the Mustard family was used to promote menstruation. It was also used to relieve pain during childbirth, as well as to cleanse the entire system after childbirth. Wallflower is a natural diuretic. Herbalists stopped recommending it after it was discovered that wallflower contained glycosides with properties similar to digitalis in foxglove. The danger was in heart failure from an overdose.

Wallflower was a plant much respected by the earlier Cherokee. This is one of the few plants that earlier Cherokee used only for the flowers and the seeds. It was administered "to hope for a new conception where the death of a newborn had been experienced." Wallflower is still used to encourage menstruation, but it is not to be used during pregnancy. Its use for cardiac insufficiency needs to be overseen by a trained herbalist or naturopathic physician. The fragrant wallflowers are popular in home flower gardens, with their spring colors of red, pink, and cream white.

Wapato (Sagittaria latifolia). In earlier years women would bathe infants with this plant after giving birth. It was also used to bathe children with fever. Timothy Coffey mentions wapato as "broad-leaved arrowhead," which is also called arrowleaf. The arrowhead-shaped leaves are distinctive and easily recognized in the North, where the plant is called swamp potato and was eaten as a food.

Watercress (Nasturtium officinale). Watercress was used on skin rashes and inflammations. It was also popular as a "spring salad" with dandelion and other greens. Today it is used for skin rashes, inflammation, and acne. In the "old Medicine" watercress was described as being used for "women's problems." Do not use during pregnancy.

Water dragon (see Swamp lily).

Water hemlock (Cicuta maculata). Water hemlock, also called spotted cowbane, was used as a contraceptive. The roots are poisonous. An elder said it was chewed for four days, but the elder did not know anyone who had used it since about 1920, when he was a young boy learning the Medicine. I do not recommend using it as a contraceptive.

The European water hemlock (C. virosa), or cowbane, was used for treating painful menstruation and migraines, but the fresh root is poisonous and acts directly on the central nervous system.

As well, the entire plant is slightly poisonous. Water hemlock is not to be confused with poison hemlock (Conium maculatum), which is also called cowbane or spotted hemlock.

Wax myrtle (see Bayberry).

Wild cherry tree (Prunus serotina). Te ta ya was used in many formulas as a blood purifier and a tonic. It was used for women with labor pains and menstrual concerns. The bark, an astringent and a sedative, was used for coughs, nervous conditions, and diarrhea. Wild cherry contains cyanogenic glycosides, but cyanide poisoning is not likely due to the low content of this compound.

Wild clover (see Red clover).

Wild cucumber (see Balsam apple).

Wild garlic (Allium vineale). Wild garlic was mentioned by an elder as used for "people who have blood rush to their faces, except when they are embarrassed." The same elder said that wild garlic was "a Johnny-come-lately plant in the Medicine." Like garlic (A. sativum), wild garlic was used to purify the blood and for treating infections.

Wild ginger (Asarum canadense). Also known as coltsfoot and snakeroot, wild ginger was used for "settling the heart and nerves." It was used in an old formula as a mild sedative for irregular or rapid heart rate. It stimulates the circulatory system and relaxes the vessels. Wild ginger was also used with dutchman's pipe (Aristolochia macrophylla) for "female conditions."

A member of the Birthwort family, wild ginger has heart-shaped leaves and a dark brown flower. It is found in moist woods or near streams. One elder said, "The roots were used in the olden days with sampson snakeroot and what you call 'star root' for discharges with pain, and was even used to get rid of worms." It was used for treating swollen breasts and pain. Wild ginger was also known as Indian ginger.

Wild golden glow (see Souchan).

Wild horehound (*Eupatorium pilorum*). The bitter leaves were used for "women with breast complaints." To my knowledge wild horehound is no longer used as an East Medicine, but as a West Medicine for several remedies that treat internal problems.

Wild lettuce (*Lactuca canadensis*). Paul Hamel and Mary Chiltoskey mentioned wild lettuce as being used for the sacred Green Corn Ceremony. It was used in earlier years as a stimulant, for pain relief, and as a calming agent for the nerves. The leaves are used in "spring greens" and as a "spring tonic." An elder said, "A good pressing of the leaves and stalks makes it a good calming and relaxation snack late at night."

Wild sarsaparilla (*Aralia nudicaulis*). A bark tea made from sarsaparilla is a very old formula used to treat coughs and colds. It is used as a blood tonic to "renew the body and spirit all year, not just as a 'spring tonic' or for ceremony." This use was verified by Paul Hamel and Mary Chiltoskey. Today sarsaparilla is used to enhance athletic performance, for treating fluid retention, and to induce sweating. As a member of the Ginseng family, it should also be mentioned that sarsaparillas are of the *Smilax* species, used with *Aralia racemosa* (Indian root) in making "mountain root beer and jams." Other names for wild sarsaparilla are sweetroot and wild licorice.

Wild sunflower (see Elecampane).

Wild yam (*Dioscorea villosa*). Wild yam was used in an old formula to relieve childbirth pains, as well as for morning sickness and pregnancy complaints. Sometimes it was used in sweats to promote perspiration. An elder called it *nu nv,* or "wild potato." Wild yam is a natural anti-inflammatory, antibacterial, and antispasmodic. A compound called diosgenin has been found to have an estrogen effect in clinical studies performed on mice. Today wild yam is used for pain in the uterus and ovaries, as well as for treating menstrual cramps. This plant is at risk of extinction in its natural environment.

Wild yam should be in every woman's Medicine bag as a salve for comfort of the breast and for treating vaginal dryness.

Willow tree (*Salix alba*). The inner bark of the white willow was popular in earlier years and was used in several formulas for general pain relief. The Willow family is a large species of small trees and shrubs. Most common in the Southeast is the eastern cottonwood or Carolina poplar and the black or swamp willow; the swamp cottonwood or swamp poplar and the southern willow are found along the coastal regions and Florida. The weeping willow *(S. babylonica)* is one of the most distinguishable willows, with its large size and weeping branches.

All of the *Salix* species' varieties contain salicin, a natural form of aspirin. Indians extracted the salicin by pulverizing the inner bark of the willow and then taking what would amount to about a half-teaspoon, or brewing that in a tea. This amount comes to about 100 milligrams, which is about one-third of an aspirin.

As an East Medicine, willow is used for treating gout, pain, backaches, and angina or heart pain. Caution is suggested because pain can also be a signal of something else going on that may need medical attention, especially with pains around the heart. Salicin is one of the plant-derived substances that I carry in my Medicine bag.

Witch hazel *(Hamamelis virginiana)*. Witch hazel was used as a female wash and douche for irritations and vaginitis, according to John Lust. An earlier formula included witch hazel with chamomile as an antiseptic wash. Witch hazel also has antibacterial and anti-inflammatory value. The German E Commission has approved witch hazel for hemorrhoids, inflammation of the mouth, rectal bleeding, wounds, and menstrual problems. It is a member of the Witch Hazel family.

Yarrow *(Achillea millefolium)*. A formula using the leaves of yarrow, witch hazel, hawthorn, and wood betony *(Stachys officinalis)* relaxes vessels and improves circulation and was used for "calming the heart." It was used in earlier years for "healing the woman with menstrual problems" and for cramps. One elder said that yarrow, an astringent, can be called "a woman's best friend." Used with black cohosh, an elder said, "it was an answer to a prayer for menstrual problems, or when menstruation was not coming." Another elder called it "blood feather," or *u gi da li*.

Yarrow is a member of the Aster, or Composite, family. My father called it "dog daisy," an Irish name; the Irish used it to stop bleeding and for treating inflammation. The German E Commission has suggested its use for venous and circulatory problems, as well as for arterial complaints. Do not use during pregnancy.

Yellow dock *(Rumex crispus)*. Distinguished by the yellow rootstock, yellow or curled dock is used in a formula to "purify the blood." It was used in earlier years in a skin ointment for "tender skin" and for women during pregnancy. Also called dock or curly dock, the plant is high in vitamin C and iron. An elder said it was used to "strengthen the lymphatic system." While I was unable to verify its use in purifying the blood, it is effective as a blood cleanser and an astringent, an anti-inflammatory and antibacterial, a tonic for the stomach, and for treating jaundice and bronchitis. Its primary use today is in formulas for treating skin sores and itching.

Yellowroot *(Xanthorhiza simplicissima)*. The roots of this plant were used in earlier years in a formula to aid in childbirth. The roots and stems are used by the Cherokee for making a yellow dye, adding color to wood strips that go into making a basket. The name *yellowroot* is also used to describe goldenseal *(Hydrastis canadensis),* which was used by Cherokee women as an antiseptic in several formulas. Goldenseal is one of the plant-derived substances in my Medicine bag.

Yellow stargrass *(Hypoxis hirsuta)*. Yellow stargrass was used in a formula brewed as a tea to strengthen the heart and the vascular system. It is not to be confused with star grass *(Aletris farinosa),* sometimes called colic root, which is used as a bitter tonic or a narcotic. Today yellow stargrass is used for treating depression and as a mood enhancer.

Yucca (see Bear grass).

Many uses of plants for East Medicine have been lost over the years. A few of those East Medicine plants are named here, in case a reader might recognize the name and know how the plant was used in earlier times by American Indians or mountain folks. These include buttercup *(Ranunculus hispidus),* trout lily *(Erythronium americanum),* meadow parsnip (*Thaspium* species), large-flowered bellwort *(Uvularia grandiflora),* small bellwort or wild oats *(Uvularia sessilifolia),* stargrass *(Hypoxis hirsuta),* hawkweed *(Hieracium pratense),* coreopsis *(Coreopsis major* or *C. stellata),* bush honeysuckle *(Diervilla sessilifolia),* hairy alumroot *(Heuchera villosa),* touch-me-not *(Impatiens pallida),* Appalachian avens *(Geum radiatum),* and yellow fringed orchid *(Platanthera ciliaris).*

If anyone recognizes these plant names and how the plants were used as East Medicine, I'd appreciate knowing that.

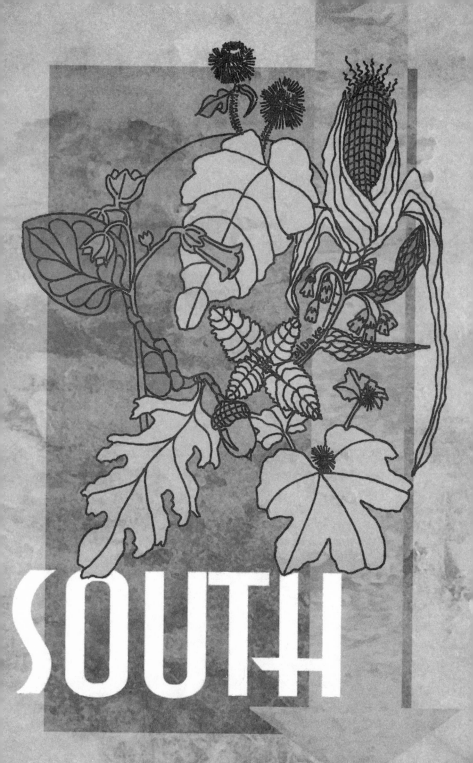

SOUTH

5

Plant Medicines of the South

South Medicine focuses on the innocence of life and the energy of youthfulness. It is the direction of curiosity and play: think of a young child, around the age of seven, playing in nature. South is Mother Earth and planting time for food and Medicine. It is enjoying the beauty of flowers and observing the movement of small animals, such as the beaver in the water or the rabbit on land. South is also the direction of warmth and protection—an image of South energies that comes to mind is a young girl or boy playing with a favorite pet or friend outside in nature. South energy is the kind of curiosity that allows us to just sit and watch ants move in single file, back and forth, as they gather food. The South Medicine protects innocence, like the skin that protects the body from injury and harm or the shield that protects a hunter from arrows.

The color of the South is green for the earth, as we recognize the value of plants and trees in this direction. It was also the color white, for the purity and innocence of a child.

Ceremonies of the South Medicine were related to small animals, with games and songs such as the Beaver Dance or the Wolf Dance that would be fun for children to participate in, as well as for adults to remember their youth. Often ceremonies of the South Medicine were about the Eagle Dance and the dance of hunters going off to join a party to gather meat for the feast. There were also decrees with the stories, offering values for children to follow for their own protection.

The Medicine of the South has many plants, barks, and natural substances to protect the skin and the body. The primary focus with

South is related to the skin and the muscular and skeletal systems. Protecting the skin barrier from infections and inflammation was important for the hunter and his family. The elder Medicine men and women knew that the body protected itself with "strong spirit and a sense of knowing what to do when cut or injured." While they did not call this internal knowing the immune system, they did know that harmony and balance was critical to having the body "take care of its own need with plant helpers."

Diseases and some injuries were considered the work of a conjurer or of some influence that was not "good Medicine" (although there was good Medicine in some conjuring, such as bringing two people together through "love Medicine." The Medicine man or beloved elder woman would provide Medicine in the form of ceremony, chants, formulas, and actions for the individual, family, and tribe to protect the integrity of the individual, the family circle, and the Universal Circle.

The protection of the skin or the spirit also included cleansing or "clearing-way." The simple act of washing the skin was realized as a way to cleanse and protect the body from some influences. The influence may be bacteria or a "spirit being that is causing harm." Washing of the skin and hair were considered sacred parts of daily life. Many formulas were used as helpers for the purpose of cleansing the skin, body, and hair. Sometimes cleansing was as simple as putting hands or feet in a body of water that had never seen fighting or bloodshed. Other times cleansing might involve a very complex ritual, with plant and bark formulas, ceremonies of song and dance, and a vision quest. This is when intermediaries, such as Grandmother Moon or powerful crystals, would also be called upon to act as helpers and healers.

Throughout my years of training and observations I kept my own "black book" of the Cherokee Medicine that was used for cuts, bruises, wounds, infections, cleansing methods and "healing ways," and plants used for infections and inflammation. Like many before me, I am concerned that this information of many generations will be lost if not recorded for future students to appreciate. As an elder said, "The sharing of this knowledge is not to be for personal gain or favor, but to be a helper to others in need and for preservation for the future."

Writing some of this information for public view was of concern to several of the Medicine elders. They were concerned that the plants might be used in a wrong way to cause harm rather than for healing. As an example, some of these plants can be harmful by just touching them, or if used without precautions or by people "not trained in how to prepare or use them," as the elders would say. Those with concerns were somewhat satisfied that I was trying to preserve this old wisdom and that my writing would be used for educational purposes. As one elder said, "Some people will just go out and grab any plant. You know, you can't just do that to a mayapple, jimson weed, stinging nettle, or Jack-in-the-pulpit. You got to know these things, or just enjoy looking at their beauty, like looking at a beautiful young woman." Because I was twenty-two years old at the time, I knew he was giving me an important message.

The Medicine of the South is about the natural environment and the helpers that tend to our cuts and abrasions; South Medicine also protects us from physical harm in the environment. It teaches the importance of support in the circle of life and the value of connection with all other things in the environment. The elder Medicine men and women understood the value of vitamins in food and medicinal plants, as well as minerals in the roots and soil.

The Medicine of the South is connected to Mother Earth and the natural environment. In this Medicine, debilities are considered gifts with challenges that provide lessons for us all. Special Medicine of the South included ceremonies for natural acceptance of whatever the Great One provided, including natural storms and disasters. However, most of the information presented here concerns plants used for healing wounds, for stanching bleeding, for cleansing, for healing, and for protecting the body from outside harm and influence or accidental injuries. Fortunately today we do not have many of the health problems of the past that plagued people who worked in rough environments. Familiarity with natural plants and substances in the wild was critical when farming and hunting, which was done by entire families among the Cherokee and other tribes.

A Cherokee elder asked me to think of a young boy playing in nature—with all its exposures—and sharing with other animals and "critters" that also live on Mother Earth. Immediately I thought of my childhood, playing on Mother Earth and running through the woods. I imagined myself making an arrow and trimming a piece of wood for a fishing pole. I felt welts from bites; allergic reactions to poison ivy; skin rash; cuts and sores; bites from ticks, spiders, and ants; stings from a wasp or a yellow jacket. I imagined burns from touching hot rocks that were being prepared for a sweat lodge. My mind created pictures of severe bleeding from a cut while I was chipping the arrow. I imagined sticking a bone fishhook in my finger and slipping on a wet rock while crossing the Oconaluftee River and fracturing my ankle. As I shared all this with the elder he said, "That is the reason we used black birch, black snakeroot, boneset, rheumatism weed. That is the reason we made a liniment of arnica, ginger, and onions, as well as burdock and dock. That is the reason we knew about willow and dogwood bark for pain. This is what Indian Medicine is really all about."

The following is a listing of plants and their uses as South Medicine.

Adam and Eve root (*Aplectrum hyemale*). As a South Medicine, the bulb and root were used to treat boils and "stubborn sores." Also known as puttyroot, Adam and Eve root is a member of the Orchid family. In addition to its value in treating sores, it is used in ceremony for "joinings," or weddings, as mentioned in the East Medicine. Traditional joining in earlier years was an event for ceremony and "a coming together of family and friends."

Adam's needles (see Bear grass).

Adder's tongue *(Erythronium americanum)*. The crushed leaves were used on "difficult wounds, or a wash was made from the leaves for sores that seem to not go away." Also known as dog's tooth violet, the bulb and roots were used in Appalachia by squeezing the juice and combining it with the crushed leaves for a skin and hair softener. Adder's tongue is sometimes called trout lily, due to its spotted leaves. It is a member of the Lily family.

Alder tree *(Alnus serrulata* and *A. glutinosa)*. The inner bark of hazel or black alder was used with other barks in formulas for skin problems. It was especially used for the itch and swelling of poison ivy and poison oak. The leaves and stems contain a thick juice that was considered a "sore Medicine" in earlier years; the juice would be rubbed on the in-flamed site of a skin problem. The bark was combined with dutchman's pipe for treating swollen feet and legs. It was combined with purple cone-flower for dressing difficult sores. Alder is a member of the Birch family.

Allspice (see Spicebush).

Aloe *(Aloe vera)*. While not a native of the Southeast, aloe vera gained popularity when introduced here in America as a soothing agent for skin lotions. The sticky substance in the thick leaves is used as an emollient, or skin softener, in skin lotions, creams, salves, and shampoos. An elder said aloe was a gift from our Indian brothers and sisters from Mexico treating on minor wounds and burns. Aloe vera penetrates the human skin al-most four times faster than water, and it provides a moisturizer under the upper layers of the skin. It is an antibacterial and anti-inflammatory and provides relief from pain. It promotes rapid healing from sunburn inflam-mation and chemical burns and makes a good ointment for treating her-pes and sores.

Earlier Cherokee used the crushed juices from several "plants of the water and fields, as well as roots," to soothe burns. These plants included arnica, adder's tongue, carrots, celery, radishes, young potatoes, and plants with bulbs that grew near water.

Alumroot *(Heuchera americana)*. Alumroot was used with wild geranium (*Geranium maculatum,* also called alumroot) to stop bleeding and for in-fection of cuts and wounds.

American spikenard (see Indian root).

Arnica *(Arnica montana* and *A. cordifolia)*. Arnica, also called mountain daisy or mountain tobacco, was introduced to the eastern Indians by a tribe from the Northwest. It was used for treating insect bites, as men-tioned by an elder. The flowers are used externally with willow on bruises only (not in places where the skin is broken). Arnica was also combined with chickweed and used for hair care. Heartleaf *(Arnica cordifolia)* flowers were considered "a choice in trading with northern tribes."

Today arnica is used for treating joint and muscle aches and pains, as well as wounds. Arnica is a pain reliever and an antiseptic and has anti-inflammatory properties. This is one of my favorite plants for treating sprains and edema, boils, and insect bites; for this use arnica is combined with purslane. It is not recommended for internal use due to its toxic lactones. There are stories of how this plant and others were used to avoid the loss of limbs due to serious wounds and infections.

Arrowroot *(Maranta arundinacea)*. The crushed dried powder of arrowroot was used in moccasins to avoid foot fungus. It is used today with comfrey and goldenseal to rid the skin of and protect the skin from fungus. Agrimony was mixed with arrowroot in a formula for skin inflammation, along with arnica and goldenseal.

Azalea, flaming *(Rhododendron calendulaceum)*. The roots and twigs of azalea were boiled and used as a poultice for treating rheumatism. It was also used with the inner bark of dogwood for treating rheumatism and the joint pains of arthritis.

Balm, melissa *(Melissa officinalis)*. The leaves and the entire melissa plant, also called bee balm, lemon balm, or balm mint, were used in earlier years by crushing the plant and putting it on wounds and insect bites.The lemon scent makes it easy to recognize this little plant, which gets its name from the Greek word for *bee*. Bee balm is found in sunny fields and along roadsides in sandy and loamy soils. The stems can reach three feet high, with white flowers growing in opposite pairs at each leaf joint. It blooms from June to September. Melissa is used today for treating herpes due to its antiviral and antibacterial properties. It is a member of the Mint family.

Balsam fir tree *(Abies balsamea)*. Balsam resin was used for treating sores and cuts. Spruce or fir *(A. fraseri)* was used for pain relief. Balsam is a member of the Pine family.

Bamboo brier *(Smilax laurifolia* and *S. pseudochina)*. The roots and bark of bamboo brier were used as a wash for burns and for sores.This is a species of vines of the Catbrier family, which has sharp briers. Bamboo brier was called "bullgrip" by tribes in South Carolina and "devil's clothesline" by northern tribes and mountain folks in Appalachia. The plant has astringent properies.

Basswood tree *(Tilia americana* and *T. heterophylla)*. The Cherokee would boil the bark of basswood, also called bee tree or linden, and mix it with cornmeal to make a poultice for treating boils and difficult sores. A lightning-struck basswood tree was also thought to be very powerful, and the tree would be used as a "power Medicine" for treating snakebites. Basswood is sometimes referred to as American basswood or white basswood. There was also a Carolina basswood. All are members of the Basswood family.

Bay shrub *(Gordonia lassianthus)*. This aromatic evergreen was used with balsam fir on difficult sores and boils. It was combined with bark from the ash tree for treating rashes. Also known as loblolly bay along the eastern coastal areas, it is a member of the Tea family.

Bear grass *(Yucca filamentosa)*. Bear grass, or Adam's needles, also known by the coastal Indians as yucca, was used in Green Corn Ceremony with broom sedge and spring amaranth. The juice was extracted by crushing the plant between two smooth, flat river rocks, to be used on sores. Earlier southeastern Indians would eat the flowers in a fresh salad, and use them with willow or rhododendron by crushing them "to rub on aching joints." Bear grass was also combined with bearberry as an astringent for soothing and healing.

Bear grass is a member of the Catbrier family. It contains saponin, which makes the plant "soapy to the feel" when it is crushed. Another plant with the common name of bear grass *(Xerophyllum tenax)* may still be used by some tribes for making baskets and hats.

Beard grass (see Broom sedge).

Bearsfoot *(Polymnia uvedalia)*. Also known as leafcup, the roots of this plant were reportedly used for treating bruises, cuts, burns, inflammation, rheumatism, and swelling. An elder remembered it used "for inflammation of sores and cuts, and as a rheumatism root remedy." It was also used with twinleaf and dwarf iris in a formula for treating skin cancer, ulcers, and difficult-to-heal sores.

Bee tree (see Basswood).

Beech tree *(Fagus grandifolia)*. Beech tree was used for treating skin rashes, itching, and poison ivy or poison oak. Called *ge tla,* the bark and leaves are used as a poultice on inflamed wounds and sores. The inner bark was also combined with bedstraw to stop bleeding. Beech is a member of the Beech family of trees.

Beet *(Beta vulgaris)*. According to Mary Chiltoskey, the Cherokee made a poultice with the wilted leaves of the beet plant for treating sores and boils. One elder said that the leaves of several "water plants"—plants such as watercress, beet, and melon—are used "to dry up boils that are from blood problems."

The beet plant is in the Goosefoot family, along with spinach *(Spinacia oleracea)*, pigweed or lamb's quarters *(Chenopodium album)*, and Virginia glasswort *(Salicornia maritina)*. The ashes of Virginia glasswort were used for making glass. These were some of the plants traded with the Cherokee for "love Medicine" and wound formulas.

Betony (see Wood betony).

Birch tree *(Betula pendula* and *B. nigra).* The inner bark of mountain or white birch and river birch was used in a formula for treating cuts, scratches, warts, and wounds. Earlier Cherokee also liked it as a hot- or cold-drink preparation. The paper birch *(B. papyrifer)* was used for its sugar, like the maple tree. The river birch *(B. nigra)* is a native of the Southeast. These species of birch are not usually mentioned for their medicinal value, like the sweet or cherry birch *(B. lenta),* which is known for its fragrant oil (oil of wintergreen) and for birch beer.

Birch bark is used today for treating warts; birch has antiviral properties due to the presence of betulin and betulinic acid. The bark also contains salicylates, which are approved for human use by the U.S. Food and Drug Administration. Birch is a member of the Birch family.

Bittersweet *(Celastrus scandens).* False or American bittersweet was used with a thorny branch to scratch the area of skin where rheumatism and aching occurred. An elder said, "I had that done to me once, and sure enough, I didn't feel any pain, but the scratch sure did hurt!" Bittersweet was also a name for nightshade *(Solanum dulcamara)*, which was used in treating rheumatism and chronic bronchial complaints.

Black snakeroot *(Sanicula marilandica).* Also called heal-all or sanicle, black snakeroot was used externally on wounds and ulcers and internally for bleeding, digestive ailments, and inflammation in the lungs, as well as for treating ringworm. An elder said, "The White people settling in the mountains called it 'self-heal,' but earlier Indians would chew on it with tobacco and put the chaw on a bad wound or snakebite." It was also used with fairywand for treating pain, arthritis, and snakebite in earlier years.

Black snakeroot was sometimes called Maryland sanicle, traded and used by northern tribes for treating severe lung problems and difficult sores. It is in the Carrot, or Parsley, family, along with angelica, caraway, hemlock, wild carrot, fennel, anise, and rattlesnake master or button snakeroot. An elder said it used to be popular with an Alabama tribe and was traded by them for its properties of "showing a man's strength and endurance with females in lovemaking." As the elder said (with a smile), "I have never tried it, but then, I didn't have to." To my knowledge this formula has been lost.

Bloodroot *(Sanguinaria canadensis)*. The Cherokee are especially careful when using this popular plant, also called redroot or Indian paint. Bloodroot is mixed in very small amounts for treating sores, eczema, and other skin problems. It was often combined with Indian root and used as an astringent, antibacterial, and anti-inflammatory. In 1751 John Bartram noted the use of bloodroot during his travels in the South. It was used as a red dye for making ceremonial masks. An elder in West Virginia called it "coon root"; the plant was valued by earlier Cherokee in that region as a "power Medicine." Bloodroot is used today for treating fungal growth, ringworm, and skin cancer.

Mountain folks knew bloodroot as "red puccon," due to the red sap from the roots. The basal leaves form a bud on the rootstock; the large, showy leaves seem to wrap around the flower, which opens during the day. The white flowers are easily identified in the shaded, rich soil of the mountains.

Bloodroot is a member of the Barberry family, along with blue cohosh, twinleaf, and mayapple; it is one of the plants at risk of extinction in its natural environment. Do not use bloodroot during pregnancy.

Bouncing bet (see Soapwort).

Broom sedge *(Andropogon virginicus)*. Broom sedge, or beard grass, was crushed for its juice, which was applied to the skin for treating "certain skin itches and bites from insects." It was combined with black-eyed Susan and beggar's lice for treating hives and skin irritations, with purslane added for healing especially difficult insect bites.

Buckeye tree *(Aesculus octranda)*. The nuts of yellow buckeye are crushed and used as a poultice for treating swelling, sprains, and infections of the skin. A salve was made for sores. The buckeye was carried in a Medicine bag and by mountain folks for good luck, which was probably learned from Europeans. In much earlier years the "upland or overhill" Cherokee—those living in upper Tennessee, Kentucky, West Virginia, Virginia, and even into Ohio—"were said to carry a buckeye seed in their Medicine bag as special Medicine." Earlier settlers carried a buckeye seed and a piece of Indian root to protect them from rheumatism, a practice likely learned from American Indians. Yellow buckeye wood is still used to make ceremonial masks.

Buckeye is a member of the Buckeye family. The buckeye seed is poisonous.

Buckthorn *(Rhamnus caroliniana* **or** *R. catharticus)*. The buckthorn shrub was called Indian cherry or yellow wood; it was used in a formula for treating itch and insect bites and as a wash for skin sores. Hazel alder

(Alnus rugosa) was added for infected conditions. The berries and bark are used from this member of the Buckthorn family. Do not use buckthorn during pregnancy or when nursing.

Bugleweed (see Virginia bugleweed).

Bullgrip (see Greenbrier and Bamboo brier).

Bull nettle (see Carolina horse nettle).

Bull thistle (see Thistle).

Burdock *(Arctium lappa* and *A. minus).* Great and common burdock were used for treating leg ulcers and swollen legs. The crushed leaves of the plant, sometimes called burr or sticky plant, were used as a poultice for treating skin irritations and sores. As one elder said, "The plant knows that it is going to cause the skin irritation, abrasion, and even slight cuts, so it gives you the leaves for healing." Old formulas combined burdock with Solomon's seal, and sometimes with yellow dock, to make a "bear or hog's lard salve, known as an itch salve."

Burdock is an excellent external antiseptic, as well as a good skin wash for treating eczema, acne, psoriasis, boils, herpes, and sores. It was sometimes used in combination with dutchman's pipe for treating swollen legs and feet. A combination of burdock, borage *(Borago officinalis)*, and chickweed is used as a natural emollient and poultice for skin sores. Today it is used to purify the blood and for treating eczema, ulcers, and arthritis.

Canker root (see Goldthread).

Carolina horse nettle *(Solanum carolinense).* Also known as bull nettle, Carolina horse nettle was used for treating the itch of poison ivy. There is also a plant called dead nettle that was used for the same purpose, as was stinging nettle.

Castor or mole bean *(Ricinus communis).* In the mountains the oil of the mole bean would be pressed from the seeds and used in an old remedy for treating warts. It was thought that the mountain folks learned this from "brown people from the south," that may have been a reference to Mexicans. The plant and seeds contain an irritating substance that can be poisonous to the blood, but the oil is safe to use. The active compound is a skin irritant with enzymes that dissolve the protein of an infected wart. It is still recognized today for its effectiveness in treating warts.

Mole bean makes an interesting plant for a home garden, with its tropical-looking, quick-growing leaves and its spiked cluster of flowers with red burrs. According to an elder, the plant got its name because it repels moles and other animals.

Catnip *(Nepeta cataria)*. Earlier use of catnip was as an insect repellent in the "planting field" or garden, to protect food and people working in the fields from insects. The essential oils in the plant act as a natural DEET, effectively repelling insects. Catnip is more effective for keeping mosquitoes at bay than most commercial products.

Chamomile *(Matricaria chamomilla or recutita)*. Today wild chamomile is known for soothing and healing the skin. It is an anti-inflammatory that is great for treating burns or sunburn. Wild chamomile protects the skin from infections due to its antibacterial and antifungal abilities; the essential oil of chamomile also helps with pain. Chamomile protects the skin from daily exposures to the environmental elements; its use was quickly adopted by the Cherokee and other tribes trading with Whites in the early pioneer years. This was a product that made the Indian women very happy, especially after working in the "planting fields" in the sun, wind, and nature's elements. It did not take long to appreciate the soothing value of chamomile in a bath and rinse for the entire body.

Indian women made a tea using the flower heads from German chamomile *(M. chamomilla)*, along with yarrow or milfoil *(Achillea millefolium)*, for regulating menstrual flow. It was also used as an anti-inflammatory. Women appreciated the applelike fragrance of the chamomile flower.

A Cherokee grandmother praised the value of chamomile as being a cure-all plant. She said that her great-grandmother would trade baskets for the seeds. She said that the seeds could just be thrown on the ground, because they needed the light to germinate. Today chamomile is used for treating blisters, eczema, and skin inflammations.

Cinquefoil *(Potentilla simplex and P. erecta)*. Cinquefoil is a mild astringent and antiseptic. Sometimes called blood root or five-finger, cinquefoil was used for treating wounds and skin irritations. There are several species of cinquefoil in the Rose family, including common cinquefoil and five-finger.

Clearweed (see Rickweed).

Colic root (see Dogbane).

Comfrey *(Symphytum officinale)*. Comfrey was used to stop the bleeding at wounds and cuts. It is one of my favorite plants for treating contusion, sprains, strains, and edema and for using as a wash and a poultice. Comfrey is rich in vitamins A and C, potassium, and phosphorus. The roots and leaves were used in a formula used to treat psoriasis and other skin problems.

While some mountain folks used comfrey in a remedy for bronchial and intestinal conditions, American Indians primarily used it with other plants for treating skin abrasions. It is important not to confuse comfrey with foxglove, because both have similarly lance-shaped leaves. Comfrey grows about five feet high, with tubular flowers that "lean down to greet you with humility." The colors of the flower range from light blue to light yellow.

To use comfrey, bring a quart of water to a boil and add 2 teaspoons of dried cut leaves. Steep for an hour. The tea can be used by soaking a cloth and laying it on the bruise, sore, or insect bite, or even on varicose veins for "comfrey comfort." Today comfrey is used externally for treating wounds. It does contain alkaloids that have been identified to cause cancer. Do not use comfrey during pregnancy or while nursing.

Corn *(Zea mays)*. The "beaten shucks" of *se lu*—Indian corn or maize— were used as a poultice in treating rheumatism. Other plants for treating pain would be mixed into the poultice, such as dogwood or willow.

Maize was also used on "stubborn boils and skin itch." An old formula included smartweed or knotweed *(Polygonium hydropiper* and *P. aviculare)* for pain. The ground powder of corn, an early form of cornstarch, was used as a drying agent. Today the unique corn-shuck dolls made by the Cherokee are very popular.

Couchgrass *(Agropyron repens)*. A wash of witchgrass or couchgrass was used with yellowroot for treating swollen legs and feet. The essential oils have an antimicrobial effect.

Cow parsnip (see Masterwort).

Cranesbill (see Wild geranium).

Crowfoot, marsh *(Ranunculus sceleratus)*. Marsh crowfoot was used as a wash for treating sores in the mouth and as a poultice for sores on the skin. Yellowroot was used with this member of the Buttercup family, which was sometimes called yellow weed. As an elder said, "Only those trained can handle this plant. The acid in the plant can cause a blister."

Crown vetch *(Coronilla varia)*. Called *ga lu ya s di* (pronounced gah lun yah se din) or "ax plant" by elders, crown vetch was used as a rub on ballplayers for treating cramps and rheumatism. The old formula is still used by the Medicine men and women for ball games at Fall Festival each year. Mountain folks used this plant "for complaints of the liver and such."

Cucumber *(Cucumis sativus)*. While primarily used as food and for eliminating excess fluid in the body, a slice of cucumber over the eyes is very soothing. Wrap a slice in cheesecloth and place it over the eyes for an hour. It can be put directly over a bruise or sore as a 12,000-year-old remedy.

As a member of the Gourd family, cucumber is relative to the melons. It is primarily water in content. As a natural diuretic it is good for treating gout and edema. Mountain folks call the skin of a cucumber "nature's ChapStick" because of the oily substance in cucumber that acts as a good moisturizer. Today cucumber is used on skin irritations and in facial-cleansing lotions.

Dayflower (see Spiderwort).

Devil's claw *(Harpagophytum procumbens)*. The tuber of devil's claw is used for "taking care of the pains and swelling of rheumatism and arthritis." The anti-inflammatory action probably helped with this degenerative condition while providing some relief from the pain. Another plant, *Proboscidea louisana*, is also referred to as devil's claw.

Devil's clothesline (see Bamboo brier).

Devil's shoestring *(Tephrosia virginiana)*. Also called goat's rue or rabbit pea, the roots of devil's shoestring were rubbed on the legs of ballplayers and runners "to give them strength for the competition." It was also combined with horse chestnut as a "special Medicine with the right chant for good fishing. The entire formula was kept secret, except for a few." The rootstock is very tough and similar to shoestrings. The plant was used as a natural insecticide and insect poison by mountain folks.

Devil's walkingstick *(Aralia spinosa)*. As a shrub or small tree, the aromatic branches of devil's walkingstick were crushed and used on old sores. A member of the Ginseng family, devil's walkingstick was used as a rheumatism remedy by American Indians. The plant was called "prickly ash" or "Hercules' club" by mountain folks, who used it as a natural astringent for treating boils.

Dock (see Yellow dock).

Dodder *(Cuscuta gronovii)*. A poultice of dodder roots was used for treating bruises. The Dodder family is a single genus of many species of twining plants. "It is a parasitic plant that grows over other plants, like long strings with no leaves, growing on clover," says an elder. Another elder referred to "love vine," or dodder, as a parasitic plant that winds around a bush with suckers that clamp down on its host "like a spider catching you in a web." Then the plant injects toxins until it abandons its own root system to live off the host plant.

There are early American Indian stories about using the plant as "love Medicine" for keeping a loved one. Dodder was used in a skin-protection formula "for the ailments of cuts and bruises."

Dogbane, common *(Apocynum androsaemifolium)*. Also called common spreading dogbane, this plant was used for treating mange on dogs. While potentially dangerous to use internally, an elder said that an old formula used the boiled leaves "for those who acted crazy."

Dog fennel *(Athemis cotula)*. Also known as wild chamomile, this plant "was used with Indian root in a formula for rheumatism and to draw blisters." Mary Chiltoskey mentioned the same uses, including "fevers of the skin." An elder called the plant "Mayweed." This plant should not be confused with chamomile *(Matricaria recutita)*, which is used as an anti-flammatory.

Dog hobble *(Leucothoe axillaris)*. Also called rheumatism plant, a formula of dog hobble, mountain laurel, and rhododendron or willow bark was used for "the old man's rheumatism." The plant probably got its name from its use in treating mange and itch on dogs. An elder said this plant was a gift from the Catawba or other eastern tribes, from areas where it grew plentifully.

Dog's tooth violet (see Adder's tongue).

Dogwood tree *(Cornus florida)*. Flowering dogwood bark was used with the the bark of birch tree, or wintergreen, for treating muscle aches and pains. A member of the Dogwood family, it was used for cleansing wounds and sores in earlier years. Dogwood was used in the old formulas as an astringent, a poultice, and as "a reed tube on a person with rheumatism pain." An elder said, "A bark tea and poultice was used for sore hands from using the shuttles and looms, which were also made of dogwood." A bath of dogwood and hophornbeam was also used for sore muscles and aches.

Dutchman's pipe *(Aristolochia macrophylla)*. The roots of dutchman's pipe were used as a poultice on swollen feet and legs. "Dutchman's pipe was used with Catawba rhododendron on the pains of feet caused by this modern disease you call diabetes." Dutchman's pipe is a member of the Birthwort family, along with Virginia snakeroot and wild ginger.

Elder *(Sambucus canadensis)*. According to Mary Chiltoskey, the leaves of American or common elder were used for treating burns, skin eruptions, hives, and as a wash for treating sores in order to avoid infection. Elder is a member of the Honeysuckle family of shrubs, woody vines, and small trees. An elder called it "elderberry," which was the preferred name among mountain folks as well.

Elm tree *(Ulmus americana)*. American elm was valued by the eastern tribes as a good Medicine for "soaking the skin for itch from insect bites." It was used in a formula with figwort, dogwood, balsam fir, and purslane. The inner bark of elm was combined with a variety of plants as a mountain remedy for treating many kinds of skin ailments. Those plant combinations included elder, goldenrod, ground ivy, soapwort, watercress, bay-berry, and elecampane. Elm is a member of the Elm family, along with slippery, or Indian, elm.

Evening primrose *(Oenothera biennis)*. The oil of evening primrose is considered valuable as an agent in several formulas for treating difficult skin problems such as eczema. Evening primrose contains gamma linolenic acid, or GLA, which is good for treating inflammation. Earlier Cherokee recognized the value of this plant for strong and vibrant hair. Today evening primrose is used for addressing allergic skin reactions and pain, as well as for improving skin, nails, and hair. In earlier years it was combined with Eastern wahoo for treating scalp itch, along with yucca leaves *(Yucca filamentosa)*, found along the coastal regions of the Southeast. Sundrops *(O. fruticosa)*, a cousin of evening primrose, was also used with evening primrose. With its beautiful cluster of yellow flowers, this plant is highly recommended for the home flower and herb garden.

Fern, bracken *(Pteridium aquilinum)*. Bracken fern was used as a wash with balsam fir, horse chestnut, and seven-bark shrub for treating burns and sores. I suspect it was effective because of bracken fern's antibiotic, anti-bacterial, and astringent content. This is a tall fern that can grow to six feet; it has lanced-shaped fronds. It was called "fire root" by one elder, who said bracken fern was used for burns and sores by several southeastern tribes.

Fern, Christmas *(Polystichum acrostichoides)*. Christmas fern was boiled or soaked in water, along with the inner bark of dogwood, to use as a wash or poultice on the skin around the aching joints of those suffering from rheumatism. It was sometimes used with cinnamon fern *(Osmunda cinnamomea)* "for wounds and the aching of rheumatism."

The fronds of the Christmas fern are five to twenty inches long; the plant prefers shady, moist areas.

Fern, highland *(Polypodium virginianum)*. A poultice made from the highland fern was used for treating swelling, wounds, and hives. The plant is better known as common polypody or rockcap fern. It has evergreen fronds about fourteen inches wide that stand upright. Highland fern grows on rocks and logs.

Fern, Indian *(Polypodium polypodioides)*. Also known as resurrection fern, this plant was used in a formula "with plantain leaves, for sores." Usually yellowish green in color and about two inches wide, Indian fern grows on trees and rocks. A common polypody *(P. virginianum)* is also used in the formula, which grows on rocks and logs. An elder said, "You gotta know these things if you are out hunting or working in the woods."

Fern, mountain wood *(Dryopteris campyloptera)*. Mountain wood fern was used with "the bark of the tree that it grows near" for treating cuts and other skin problems. The fronds of the mountain wood fern grow about two feet in length in a double-pinnate shape.

Fern, rattlesnake *(Botrychium virginianum)*. This evergreen fern, found in thick, dry woods, produces a single frond that is usually under two feet in height. The small fern cluster on the long stems looks like the head of a rattlesnake. The juice of the frond would be put on insect bites and stings. An elder said the frond "was a sign that a ginseng patch was nearby." Rattlesnake fern is a member of the adder-tongue Fern family.

Fern, wood *(Dryopteris marginalis)*. Also known as marginal shield fern, this evergreen is about six inches across and twenty inches in height. It was used in a formula for treating rheumatism. An elder said, "The wood fern would be looked for when rheumatism would be kicking in, such as when the weather was cool and damp—you know, when the pain was ready for some fern Medicine."

Figwort *(Scrophularia nodosa)*. Known popularly as heal-all, figwort was used in an ointment with dogwood and bear grease in earlier years for treating cuts, scratches, and burns. This plant was favored for its ability to heal the skin. The plant is a diuretic and is used as a natural laxative. It has also been used for treating rashes and venereal warts.

Five-fingers (see Cinquefoil).

Fly poison (see Itchweed).

Forget-me-not *(Myosotis scorpioides* and *M. sylvatica)*. There are interesting stories about how this plant got its name. This story, an American Indian or German tale, comes from a time when plants and people could talk to each other. A young Indian in love with his young maiden is swept away in the waters during a storm. He yells out to this plant to please tell his love to "forget me not"! The plant tells others, and the name sticks.

Myosotis sylvatica is a beautiful garden plant that has sky-blue flowers with white centers, considered to be "flowers of love."

Earlier Cherokee would say this little plant is for treating snakebites and insect stings. Concerns have been expressed in the herbal literature about the hepatoxicity of this plant when taken internally. It is a member of the Borage, or Forget-me-not, family.

Four-o'clock *(Mirabilis nyctaginea)*. This plant was sometimes called pretty-by-night or wild four-o'clock. Paul Hamel and Mary Chiltoskey mention beating the root of this small plant on rocks and using the ooze or juice on boils. Crushed dried roots were used as a "special Medicine" for vision-seeking by eastern and western tribes. A Lakota Sioux friend of mine used this plant for treating children with sores in the mouth, the same way earlier Cherokee used alumroot.

Mirabilis jalapa has different-colored blooms of fragrant flowers on the same plant. These are great plants for home flower gardens. The flowers open in the late afternoon and close in the early morning.

Garlic *(Allium sativum)*. This cure-all plant can still be used as a natural insect repellent by rubbing it on the skin to keep mosquitoes, gnats, and other little pests away. Along with being nature's insecticide, it can also be used for treating infected areas of the skin. Garlic is said to stimulate the immune system and to help combat cancer. Today it is used for treating fungal infections, inflammation, and bacterial problems. Do not use garlic medicinally while nursing.

Goat's beard *(Aruncus dioicus)*. An elder said the fresh roots of goat's beard were crushed to make a juice pulp for use in treating insect stings and for pain relief. I tried it and was pleasantly surprised that it worked. This use was verified by Paul Hamel and Mary Chiltoskey, who also mentioned its use for treating swollen feet.

Goat's rue (see Devil's shoestring).

Golden glow *(Rudbeckia laciniata)*. This plant, a cousin to black-eyed Susan *(R. hirta)*, was "used as a wash on sores, and used by the old ones for snakebites." In West Virginia and Kentucky it is called coneflower and is used there for the same purpose by mountain folks. It is also combined with balsam fir and American chestnut *(Castanea dentata)* for use in treating difficult sores and skin cancers.

Goldenrod *(Solidago odora)*. American Indians have used the flower-head blossoms of goldenrod for treating sore throats by chewing and swallowing the juice; the roots were used as a poultice for treating toothaches. It was also used as a yellow dye.

Cherokee use the flower blossoms for treating bee stings and swelling. The plant is an anti-inflammatory. It is a good astringent as an "Indian Band-aid," along with plantain, used for treating wounds and inflammation. Goldenrod was introduced to America by Europeans; it was quickly naturalized here on Turtle Island.

Goldenseal *(Hydrastis canadensis)*. Goldenseal is also called Indian paint. It is used for treating many complaints and skin problems, but it is especially useful for healing cuts and wounds. It is used as an antiseptic and astringent for treating ringworm. Mixed with bear grease and the juices from the inner barks of several different trees, goldenseal was used as nature's insect repellent in earlier years. Today it is used as an eyewash, for treating ear discharge and mouth sores, for cleaning wounds, and for treating inflammation and itching skin. It has antibacterial properties as well. Goldenseal is at risk of extinction in its natural environment.

Goldthread (Coptis trifolia). John Lust reported that goldthread was called "canker root" by the mountain folks; some also called the plant "golden-club." Goldthread was used as a wash for treating sores. Found in the damp and cool woods, it was thought to "be cooling to the skin for skin irritations and burns."

Gourd (Lagenaria vulgaris). Gourds were dried and then cleaned for use as ceremonial rattles. The seeds of the gourd would be saved for use in a poultice for treating boils. The seeds would be crushed and made into a mush or a powder, then placed on a boil to "draw out the poisons."

Greenbrier (Smilax rotundifolia). Also known as bullgrip, greenbrier was used for treating muscle twitches and cramps. An elder said, "A scratch would be made by the Medicine man and greenbrier would be put on it in ceremonies for ballplayers."

Heal-all (see Woundwort and Figwort).

Heartweed (see Lady's thumb).

Hemlock tree (Tsuga canadensis and T. caroliniana). The inner bark of Eastern hemlock and Carolina hemlock was used along with purslane (Portulaca oleracea) for treating stubborn sores and swelling from insect bites. It is used as a natural astringent and anti-inflammatory, as well as a natural diuretic. An evergreen, hemlock is a member of the Pine family. This tree is not to be confused with poison hemlock (Conium maculatum), also called cowbane or spotted cowbane.

Holly tree (Ilex opaca). The leaves of American holly were used in earlier years to scratch cramped muscles. An elder said that the practice of "scratching" for cramps was a similar technique used by the old Medicine men and women for treating rheumatism, and for ceremonies with ballplayers. An evergreen tree, holly is a member of the Holly family.

Hophornbeam tree (Ostrya virginiana). A warm bath made from the crushed leaves of hophornbeam can be used for treating sore muscles, and a bark tea taken internally "to improve strength." Hophornbeam was also used with magnolia bark for treating "internal cramps and aches." Some mountain folks called the tree "ironwood" because it is so hard. The wood is excellent for making tool handles and fence posts.

Horehound *(Marrubium vulgare)*. American Indians used horehound for treating wounds, in a formula that included yellowroot and many other astringent plants and barks with tannins.

Horse chestnut tree *(Aesculus hippocastanum)*. Indians taught the mountain folks how to use the horse chestnut seed for treating hemorrhoids. The young horse chestnut bark and nuts were used for treating skin sores. It was also used for treating "weak veins and bruises, like varicose veins." The seeds and young bark are the usable parts of this tree; older bark and the leaves are poisonous.

An elder called the plant "fishing buckeye" because in earlier years the seeds were crushed and placed in a favorite fishing hole. Supposedly this interfered with the fish's lateral nerve line, which made for easy catching.

Today horse chestnut is used for treating varicose veins and vein inflammation. James Duke, Ph.D., recommends using this plant and witch hazel as strong antioxidants and astringents for smoothing wrinkles. Horse chestnut is a member of the Buckeye (Horse Chestnut) family.

Horse gentian *(Triosteum perfoliatum)*. The horse gentian plant was crushed and the juice was used on swelling areas. Horse gentian was also mentioned by Paul Hamel and Mary Chiltoskey as an emetic, used for purging. Also known as feverwort or fever root, it was used in traditional sweats, especially in earlier years.

Horsetail *(Equisetum arvense)*. Horsetail, also called shave grass, was used with goldenrod as a wash for treating skin irritations, wounds, boils, and inflammation. It was also used with spearmint *(Mentha spicata)* for treating itch. Horsetail was used to make blowguns, but the tubes have been reported to be poisonous to children. Horsetail has been used as an astringent and an anti-inflammatory. Today it is used as a septic to stop bleeding.

Indian apple (see Mayapple and Jimson weed).

Indian balm tree *(Populus candicans* or *P. balsamifera)*. Also known as balm of Gilead and poplar, the buds of Indian balm were made into a salve for treating wounds. Earlier Indians would rub the tree resin on a sore or cut and use it on the back or chest for pain relief. The inner bark was used in a tea for treating pain, and the needles were used in a traditional sweat lodge clearing-way, a ceremony for clearing the mind and receiving messages from the spirit world and the ancestors. Mountain folks prefer to call this tree "balsam poplar."

Indian hyssop (see Vervain).

Indian physic *(Gillenia trifoliata* or *G. porteranthus)*. Also called bowman's root or American ipecac, Mooney reported that Indian physic was used by the Cherokee for treating bowel complaints. An elder said the leaf wash was used for treating swelling, and the "dried roots were crushed and steeped in a tea with peppermint to purify the blood, especially for skin allergies and wounds where there was a loss of blood and infection."

Indian plantain (*Cacalia atriplicifolia*). The leaves of Indian plantain would be rubbed together to release a juice in an old formula for treating skin cancers. The plant would be used by bruising the leaf and applying it directly to a wound or cut. Indian plantain was combined with turtle-head (*Chelone glabra*) and placed as a salve on sores and skin eruptions. It was also combined with spotted pipsissewa (*Chimaphila maculata*) in a wash for treating skin cancers. Plantain was combined with Carolina poplar for treading scalp sores, lice, and wounds.

Indian poke (*Veratrum viride*). Also called devil's bite, bugbane, and American hellebore, Indian poke was used in an ointment for treating rheumatism. It was also used for treating pain and was combined in a formula for treating skin conditions. In the old days the Cherokee would combine it with bear grease for dressing wounds and put the root powder on sores for healing. An elder reported that "it was used for pain when you couldn't get dogwood or willow." The young leaves were not used because they were considered poisonous. Consult only with those trained in the safe dosage and preparation of Indian poke.

Indian root (*Aralia racemosa*). Also known as American spikenard or Hercules' club, Indian root was applied to cuts and wounds. The roots were crushed and used for treating burns, boils, and sore eyes. It was combined with many other plants for treating skin problems, including agrimony for wounds and bearberry for sores. Krochmal mentions Indian root as being used for treating backaches and as a poultice for sores and inflammation of the skin. It was also considered "a life root for ailments of elders. Everyone used to know about this plant."

Indian tobacco (*Lobelia inflata*). Indian tobacco was used for treating ringworm and insect bites, with chickweed added for soothing. According to John Lust, Indian tobacco was also used to treat the itch of poison ivy. Today it is used in treating asthma and muscle spasms.

Itchweed (*Amianthium muscaetoxicum*). Also called fly poison, itchweed was used in treating toe and foot itching and as a "poison for the little boogers that fly around you while you are trying to work in the fields." In the mountains, "a light syrup would be put on the bulbs to kill flies." Itchweed was considered poisonous to cattle.

Ivy (*Hedera helix*). The elders mentioned ivy as being used in earlier years for addressing skin problems and respiratory conditions. James Duke,

Ph.D., discovered that this particular ivy has saponin compounds that are active against bacteria and fungi as well as bronchitis. *Hedera helix* is a cousin to catnip but has small purple flowers.

Jewelweed *(Impatiens capensis* or *biflora)*. Also called touch-me-not, jewelweed was used for treating the rash and itch of poison ivy, insects, and stings from plants. I call jewelweed "Joi weed" after my niece, because of the quick reaction of the seeds when touched: they tend to snap out quickly with strength and purpose.

Jimson weed *(Datura meteloides)*. As young Cherokees we were told to stay away from this plant. People were known to smoke jimson weed, what some called "crazy" or "locoweed." The roots and leaves would be made into a poultice to apply to burns, bruises, and cuts. In earlier years the seeds would be crushed and mixed with bear grease to apply to "boils and difficult sores, for good results."

My father pointed out jimson weed to me one day when we were stringing television cable on a mountainside. He called it "devil's trumpet." He said his mother told him to stay clear of this dangerous plant. The varying concentrations of certain alkaloids can have a contrary effect on the heart. This plant was sometimes referred to as mayapple.

Knotweed (see Smartweed and Lady's thumb).

Lady's thumb *(Polygonum persicária)*. Also known as knotweed or heartweed, according to Mary Chiltoskey the Cherokee used the crushed leaves of lady's thumb for treating poison ivy, urinary infections, and pain. I was able to verify its use in dressing wounds, bruises, and cuts, but as an astringent it is also irritating to sensitive tissue. An elder said that "some people have an allergic reaction to it, just like goldenrod." The elder also remembered it being used in a formula with toadflax or bastard toadflax *(Comandra umbellata)* on "difficult sores and oozing cuts."

Larkspur *(Delphinium ajacis* and *D. tricorne)*. Also called field larkspur, this member of the Buttercup, or Crowfoot, family is well known in the western part of the country as *Delphinium consolida*. Along with locoweed (jimson weed), it is known for causing death to grazing livestock. It was used by American Indians to rid the body of parasites in dogs and humans, as well as for getting rid of lice, nits (eggs), and itch mites.

Larkspur has beautiful flowers and is considered a good plant remedy to stanch bleeding. My Uncle Grady first pointed out this plant to me and said it was used for treating wounds during the Civil War, which is how earlier Cherokee used it. Larkspur has an alkaloid compound, delphine, which has a paralyzing effect on the central nervous system, making its safe use questionable. The unusual flower has a spur, which makes it different from other plants in the Buttercup family.

Laurel (see Mountain laurel).

Leafcup (see Bearsfoot).

Licorice *(Glycyrrhiza lepidota).* Also called American licorice, this plant is still popular today for treating viral infections such as herpes, along with melissa or lemon balm. An antiviral compound in licorice, glycyrrhizin, inhibits viral replication. Licorice was used in earlier times on "skin conditions of the face, itching and irritated feet [athlete's foot], on the scalp for dandruff and itch, and for the itching of hives."

Lily, swamp *(Heteranthera reniformis).* Called mud plantain, the root of swamp lily was used for treating inflammation associated with sores, wounds, and ulcers. An elder called it *ge ga a ste ske* and said it was used with a "special chant to the water for healing of the wound and the spirit."

Lily, Turk's cap *(Lilium canadense).* The plant tubers of Turk's cap lily were used for treating rheumatism. Eastern tribes in the Carolinas gifted the Cherokee with this lily and others that grow plentiful in the wetlands. Those gifts included the Michaux's, or Carolina, lily, and one that an elder called "pot-of-gold lily" *(L. iridolae),* a beautifully spotted yellow, orange, and brown lily that is rare today. In addition to the Turk's cap and the Carolina lily, there is a blackberry lily *(Belamcanda chinensis)* with showy orange flowers, a great plant for a home flower garden.

Linden (see Basswood).

Lizard's tail *(Saururus cernuus).* A poultice for treating rheumatism and pain was made from the roots of this plant, also known as swamp lily or water dragon. The plant grows in wet places and carries a long spike and a large white flower at the end of the spike. The roots of lizard's tail were dried and carved into beads for necklaces that were used for sacred purposes and for ceremonies.

Lobelia (see Indian tobacco).

Lousewort *(Pedicularis canadensis).* Sometimes called wood betony, the root juice of lousewort is used with lobelia, or Indian tobacco, in dressing sores. It was also used for treating cuts and wounds. Lousewort is not to be confused with another wood betony, *Stachys officinalis.*

An elder said it was used by earlier Indians for internal swelling, because it "relaxed the inners."

Magnolia tree *(Magnolia glauca).* The magnolia tree bark was a gift of the Creek Indians, according to an elder who referred to it as "creek bark strips." This indigenous plant was used as a rheumatism remedy. It is also called Indian bark or swamp sassafras. There is also a sweetbay, or swampbay, magnolia *(M. virginiana)*. All are members of the Magnolia family.

Mallow *(Malva neglecta* and *M. silvestris)*. Paul Hamel and Mary Chiltoskey note that the flowers of round-leaved mallow were used in an oil mixture for treating sores. Common, or wild, mallow *(M. silvestris)* was used for treating inflammation. The leaves were also eaten in green salads. The colorful pink flowers growing from the leaf axes have a distinctively raised, purple center.

Maple tree *(Acer rubrum)*. The bark of red maple is used in poultices for treating skin abrasions. Sugar maple *(Acer saccherum)* was used for basket making, with strips of red maple used for varying the texture and color. A drink was made from the inner bark for treating cramps and dysentery and for calming the nerves.

Marigold *(Calendula officinalis)*. Also called pot marigold, marigold is used as an astringent and for its antifungal value on skin infections, bites, sores, burns, and itching. It was an addition to the Medicine bag that was used in earlier years for treating severe cuts and wounds. It was sometimes combined with Indian physic *(Gillenia trifoliata)* for treating insect stings and swelling. It is an astringent and anti-inflammatory, useful for dressing wounds and sores on the skin and in the mouth. It was also used for treating burns.

My Uncle Grady and my father told stories of a family member who served as a Cherokee scout in the Civil War. He was well known for his abilities with plants, but in particular for his use of this plant and others to stop bleeding. Earlier Cherokee called marigold "eye" flowers, or *a ga do li*. Difficult skin conditions and sores were treated with a combination of marigold, queen-of-the-meadow, white snakeroot, and coltsfoot in an old mountain remedy. Today marigold is mixed with aloe gel to soften the skin.

Marsh crowfoot (see Crowfoot, marsh).

Marsh mallow *(Althaea officinalis)*. Marsh mallow grows about four feet tall, with heart-shaped leaves and beautiful five-petaled white to pink flowers with purple anthers that bloom from July to October. While originating in Europe, marsh mallow is found in freshwater marshes. The Cherokee learned the medicinal value of marsh mallow from another tribe; they boiled the plant and used it to soothe the skin and mucous membranes. It was also used as a gargle for sore throats. Today it is used for treating skin inflammation. Marsh mallow has anti-inflammatory and antiseptic properties.

Masterwort *(Heracleum canatum)*. Also known as cow parsnip, the leaves of masterwort were used in a formula for making a poultice to treat sores and difficult skin problems. It was probably a more recent addition to the Medicine bag, because there seemed to be no mention of it in earlier records or with the Cherokee elders.

Mayapple *(Podophyllum peltatum)*. Also known by the mountain folks as "Indian apple" and "mandrake," mayapple was used with common milkweed *(Asclepias syriaca)* as a treatment for warts. The sap of dandelion was also used with mayapple on warts. The mountain folks were aware that the mayapple plant is poisonous, except for the ripe fruit.

Mayapple grows abundantly in damp wooded areas in the Appalachian and Smoky Mountains. The plant has distinctive umbrella-shaped leaves with a single white flower that blooms in May and a yellow berry that is ripe in July and August. The rhizomes were used as a laxative. The Penobscot of Maine used it for certain cancers, along with periwinkle. Today mayapple is used to treat plantar warts and as a treatment for cancer and tumors.

Milkweed *(Asclepias syriaca)*. The milky sap of common milkweed was used with mayapple for treating warts. The plant's effectiveness is probably due to its ability to inhibit the virus of the wart. It was used in a formula for "irritated skin, and on the face for smooth skin." An elder called the plant "glider plant" because the bristles glide the seed in the wind.

Moss *(Cladina subtenis)*. This plant, sometimes called reindeer moss, was used for treating "the pain of insect stings, sometimes mixed with tobacco that would be chewed in your mouth and placed on the sting."

Mountain daisy or Mountain tobacco (see Arnica).

Mountain laurel *(Kalmia latifolia)*. The leaves of laurel, or calico bush, are used in a wash for treating skin rashes and as a lotion for other skin conditions. It was also used as a poultice with dogwood or willow bark for treating rheumatism and bruises. An eastern Carolina cousin was the white wicky *(K. cuneata)*, a plant about half the size of the mountain laurel and also carrying white flowers. The roots of mountain laurel were used for making cooking spoons. Mountain laurel is a member of the Heath family.

Mouse ear *(Gnaphalium uliginosum* or *Hieracium pilosella)*. This plant was used in a formula for treating cuts and wounds, as mentioned by a Medicine elder. This is an old remedy that included beech bark or white willow bark and yellowroot.

Nettle, stinging *(Urtica dioica)*. The sting from the nettle plant can help induce increased bloodflow and reduce inflammation; this was the way in which nettle was sometimes used for treating a person with rheumatism. Nettle was included in a spring tonic, along with sassafras. Boiling the plant removes the skin-irritating substances and produces a broth rich in vitamins A and C, iron, and protein. Wilted nettle leaves mixed with dandelion leaves and other greens such as collards makes a great salad. Stinging nettle was also used as a treatment to stimulate the scalp and was very well liked in hair grooming by earlier Cherokee. It was also combined with chickweed as an astringent for healing wounds and for treating eczema. One does need to be aware that some people experience allergic reactions to this plant.

Nightshade *(Solanum dulcamara)*. Also called bittersweet, nightshade was combined with yellowroot and yellow dock for treating sores and skin conditions. This is an old remedy that is probably not used today. Yellowroot contains alkaloids that are considered toxic.

Oak tree *(Quercus alba* and other species). The inner bark of white oak was used for treating burns and skin sores and soothing inflammation. Oak splits are used with river cane for making baskets. Chestnut or rock chestnut oak *(Q. prinus)* and black or yellow oak *(Q. velutina)* contain high levels of tannins, which made them useful in the tanning of leather. They are members of the Oak family.

Pansy *(Viola tricolor)*. Pansy was used for treating skin sores, especially those of children. It was also used in treating rheumatism, along with willow bark. My father called pansy "Johnny jump-up." My mother remembered it being called "heart's ease." I have special memories of working in the flower garden with my mother and grandmother while learning the names and stories about the plants and their uses as Medicine helpers. Learning about pansy is one of those special memories.

Passionflower *(Passiflora incarnata)*. The crushed leaves of maypop, or passionflower, were used to treat bruises. It was also used in treating boils, cuts, and inflamed wounds. The juice of the ovate yellow fruit was used for soothing sore eyes. The young leaves and top of the plant are still used by some for dressing burns and skin problems. Today passionflower is used for its calming effects.

Pawpaw *(Asimina triloba)*. The common, or American, pawpaw is a shrub or small tree used for getting rid of head lice. A mixture of stinging nettle and yellowroot was included in the formula. The seeds were crushed into a powder and added to the roots of the other two plants.

Pennyroyal *(Hedeoma pulegioides).* American pennyroyal was primarily used for treating headaches and itching eyes. The Cherokee found it to be a good insect repellent; they crushed the leaves and rubbed them on hands, arms, and face. The essential oil is used today for animal flea collars and as a mosquito repellent. Mountain folks referred to English, or European, pennyroyal *(Mentha pulegium)* as being used "to keep the peasants and the pesty away in the old days." My Uncle Grady remembered it being used with children in the mountains for lowering fever. The essential oil of pennyroyal is a volatile oil that contains ketones and pulegium, which are toxic.

In earlier years pennyroyal was used as a strong uterine stimulant by those specially trained in pennyroyal's Medicine. My father called it "mosquito plant," and he remembers it being called "squaw mint" by mountain folks. He would crush the leaves and rub it on our arms and neck while we worked outside on cable lines. As a natural antiseptic, pennyroyal is useful for treating skin scratches and cuts, as well as for easing itching. The plant grows about a foot high with blue flowers. It is a member of the Mint family.

Pepper (*Capsicum annuum* and other species). The plant and seeds of pepper or cayenne are used as a stimulant for the elderly and a poultice for treating sores on feet. Today we better understand pepper's ability to block pain signals in the skin, which is why it is used for treating shingles and is an element in creams for treating arthritis.

Pepper grass *(Lepidium virginicum).* This plant is not very well known or used by most American Indians, but the Cherokee would crush the roots and mix it into a paste along with the dried leaves of an astringent plant to treat stubborn boils and sores. The use of spotted wintergreen *(Chimaphila maculata)* was noted with pepper grass, as were astringents such as goldenseal and fringetree *(Chionanthus virginicus),* for treating skin inflammation and sores on the skin and in the mouth.

Phacelia, common *(Phacelia purshii).* The phacelia plant was used on swollen joints. The small-flowered phacelia, or *oo ste s gi,* was used as a cooking green, along with dandelion and other wild greens. There is a white-fringed phacelia *(Phacelia fimbriata)* that can cover a mountainside and looks like snow among green.

Pine tree *(Pinus virginiana, P. palustris, P. strobus,* and *P. taeda).* The pine was considered a "gift that is always giving from the Great One." Common pines such as jack pine, scrub pine, spruce pine, and Virginia pine were included in "a wash for skin ulcers and sores." The sap would also be used on stubborn sores that had difficulty healing. While longleaf pine

(P. palustris) was used for making turpentine, the same sap was used on sores. The sap of loblolly pine *(P. taeda)* was used for treating skin problems. Eastern white pine *(P. strobus)* was crushed and soaked for dressing wounds. The sap was used on sores, according to Arnold Krochmal.

Pine bark is considered a sacred South Medicine. It is often named in Cherokee myths as an agent for sending messages to the spirit world, and pine is included in several healing formulas. The trunks of pine trees were also used by American Indians in earlier years as "long canoes."

Piney weed *(Hypericum hypericoides* and *H. gentanoides)*. Piney weed, or "St. Andrew's cross" as it was called by mountain folks, was used as a snakebite remedy. The root was chewed and then applied to the bite, and then some of the root was spat upon the snake. A prayer-chant would be used for "calming, and to clear the spirit of the snake so as to avoid bad dreams."

Pipsissewa *(Chimaphila umbellata)*. External use of pipsissewa was for treating skin problems and rheumatism. It was called "pip" by mountain folks, who used it for treating edema and inflammation.

Plantain *(Plantago major)*. Common plantain, sometimes called Indian Band-aid, was used by many American Indian tribes for treating rheumatism and swelling. It was used with horehound for treating snakebites to humans and dogs. The earlier Cherokee would crush or bruise the leaves and apply them directly on a cut or a "scratch from the poisonous prickly plants" as a natural antiseptic and for "quick healing when out in the mountains." Lance-leaf plantain *(P. lanceolata)* is also used on wounds. The narrow-leaf plantain *(Hosta japonica)* would be rubbed on the arms, legs, and feet for protecting against no-see-ums, tiny insects that have a ferocious bite. Sometimes blood leather *(Gyrophora dillenii)* would be used along with plantain in treating deep cuts or wounds to stop bleeding.

Poison ivy *(Rhus radicans)*. An elder mentioned that "there is value even in poison ivy as a Medicine. The juice would be crushed between two rocks from the leaves and mixed with another plant to relieve itch and for ringworm." Another elder said it was mixed with jewelweed *(Impatiens biflora)*, a practice that was learned from another tribe.

The oil called urushiol in the poison ivy leaves and roots can cause a rash that is probably the most common plant allergen today. It takes very little oil to cause a reaction. Poison ivy rash is spread by direct contact with the plant oil, not by breaking the blisters or touching the rash. It is good to know how to identify poison ivy in the woods. The leaves are bright and shiny in early spring and bright orange in fall. The small white flowers appear in clusters, with white berries appearing in early fall.

My grandmother would put the fresh juice of catnip leaves on an area exposed to poison ivy and prepare a mugwort rinse, or use baking soda or aloe leaf. The old remedy used by mountain folks to combat the effects of poison ivy was jewelweed. The inner bark of jewelweed was used for making a dye, along with red maple and red oak.

Poke (*Phytolacca americana*). The roots of pokeweed were usually boiled with several other plants in a formula that was administered for treating minor skin irritations. The dried root was used for treating ringworm and skin infections as an anti-inflammatory. The mountain folks used a poultice of pokeberry juice for treating rheumatism. Today poke is used to treat boils and sores. While it is used as an internal tonic for clearing up skin impurities, it can be extremely toxic.

Poplar, tulip (*Liriodendron tulipifera*). Tulip, or yellow, poplar, called *tsi yu* in Cherokee, was part of a formula made into a paste as a poultice for skin conditions such as rashes. Other elements of the formula included pine, broadleaf plantain, willow tree bark, and possibly an astringent, depending on the condition that was being treated. Queen Anne's lace (*Daucus carota*) is one of those plants added to the formula when it was to be used as a wash to treat swelling. Prickly ash (*Zanthoxylum americanum*) would be added for swollen joints.

Poplar was used in earlier years for building canoes and for making ceremonial masks called "booger" masks. Today poplar is used for treating sores and skin rashes. Poplar contains alkaloids that are microbial; concerns are expressed about its potential toxic effects. It is a member of the Magnolia family.

Prickly ash (see Devil's walkingstick).

Puffball (*Lycoperdon periatum*). The dried mushroom snuff in the "puffball" was used for treating sores and earaches. Paul Hamel and Mary Chiltoskey mentioned devil's snuffbox (*L. pyriforme*) as a dried snuff used for treating sores.

Pumpkin (*Cucurbita pepo*). While pumpkin seeds have been used for treating intestinal worms and parasites, an elder remembered the seeds being crushed for the oil to be used on "difficult wounds and sores." Indigenous to America, pumpkin was used in earlier formulas for intestinal and bladder problems. Today that list also includes prostate complaints.

Puttyroot (see Adam and Eve root).

Queen Anne's lace (see Wild carrot).

Rabbit pea (see Devil's shoestring).

Ragweed (Ambrosia trifida and A. artemisiifolia). The common and great ragweed leaves were rubbed together and applied to insect stings or bites. Mary Chiltoskey verified mountain folks' use of ragweed to treat infected toes. Of course in earlier years it was common to not wear shoes, so cuts and scrapes would easily become infected. People who lived closer to nature had knowledge of little things one could do and plants that would be "helpers." Ragweed was one of those plants; another was richweed (Pilea pumila)—otherwise known as toe itch—a plant from which the stems would be rubbed between the toes to stop the itching. According to Mary Chiltoskey, another plant used for toe itch was staggerbush (Lyonia mariana). It was used in a formula with "goldenrod in the old days for itch and stings. Today we use garlic."

Rattlesnake plantain (Goodyera pubescens). Rattlesnake plantain, also called ratsbane, was used with rhododendron or mountain laurel for treating difficult sores. I have heard it called canker root, but do not know anyone who used it for that purpose. In recent years rattlesnake plantain has been recognized for treating skin irritation and rashes, in combination with goldenseal.

Rheumatism root (see Twinleaf and Dog hobble).

Rhododendron (Rhododendron maximum and R. catawbiense). The crushed inner bark of Catawba or purple rhododendron, sometimes known as great laurel, was used for "pain poultices, along with laurel bark by those who knew how to prepare it right."

Richweed (Pilea pumila). The bark of richweed was peeled from the stem and the stick was rubbed between the toes for alleviating itch. This plant was referred to by an elder as "clearweed," used with corn silk as an appetite depressant.

Rosemary (Rosmarinus officinalis). This favorite plant of the kitchen was used in a formula for treating sores and wounds. Today it is used for addressing chronic circulatory problems, rheumatism, and muscle spasms. It is considered effective in treating fungal and bacterial infections.

Rue (Ruta graveolens). Common rue grows as a bush in fields. It is popular in the Appalachia area for use in treating deep cuts and wounds. Rue was used as a poultice with Indian tobacco on sore joints. Mountain folks would smoke rue with tobacco as a sedative for relief from the aches and pains of rheumatism and neuralgia. Today it is used for treating bruises, arthritis, and muscle disorders. It is also used with insect bites "that are too stubborn to heal with burdock."

Saffron *(Crocus sativus).* The crocus was used for treating hives on children. It was also used to treat skin rash. It is uncertain how crocus got to this country from India and the Mediterranean, or when it arrived here. The Dutch crocus *(C. vernus)* is the variety most commonly found in home flower gardens.

Sage *(Salvia officinalis).* While sage was used in ceremonies and as "special Medicine," it also had a common use as an astringent in a formula for a skin wash and care for skin irritation. It is an old remedy for dandruff, along with goldenseal, to "give the hair strength" as well as for preventing hair loss. Sage is also taken internally to treat muscle spasms. A blue sage *(Salvia azuera)* was traded with coastal Indians. There is also a lyre-leaved sage *(Salvia lyrata)* found in the mountains that was used in earlier years as a skin "conditioner and wash."

　　Sage is most often called red, white, garden, or wild sage. It is a member of the Mint family, along with purple and blue sage.

Sarsaparilla *(Smilax officinalis).* The crushed root of sarsaparilla was used to treat ringworm and other "special" skin conditions. It was also brewed as a tea for drinking, sometimes along with other plants or barks. Sarsaparilla is in the Lily family. There is also a wild sarsaparilla tree *(Aralia nudicaulis)*, probably better known in Appalachia as sweetroot or wild licorice owing to its sweet taste.

Sassafras *(Sassafras albidum).* Called *ka sta ste,* sassafras was used as a poultice for treating wounds and sores. It was also used in a spring tonic for "strength for hunting and for protection of the family." Sassafras is a member of the Laurel family.

Self-heal *(Prunella vulgaris).* Also called heal-all and woundwort, self-heal is a common weed in lawns and fields. The Cherokee called it *ga ni qui li ski.* Self-heal has a creeping rootstock; it grows a foot or more in height, with a hairy stem with opposite leaves that are lance-shaped and a purple flower with two lips in a spiked terminal.

　　Self-heal was a popular plant for southeastern American Indians. It was used for providing flavor in medicinal formulas, and the greens were eaten with dandelion greens for nutrition. Its "power given by the Great One" was as a powerful astringent for healing sores and wounds. It also has value as an antibacterial and was used as a wash for skin problems.

Senega *(Polygala senega).* Senega, or senega snakeroot, was used for treating wounds and snakebites in earlier years. It was also used in several formulas that have been lost today. Along with senega, black snakeroot *(Actae pachypoda)* is still used today for treating skin itch and similar problems.

Senna *(Cassia* or *Senna marilandica).* The leaves of wild senna are crushed or "bruised and placed on difficult sores." The usual reference on senna would indicate its use for constipation. However, several elders said it was used for treating sores, along with goldenseal and other antiseptic plants. Do not use senna during pregnancy or while nursing.

Seven-bark shrub *(Hydrangea arborescens).* Also known as wild hydrangea, seven-bark shrub was used as an antiseptic and a stimulant for treating difficult sores, swollen areas, and rheumatism aches; it was mixed with willow for pain relief externally and internally. The use of seven-bark shrub and wintergreen was also a popular rheumatism formula, sometimes mixed with self-heal.

Sheep sorrel *(Rumex acetosella).* The spear-shaped leaves of common sorrel were used for treating skin itch and rashes. The name *sorrel* likely comes from a French word meaning "sour." Sheep sorrel is a member of the Smartweed, or Buckwheat, family, along with garden sorrel and curled dock.

Shepherd's purse *(Capsella bursa-pastoris).* This plant blooms most of the year. The newest growth is used to stanch nosebleeds and to treat cuts and wounds.

Shinleaf *(Pyrola elliptica* and *P. rotundifolia).* Sometimes called wild lily-of-the-valley, shinleaf was used for its astringent properties in mouthwashes and vaginal douches, according to John Lust. The Cherokee and the mountain folks favored using the leaves for treating insect bites, sores, and other skin conditions. Shinleaf was one of those plants that could be used in a formula or could simply stand alone as a good healing agent.

Slippery elm tree *(Ulmus rubra).* The inner bark of slippery elm is used for treating skin problems. This member of the Elm family is a natural antiseptic.

Smallflower buttercup *(Ranunculus abortivus).* A poultice of smallflower buttercup was applied to boils. A Medicine elder said this plant was used in a very old formula for treating difficult sores and boils. That formula is no longer known.

Smartweed *(Polygonum hydropiper).* Also called knotweed, smartweed was combined with wintergreen to make a good remedy for treating skin conditions and swelling. It was also part of a formula for treating snakebites, along with Senega snakeroot *(Polygala senega)*. An elder said smartweed was called *ta wa se lu* by his grandfather, who used it on old sores and wounds "too stubborn to heal, along with creeping sourgrass *[Oxalis corniculata]* for skin cancers." This use was verified by Paul Hamel and Mary Chiltoskey. Mary mentioned the use of buffalo nut *(Pyrularia pubera)* combined with smartweed for treating sores.

Snakeroot, Virginia *(Aristolochia serpentaria)*. Virginia snakeroot was used for making poultices to treat skin conditions and wounds. This was one of the most popular of all the snakebite remedies. Virginia snakeroot is also used as an agent for pain relief in several formulas.

Soapwort *(Saponaria officinalis)*. Soapwort was used in an external wash for treating skin problems. John Lust reported that soapwort was used for alleviating dermatitis and itching skin. Paul Hamel and Mary Chiltoskey called soapwort "bouncing bet" and said it was used as a poultice for treating boils. Today soapwort is known as a remedy for aches, boils, and severe skin problems and for treating conditions of the scalp.

Solomon's seal *(Polygonatum biflorum)*. The roots of Solomon's seal were used for treating skin irritations, including poison ivy and poison oak. It was a remedy for boils and difficult skin sores, sometimes combined with violet and dogwood. A poultice of Solomon's seal and woundwort was employed "for stubborn wounds and difficult skin conditions that would not easily or quickly heal otherwise."

Sorrel *(Oxalis violacea)*. Also known as wood sorrel, this simple little plant has shamrock leaves and small purple flowers. A salve made of sorrel, an astringent, and creeping sourgrass *(Oxalis corniculata)* for "healing old sores." There was mention of the inner bark juice of "sweetgum" (for treating itch) being included in this salve formula. A wood sorrel *(Oxalis montana)* in Appalachia has shamrock-type leaves and white flowers with beautiful pink stripes and a yellow center.

Today sorrel is used as a natural antiseptic. My father and Uncle Grady remembered it being called "shamrock sorrel" or "fairy bells."

Speedwell *(Veronica serpyllifolia)*. Speedwell would be used alone for treating boils, according to Mary Chiltoskey. An elder said speedwell was known as "moccasin weed" and was applied to swollen or sore feet for "itch and comfort after the long journey." He asked, "How do you think that Junaluska could walk all the way to Washington to see the president if he didn't have speedwell as his friend?"

Spicebush *(Lindera benzoin)*. The plant, used for treating hives and swelling, was noted by Paul Hamel and Mary Chiltoskey as an old remedy. While unable to verify its use in the herbal literature, an elder remembered spicebush being used to treat gastrointestinal complaints.

Spiderwort *(Tradescantia virginiana)*. A poultice of spiderwort (or dayflower) root was used on cancers in earlier years and is still used for treating insect bites. An elder said spiderwort was also used for treating skin complaints, along with wild oats.

Spotted cranesbill (see Alumroot).

Staggerbush *(Lyonia mariana)*. Paul Hamel and Mary Chiltoskey mentioned staggerbush as a plant remedy for toe itch and ulcers. An elder remembered staggerbush as being effective in a formula with several tree barks for treating itch.

St. John's wort *(Hypericum perforatum)*. St. John's wort was used in a formula for treating cuts and burns. It was also used with pineweed *(H. gentanoides)* for treating "wounds of the skin." John Bartram mentioned it in his memoirs in 1751 as an ingredient—along with pennyroyal, hemlock, and henbane—in an ointment for treating bruises and strains. St. John's wort is a member of the Mangosteen, or St. John's wort, family. Today St. John's wort is used to treat mild depression and as a mood-enhancing agent.

Strawberry *(Fragaria vesca)*. The leaves of wild, or mountain, strawberry were used on skin rashes, along with goldenseal.

Sumac *(Rhus glabra)*. The bark and roots of sumac have been used for treating skin ulcers. Both *R. typhina* and *R. vernix* were mentioned as being used for treating sunburn and ulcers.

Sunflower *(Helianthus annuus)*. The oil of common sunflower was used for treating skin problems and for rheumatism. While sunflower is a sacred plant, with several traditional stories talking about its "spirit power," it's nice to see that it also had a humble use as a helper plant.

Swamp lily (see Lizard's tail or Lily).

Sweetgum tree *(Liquidambar styraciflua)*. Sweetgum, or *se la le,* grows to almost 125 feet in height; the fruit is spiky and round. The leaves, bark, and buds of the sweetgum tree are used for treating cuts, and the antiseptic wash is used for treating skin and scalp conditions. It was also used for dressing sores, ulcers, and wounds, according to Paul Hamel and Mary Chiltoskey. Sweetgum is a member of the Witch Hazel family.

Sycamore tree *(Platanus occidentalis)*. The crushed inner bark of American sycamore was used with birch, willow, and other tree barks as a wash for soaking problem skin areas. This was especially true of skin conditions that were difficult to heal.

Tansy *(Tanacetum vulgare)*. The entire tansy plant, with its strong camphor-like aroma, was used "in earlier days as an insect repellent while working in the planting fields. The plant itself is poisonous, but it was still used in an earlier formula." Do not use tansy during pregnancy.

Thistle *(Cirsium pumilum* and *C. altissimus).* Called bull thistle, the roots of this plant were used for making a poultice for treating bruises and boils. Mary Chiltoskey notes that a poultice made of thistle was also used for treating sore jaws. An elder said, "When a man had a difficult fight while being bullheaded, he usually looked for bull thistle to help him out with bruises." *Cirsium repandum* was used by earlier Cherokee and the Lumbee Indians to treat insect bites, according to an elder.

Thunder plant *(Sempervivum tectorum).* Also called houseleek, thunder plant was used for treating insect bites and stings, sometimes with plantain.

Tickseed *(Desmodium perplexum).* Also known as devil's shoestring, tickseed was used as a warm bath of "scent and calm healing" for alleviating cramps and soreness after a long journey. Wild cherry bark was included in the bath for ballplayers after taking the "plunge," or jumping into the cold river water.

Toadflax *(Comandra unbellata).* The juice of toadflax was mixed with Indian moccasin, or pink lady's slipper, and used for treating sores and wounds. According to my father, toadflax was used in animal stalls because vermin and animals will not eat it.

There is also a toadflax in the Figwort family that is used as a diuretic, as well as a yellow toadflax *(Linaria vulgaris)* used in the Southeast to aid in digestion. This was mentioned by a Lumbee elder who used to make trips to the Smoky Mountains to visit with Cherokee Medicine elders.

Tobacco *(Nicotiana rustica).* In earlier years wild tobacco was used on bites and stings for assisting with pain relief. It would be chewed and "the chaw placed on the sting, or just place a piece of the tobacco leaf with the juice of inner bark, and it took the sting right away." When I asked which inner bark, the elder replied, "Well, if you don't know that, then you shouldn't be in the Medicine." Tobacco leaves contain nicotine, a toxic alkaloid.

Turtlehead *(Chelone glabra).* Also known as rheumatism root or snakehead, turtlehead was used for treating boils and other open skin conditions. (We are uncertain today how this plant was used in treating rheumatism.) One elder remembered the mountain folks using it for expelling worms and parasites. The name comes from the small turtlelike snout that protrudes from the flower cap. Pink turtlehead *(C. lyonii)* is a beautiful garden plant, a brushy perennial with large leaves and the distinctive pink flowers. Pink turtlehead looks great massed with phlox and goldenrod at the edge of a wetland or marshy area.

Twinleaf *(Jeffersonia diphylla).* Twinleaf was prepared as a poultice in a formula for treating sores and inflamed areas of the skin. Some Indians and mountain folks called it "yellowroot" or "rheumatism root" and used it as an antispasmodic and a tonic.

Vervain *(Verbena officinalis)*. While introduced by Europeans, vervain became known as Indian hyssop. According to John Lust it was a popular roadside plant used for treating skin conditions. It was used with woundwort in a formula that included laurel or willow bark for difficult skin sores. One formula included burdock and comfrey. Vervain is also called American vervain or wild hyssop *(V. hastata)*.

Vetch, Carolina *(Vicia caroliniana)*. In earlier years the Cherokee Medicine man or woman appointed for ceremony would have a salve formula that included vetch mixed with bear grease. The ballplayers would be rubbed with this special formula to help their muscles be strong, as well as for alleviating cramps and twitching. A plant called crown vetch *(Coronilla varia)* is used in Europe as a salve or poultice for treating rheumatism.

Violet *(Viola pedata, V. rotundifolia, V. sororia,* and *V. blanda)*. Bird's foot violet, round-leaved violet, common blue violet, and sweet white violet were used for treating wounds and sores. Along with pansy *(V. tricolor)*, they are members of the Violet family. Violets were used as an anti-inflammatory on stubborn boils and infected sores, a use verified by Paul Hamel and Mary Chilstoskey.

Violet wood sorrel (see Sorrel).

Virginia bugleweed *(Lycopus virginicus)*. The root of bugleweed, which has also been referred to as water horehound, was chewed and put on snakebites, as well as spit on the snake "to avoid the snake coming into your dreams." It was used "with cow's milk and given to dogs bitten by snakes, then it would be spit on the snake." Bugleweed is a member of the Mint family.

Walnut tree *(Juglans nigra)*. Several elders confirmed that a wash made from the bark of the black walnut was used for treating difficult sores and "to kill the poison." Black walnut was valued by earlier Cherokee for its use with wild garlic in treating fungal infections and for treating skin inflammation using the leaves, stems, and roots (although I certainly do not recommend bothering the tree's roots). Black walnut is a member of the Walnut family.

Watercress *(Nasturtium officinale)*. This member of the Mustard family was used along with goldenseal for treating acne. It was used with yarrow for treating skin conditions, and was drunk as a "tonic water."

Water dragon (see Lizard's tail).

Water plantain *(Alisma subcordatum)*. The roots of water plantain would be crushed and the juice applied to difficult sores and wounds. Water plantain was used in a formula with alumroot for treating intestinal problems. It was also mentioned for its use in treating bruises, swelling, inflammation, and ulcers. Water plantain and watercress were reportedly used in earlier years with sage as a wash to prevent hair loss, as well as to brighten and strengthen the hair.

Another plant called water plantain *(A. plantago-aquatica)* was reported by a Chinese friend of mine as being used for lowering blood pressure, blood sugar, and cholesterol levels. Both of these plants are considered poisonous when the rootstock is fresh.

Wild carrot *(Daucus carota)*. Also known as Queen Anne's lace, wild carrot is used as a poultice for treating cuts and bruises. Dutchman's breeches is used with wild carrot for treating skin disease, along with purple coneflower *(Echinacea purpurea)* when "the condition is stubborn and difficult to heal." An elder referred to wild carrot as a "beggar that clings to anything it can to get a free ride." Do not use wild carrot during pregnancy.

Wild chamomile (see Dog fennel).

Wild geranium *(Geranium maculatum)*. Also called alumroot or American cranesbill, the dried root powder of wild geranium is used to stop bleeding at cuts and wounds. A poultice of wild geranium was used on difficult skin sores, itches, and wounds. In Appalachia it was used in a formula for treating venereal disease, as well as for treating sore throats and diarrhea in Appalachia. Wild geranium should not be confused with *Heuchera americana*, a member of the Saxifrage family that is also called alumroot and used as an astringent.

Wild geranium is a member of the Geranium family. It is still an important part of the Medicine bag today.

Wild hydrangea (see Seven-bark shrub).

Wild indigo *(Baptisia tinctoria* and *B. australis)*. This long-stemmed plant that stands about three feet tall has blue-green leaves and yellowish flowers. It is found in woodlands and fields and along coastlines from Canada to the Carolinas. Wild indigo was used by southeastern Indian tribes as an antiseptic for treating cuts and wounds and as a gargle. Do not use wild indigo during pregnancy.

Wild lily-of-the-valley (see Shinleaf).

Wild strawberry (see Strawberry).

Willow tree *(Salix alba* and *S. discolor)*. Willow bark was very popular for its use in relieving pain, as a topical treatment for skin problems, and to reduce fever. Willow contains salicin, which converts to salicyclic acid, the active ingredient in aspirin. While it was not used on open wounds, it was used as an astringent for treating old sores. Today willow is used for treating fever, inflammation, pain, and rheumatism. It is a member of the Willow family.

Wintergreen shrub *(Gaultheria procumbens)*. The compound methyl salicylate, used for treating joint and muscle pains, is made from the leaves and bark of wintergreen. This plant is a favorite of deer and other animals for feeding on, especially in the winter. The Cherokee referred to wintergreen as rheumatism root. It was also known as checkerberry or teaberry, a good flavor in chewing gum.

Witchgrass (see Couchgrass).

Witch hazel tree *(Hamamelis virginiana)*. A small tree, witch hazel is a popular astringent in compresses for treating bruises and strains. The distillation is made from bark, twigs, and leaves mixed with alcohol and water. Earlier Cherokee used the leaves as an astringent for dressing minor cuts and to reduce inflammation, as well as "for blood vessels that stick out from the upper legs [varicose veins]." Witch hazel was also used in earlier years as a remedy for hemorrhoids and bleeding. The wood of witch hazel was strong enough for use as a bow. Witch hazel branches have also been used as dowsing rods for locating water.

Wood betony *(Stachys officinalis)*. Betony, or wood betony, was used in earlier years as an astringent on cuts and wounds and as a mouthwash. Mountain folks used it as a gargle for sore gums and as a mouthwash. My father told me wood betony was useful for lowering blood pressure or the "feelings of flush and redness in the face." He would joke that for an Irishman like him with light skin and red hair it might be difficult to presume redness in the face was caused by high blood pressure. There is also a wood betony listed in South Medicine as lousewort.

Wood sorrel (see Sorrel).

Woundwort *(Stachys palustris)*. The woundwort plant belongs to the Mint family. It was used as a natural antiseptic and to stop bleeding of wounds. It is also called all-heal and used for female health concerns and in birthing. Woundwort acts as a disinfectant, and so is good for treating topical skin problems and wounds. Several plants have the common name of woundwort; all are used for healing wounds and skin conditions. Today woundwort is also used in treating joint pain.

Yarrow *(Achillea millefolium)*. This well-known field plant with its clustered heads of flowers is still used as a poultice for cuts and wounds.

Yarrow was known to the Cherokee as "snakegrass" or *i ma dah;* it was used to reduce fevers and stop bleeding and as a poultice with wintergreen or birch for treating rheumatism. Yarrow is an astringent and an anti-inflammatory. It was used to stimulate appetite for elders and those who were sick. The Cherokee also used yarrow to treat edema and gout, as well as in a formula with chamomile as a cream for the face and skin during cold winters. Today yarrow is used to stop bleeding at cuts and wounds.

There is some concern about allergic reactions on the part of some folks. My father called yarrow "devil's plaything." Uncle Grady said that one of our family members gained recognition during the Civil War as an Indian scout who could stop bleeding. That was certainly a time when the knowledge of other American Indian remedies and formulas was needed. Do not use yarrow during pregnancy.

Yellow dock *(Rumex crispus* and *R. patientia).* Sometimes called dock or curled dock, yellow dock was combined with bear grease or other salves to treat skin problems and itch. A poultice is still used for treating sores, ulcers, and skin problems, and yellow dock is combined with common sorrel *(R. acetosella)* for skin itch. An elder referred to dock as *oo na sa ste ske.* Dock and sorrel are members of the Smartweed, or Buckwheat, family.

Yellowroot *(Xanthorhiza simplicissima).* Called *da lo ni,* or "yellow plant," in Cherokee, yellowroot is used in a formula "for skin itch and irritation problems." The soft inner bark of the branches and roots are boiled to make a wash for many skin ailments. For other plants known as yellowroot, see the entries for twinleaf and goldenseal.

Many uses of plants as South Medicine have been lost over the years, as fewer young people took on the study of Indian plant Medicine. Luckily that situation is changing now, and the Medicine elders are being sought for sharing their knowledge. If the reader knows of the use of other plants in the South Medicine, I would certainly appreciate hearing about them.

Here is a listing of plants that may have been lost in terms of how they were used for skin and related conditions: spring beauty *(Claytonia virginica),* trailing arbutus *(Epigaea repens),* dutchman's breeches *(Dicentra cucullaria),* Fraser's sedge *(Cymophyllus fraseri),* silverbell *(Halesia carolina),* foamflower *(Tiarella cordifolia),* brook lettuce *(Saxifraga micranthidifolia),* stonecrop *(Sedum ternatum),* wood anemone *(Anemone lancifolia),* robin's plantain *(Erigeron pulchellus),* false

Solomon's seal *(Smilacina racemosa)*, black locust *(Robinia pseudoacacia)*, doll's eyes or white baneberry *(Actaea pachypoda)*, witch hobble *(Viburnum lantanoides)*, umbrella magnolia *(Magnolia tripetala)*, fire cherry *(Prunus pensylvanica)*, daisy fleabane *(Erigeron philadelphicus)*, serviceberry *(Amelanchier laevis)*, galax *(Galax aphylla)*, thimbleweed *(Anemone virginiana)*, Spanish bayonet *(Yucca smalliana)*, yellowwood *(Cladrastis kentukea)*, wild potato vine *(Ipomoea pandurata)*, flowering spurge *(Euphorbia corollata)*, mountain camellia *(Stewartia ovata)*, Michaux's saxifrage *(Saxifraga michauxii)*, grass of Parnassus *(Parnassia asarifolia)*, starry campion *(Silene stellata)*, summer sweet *(Clethra acuminata)*, downy aster and white wood aster *(Aster pilosus* and *A. divaricatus)*.

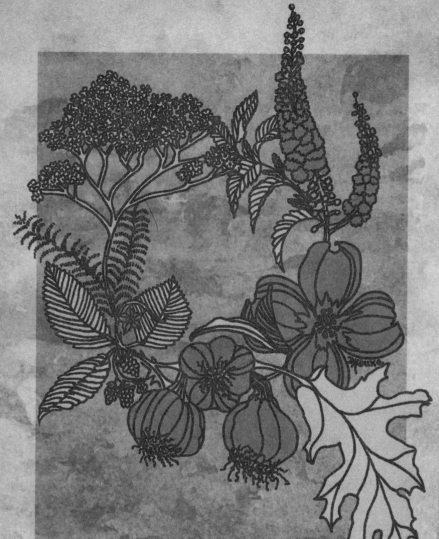

WEST

6

Plant Medicines of the West

In earlier Cherokee Indian Medicine, West Medicine teachings focused on the internal aspects of the physical body. The Medicine included many plants for building strength and endurance. The primary focus of West Medicine is on systems of the physical body, including the digestive system, the endocrine system, and the urinary functions, and the internal infections that can cause unwellness. Describing the realm of West Medicine, an elder said, "Everything that is going on inside that cannot be seen with the eye, but causes the body to be ill or act strange, both physically and spiritually."

The plants and trees used for addressing internal ailments or complaints were originally created from watching animal behavior. The Cherokee stories tell of a time when animals and plants could talk to humans. I am sure that observable actions of animals were a good teacher about how certain plants and trees were used. As an elder Medicine man said, "The plants and trees talk to you and tell you what they are there to be a helper for; you just gotta' know how to listen." Another said, "You either got better or you died, but Mother Nature always had something to cure you or relieve pain as a helper."

Some conditions associated with the West, such as internal worms and parasites, were sometimes considered to come from negative influence or conjuring by someone or something in nature, probably because of an action one has taken outside of the way of right relationship, as when a hunter takes an animal's life without proper prayers. And sometimes it was just a matter of intestinal worms coming from meat not being cooked well. In an earlier time our needs were different from what they are today with regard to health and wellness. Our lives were more directly related to nature. The exposures were more about getting bitten by a snake or cut with a tool or weapon. It was reasonable to eat contaminated meats and foods with some type of parasite or spores. Intestinal worms and parasites were more of a problem of that time. On the other hand, we ate fresh fruits, vegetables, leafy foods, and berries and nuts. Washing the fruits and vegetables was as much for ceremony and thanks-giving as it was for food safety and disease prevention. As an elder said, "Food was sacred. It was as much Medicine as it was sustenance."

Earlier American Indians were guided in a sacred way by choice, influence from the environment, and their way of life. As one elder said, "Most folks think it was simpler back then or in the old days. Not so, 'cause there were plenty of animals out there also looking for food. The exposure and elements were sometimes very harsh. The stresses were different than today, but they were still stresses to survive. We did not have doctors and hospitals as we do today. That is what is different, but I don't know that is better. In any time, people just do the best they can."

As in an earlier time, we seek helpers for protection and resolution. The Medicine man or woman "knew things, 'cause they were taught. They were helpers, just as the plants were helpers. That is how we survived as a tribal people." The seeking of guidance was to assure our safe journey in this life, especially with the choices we made, because everything we did affected every other member of our family, clan, and tribe. The focus then was more on "good Medicine" choices, rather than on treatment modalities, symptoms, prescriptions, and personal satisfactions. As one elder said, "Instead of insurance and managed care, we managed ourselves the best way we could."

Before there were doctors, the "Medicine" involved choice of natural plants and substances based on trial and error or what worked to restore health or relieve pain. The knowledge of body systems and what plants to take for rebalancing the organs held by the elder Medicine men and women was amazing to me. In the old way there was a secret Medicine Society of codes so strict that many would not be able to follow them today, including ceremonies and sacred reminders of the way of right relationship. Instead of "do no harm," the Medicine person's guiding principle was to harm no one or anything in our Universal Circle and to be a protector and helper to everything on Mother Earth as we give thanks to the Great One.

The Medicine of the West was described to me as being "animal Medicine." Several Cherokee myths tell about conditions caused by animal spirits, or "the animal in humans." For the Cherokee, the bear is the animal most often associated with the direction of the West. (For other tribes it is the buffalo.) The color of the West is black, the direction of death or passing and the "darkening land." The key principle is balance. In the West Medicine, water and cleansing were very important. In the old stories, Bear was a friend to the water spirits. The bear represents strength and endurance, while the water represents healing and cleansing. The West Medicine is intended to restore a person's physical strength and endurance.

The following is a listing of plants and their uses as West Medicine.

Adam's needles (see Bear grass).

Adder's tongue *(Erythronium americanum)*. Also called dog's tooth violet and trout lily, adder's tongue was used in a formula for gout, sometimes combined with Indian root. The bark is antiseptic and was used in a wash externally and internally, sometimes with blackberry. It is a member of the Lily family. It was also combined with honeysuckle *(Lonicera japonica),* sometimes called woodbine, for treating gout, as well as for general use as an antimicrobial agent. The old ones would say it's time to go fishing for brown trout when the trout lily blooms.

Agrimony *(Agrimonia gyposepala* and *A. parviflora)*. The earlier Cherokee used the roots of agrimony, or liverwort, for reducing fever. A member of the Rose family, this "heal-all" plant was used by the Cherokee to calm the system, often in combination with peppermint. Its astringent quality was especially helpful for gastric problems.

Agrimony was called "church steeple" by the mountain folks, probably because of the tall spikes of flowers. It is an antibiotic, anti-inflammatory, and astringent with tannin content. Today it is used for treating gallbladder problems. It is also prepared as a tea for treating diarrhea, and the dried plant is used to treat sore throat.

Alder shrub *(Alnus serrulata)*. A tea of common, or tag, alder is used for pain and fever. In earlier years it was used as a tonic to strengthen the body. It was used with other barks, including balsam fir and pine, as a formula for intestinal problems. It was prepared as a tea for treating jaundice and conditions of the kidneys. Sometimes creeping sourwood *(Oxalis corniculata)* was added for nausea and diarrhea. This shrub or small tree is usually found near the edge of water. It is a member of the Birch family.

Alfalfa *(Medicoga sativa)*. Alfalfa was introduced to the Cherokee by other Indians, who called it "buffalo weed." It was used as a mild laxative and a natural cleanser, as well as a diuretic. It was also used to improve the appetite of elders "and sickly children, to give them strength."

Aloe *(Aloe vera)*. The soft substance from the aloe leaves is used as a laxative for acute, not chronic, constipation. This plant was introduced by European settlers. A plant called false aloe *(Agave virginica)* was used as a general purpose antiseptic in earlier years. Today it is used internally for colitis, constipation, diabetes, and stomach ulcers. Do not use aloe during pregnancy.

Alumroot *(Heuchera americana)*. Sometimes called American sanicle, alumroot was crushed or chewed by the Cherokee as an astringent for treating diarrhea. Blackberry would be added as a juice when it was in season. It was also used as a cleansing for the liver, as well as with wood fern *(Dryopteris filix* or *D. marginalis)* for ridding the body of parasites and worms in the intestines. It was used for addressing bowel complaints.

American senna (see Senna).

American spikenard (see Indian root).

Angelica *(Angelica archangelica)*. This plant was only collected by those who knew it well; it would be easy to mistake angelica for water hemlock, which is extremely poisonous. Angelica was a favorite of one Medicine man for "inviting a new appetite to elders who had troubles with cramping and gas, and little interest in food 'cause of what it does." It was also used as a diuretic, along with chamomile and goldenseal. During his tour in South Carolina in 1788, William Bartram mentioned the aromatic scent of *Angelica atropurpurea* as being similar to anise seed. He also made mention of the Cherokee trading with southern Indians for such herbs for treating stomach disorders, back pain, and intestinal worms. There are myths about angelica's ability to create positive occurrences in one's life. An elder called it a "spirit plant" that was used for "good hunting." Another elder said that angelica was used "in the olden days for pain in the joints [arthritis]." Do not use angelica during pregnancy.

Anise *(Pimpinella anisum)*. Also called sweet plant, anise was used to improve digestion and appetite for elders, along with ginger and other substances for settling the stomach, such as mint tea. In recent years cinnamon *(Cinnanomum zeylanicum)* has been combined with anise in cooking to settle an upset stomach and indigestion. This is especially true for the elderly. Today anise is also combined with wormwood *(Artemisia absinthium)*, angelica, and Indian root to stimulate digestion and for addressing gallbladder complaints.

Anise is a member of the Carrot, or Parsley, family. It is not to be confused with anise root *(Osmorhiza longistylis)*, which is in the same family. Today anise is used for treating intestinal gas and spasms.

Apple tree *(Malus sylvestris)*. The inner bark of wild apple tree was used for addressing gallbladder complaints and constipation. The bark was also used as a yellow dye. A formula with white pine and balsam fir was prepared in a tea by the Medicine man or woman for the ballplayers, to give them "wind" strength. Apples contain pectin, which acts as a stool softener.

Arbutus (see Terrapin's foot).

Arrowhead *(Sagittaria latifolia)*. The Cherokee used the leaves of arrowhead, or *di ga da tla dah,* to make a tea for "fever of the body" after an accident or illness, especially with children. It is a member of the Arrowhead, or Water Plantain, family.

Asafoetida *(Ferula foetida)*. While not a native plant of North America, asafoetida found its way into the Medicine bag for treating stomach cramps and spasms, colic, and gas, and for getting rid of parasites and worms. Other names included colic root and cramp root. Asafoetida is known as an antispasmodic and a laxative.

Ash tree *(Fraxinus americana)*. Ash, or white ash, is called *su co no huh* in Cherokee. It was used by southeastern tribes as an astringent, and a tonic for the intestines and the liver was made of the inner bark. One Cherokee formula mixed seven different barks of trees as a "cure-all" tonic for weak stomachs, especially for ballplayers and hunters. White ash, *tsu ga no nv,* was one of the firewoods used in earlier years for tribal gatherings. White ash was used in recent years for making baseball bats and handles for tools. Another variety, called red, green, or water ash *(F. pennsylvanica)*, and Carolina or pop ash *(F. caroliniana)* is found along the Carolina coast.

Asparagus *(Asparagus officinalis)*. Asparagus was used as a food and for medicinal purposes by the Cherokee and other tribes. It was a good diuretic and thought to help with inflamed kidney and other urinary tract problems, as well as to help with constipation. The Cherokee and the Creek used asparagus as a food medicine for treating gout, while the Catawba used it for settling the "rough stomach after a rough travel."

Aster *(Aster novae-angliae* and *A. linariifolius)*. The leaves of aster were used in a tea for treating diarrhea. The roots were used for fever and as a poultice for pain. My grandmother Edna Rogers called this flower, which has a purple daisylike flower and a yellow center cone, "the last rose of summer." Mountain folks used the creeping rhizomes by boiling them to make a decoction for treating intestinal problems and skin conditions.

Balm, melissa *(Melissa officinalis)*. The value of melissa cannot be overstated in terms of its use as an antiviral, antibacterial, carminative, antispasmodic, and mild sedative. Lemon, or melissa, balm was used in several formulas as a "calming agent for the physical body, mind, and spirit."

Balsam poplar tree *(Populus balsamifera)*. Balsam poplar was also known as balm of Gilead; the inner bark was used in formulas for treating gout and infections in the intestinal tract and kidneys. Sometimes the formula included lady's slipper, or Indian moccasin, and toadflax, or bastard toadflax *(Comandra umbellata)*. Sometimes the bark of Fraser fir *(Abies fraseri)* would be included in a formula to rid the body of intestinal worms. The needles were used over hot coals in traditional sweats.

Barberry shrub *(Berberis vulgaris)*. Barberry was introduced by Europeans as being good for the liver. American Indians used in it a formula for treating diarrhea. The plant contains berberine salts, a mild laxative. Barberry is also used for treating inflammation of the gallbladder and as a bitter to reduce gas and indigestion. Today it is used for addressing diarrhea and fever and used in traditional sweats. Barberry is a member of the Barberry family, along with twinleaf, blue cohosh, umbrella leaf, and mayapple, or mandrake, and is found in the Smoky Mountains and Appalachia. It is not recommended for use during pregnancy due to its effect of stimulating the uterus.

Basil *(Ocimum basilicum)*. Basil was used for treating gas pains and nausea and to reduce fevers. It was one of those plants introduced by the White settlers, who used it with cinnamon *(Cinnamomum zeylanicum)* for cooking meats and fish. Basil was mixed with peppercorns as a remedy to reduce fever. The Cherokee in Kentucky and West Virginia similarly included basil in an old formula for reducing fevers and as a carminative or substance to relieve gas from eating beans. A wild basil *(Clinopodium vulgaris)* is commonly found in Europe.

Bayberry shrub *(Myrica cerifera)*. The leaves and stems of bayberry, also known as southern wax myrtle, were boiled in water for a fever-reducing remedy. It was also used in a formula with other tree barks for eliminating intestinal worms. The elder I spoke with remembered it being used with alumroot *(Heuchera americana)* as a treatment for thrush. Bayberry was used for wax to make candles. It is a member of the Bayberry family.

Bean *(Phaseolus vulgaris)*. Beans, or *du ya,* such as kidney, navy, pinto, string, and wax beans, are used as natural diuretics. In earlier years beans were a staple food for American Indians, along with corn and wild greens. Mashed beans with gingerroot were used with elders to help them keep their systems "cleansed." According to James Duke, Ph.D., beans are good for diabetes and controlling blood sugar, and they have natural phytoestrogen benefits.

Bearberry shrub *(Arctostaphylos uva ursi)*. Bears favor the fruit from this evergreen shrub, which was used as an astringent and diuretic by the Cherokee, Creek, and Catawba Indians. Bearberry was used to treat gout and kidney stones. It is also used for treating urinary complaints, except during pregnancy or if there is a digestive problem. The unique pitcherlike flower has five points, with fruit that turns to purple-red berries. It is used now for keeping the urinary tract clear and reducing fluid buildup. It is a member of the Heath family along with several other berry plants, including teaberry, cranberry, and blueberry, as well as mountain laurel and terrapin's foot.

Bear grass *(Yucca filamentosa* and *Y. arborescens)*. Southeastern Indians used Bear grass, or yucca, to treat what we now call diabetes. It is uncertain how it was prepared. Another yucca found in the Smoky Mountains is Spanish bayonet *(Yucca smalliana)*. Mountain folks called it "Adam's needles" and used it to make great sun hats. The leftover leaf parts were ground into a tea for treating liver and gallbladder problems. Do be careful in handling bear grass because the sharp needles will sting you. This plant produces a tall stalk with clusters of bell-shaped white flowers.

Beard grass *(Andropogon virginicus)*. Commonly known as broom sedge, beard grass was steeped to make a bath solution for treating frostbite and for alleviating itch and sores, according to Mary Chiltoskey. It was used as dye and also included in the Green Corn Medicine formula, probably as a stimulant.

Beardtongue, hairy *(Penstemon laevigatus* or *canescens)*. In earlier years a tea of hairy beardtongue was used for treating cramps. The beautiful lavender flowers are about fifteen inches tall and can be seen at Mile High, a point along the Blue Ridge Parkway in North Carolina that some elders call "Spirit Mountain." The elongated whorl of flowers that bloom from April to July extend like a tongue with fine hairs, similar to a beard.

Common beardtongue *(P. barbatus),* with its erect spike of pink flowers, looks great in a home garden. Pale beardtongue *(P. pallidus),* with white flowers, was used in earlier years for treating snakebites and toothaches.

Bedstraw *(Galium aparine, G. triflorum,* and *G. verum).* Bedstraw, sometimes called cleavers or goosegrass, was used as a diuretic and antispasmodic by American Indians and mountain folks alike. As a tea it also helped with the pain of gallstones. The crushed leaves were used to stop bleeding, both internally and externally. Mountain folks used bedstraw for treating epilepsy. The pleasant honeylike aroma made bedstraw popular for placing in pillows and beds in earlier years.

Bedstraw contains glycosides and tannins that make it a good, mild diuretic and a means for relaxing the urinary tract. Bedstraw also stimulates the lymphatic system to eliminate toxins. This hairy plant with rings of leaves around the stem is a member of the Madder, or Bedstraw, family. The hairy fruit sticks to clothing. Uncle Grady called bedstraw "clabber grass," an Irish name for the plant. An elder said that "cleavers was called goosegrass, and the bristles hooked on to anything to carry it to a new home." The same elder mentioned lady's bedstraw *(G. verum)* as being used for treating urinary conditions.

Bee balm *(Monarda didyma).* Sometimes called Oswego tea, bee balm was used for treating colic, fever, and headaches and as a calming agent. Bee balm contains thymol, which is valued as an antiseptic in commercial products. Earlier formulas for colds and cuts included bee balm, but it was valued as a West Medicine for "headaches caused by the internal infections" and was used for that purpose in an old formula with birch and willow. It was also used as an antispasmodic and a diuretic and for improving digestion.

Beech tree *(Fagus grandifolia).* The nuts of American beech were chewed to rid the body of worms, according to Mary Chiltoskey. A tea made from the bark and small twigs of beech and the bark of balsam was used as an astringent to "to flush the system." Called *ge tla* in Cherokee, beech was considered an "ancestor tree," a tree native to our part of the mountains and North America. Beech was one of the council-fire woods, the *gu sv,* used in earlier years for tribal gatherings. The beech nuts were used to attract small game such as squirrels and some birds, as well as for attracting bear in the eastern mountains.

Beggar lice *(Hackelia virginia)*. The roots of beggar lice were used in a formula for treating kidney problems. In earlier years it was mixed in a formula for "sores that just would not go away." It is used for itchy skin and itching at the genitals. Today we know that beggar lice prevents the formation of kidney stones by decreasing calcium and increasing citrate in the urine. It should not be confused with beggar's ticks *(Bidens aristosa)*.

Belladonna *(Atropa belladonna)*. Belladonna, or deadly nightshade, was primarily used in a very diluted form as an antispasmodic. Only those with special training would prepare a belladonna remedy, "'cause you have to know how it can affect someone." The leaves were used to calm the intestinal tract; however, plant alkaloids induce a narcotic action that affects the central nervous system, making the plant deadly poisonous. This plant highlights how careful earlier Cherokee and other Indian tribes were with plants that can have harmful effects but can still be "good Medicine."

Benne plant *(Sesamum indicum)*. Also called sesame, the leaves of benne were crushed for the oil, which was used as a cathartic to increase peristaltic motion to cleanse the system. Paul Hamel and Mary Chiltoskey reported that the leaves and seeds were used for dysentery and "flux." It's my understanding that this plant is native to Africa and made its way to Georgia and the Carolinas possibly during the early slave trade. The leaves and seeds were used for treating diarrhea "and anything with the bowels and the insides," as an elder put it. The seeds were known for their oil and used in a manner similar to the castor bean, especially in administering to children.

Bethroot (see Trillium).

Bilberry *(Vaccinium myrtillis)*. Sometimes called huckleberry, or *ka wa ya* in Cherokee, bilberry is used for treating "weakness of the old ones" and for elders who experience low blood sugar. In earlier years a formula for this condition was called Indian remedy. Bilberry was also made into a tea with thyme and strawberry leaves for treating diarrhea. Part of the Heath family, bilberry was used with cranberries or "bearberries to make a soothing tea." Today we know that it contains anthocyanosides that stimulate the production of mucus and protects the lining of the stomach from digestive acids. Like its cousins blueberry and huckleberry, bilberry prevents blood clots and breaks down plaque deposits in the arteries to prevent strokes.

Birch tree *(Betula alba* and *B. lenta)*. The inner bark and the young leaves of sweet birch, or mountain birch, were valued by several tribes for treating kidney stones. The oil was used for flavoring. The oil of wintergreen and wild cherry bark were other taste treats for Indian children. The children also enjoyed birch beer. Today birch is used to treat bladder infections, digestive problems, gout, and kidney stones and for pain relief. Birch, or *a ti sv gi,* was one of the council-fire woods used in earlier years for tribal gatherings.

Bird's foot violet *(Viola pedata).* Bird's foot violet was used to treat kidney and urinary problems. This small woodland plant was treated with respect by the earlier Medicine men and women, who said it was a special gift from the Great One when He (or She, depending on which Medicine person you talk to) came down to Mother Earth to talk with the birds about arguing among themselves. This little plant was to honor the little birds and be a Medicine for the little winged ones, as well as for the benefit of the humans who were given the responsibility to protect Mother Earth.

Bittersweet *(Celastrus scandens).* "A chew on the bittersweet bark is good to settle the stomach." American Bittersweet was also used for treating bowel complaints and was combined with raspberry leaves, along with field horsetail *(Equisetum arvense),* for treating kidney ailments. Horsetail was used by itself as a remedy for constipation.

Bitter weed *(Helenium tenuifolium).* The flower and roots of bitter weed were used in a special formula for "the serious problems of what you call diabetes." Bitter weed is a member of the Aster, or Composite, family, along with sneezeweed and sunflower. Bitter weed should not be confused with bitter root, which was used as a laxative.

Blackberry *(Rubus villosus).* A tea is made from the bark of blackberry and used for diarrhea and kidney complaints. The roots have a high tannin content, which accounts for blackberry's gift as an astringent. Several Indian tribes besides the Cherokee found the value in blackberry for treating diarrhea and dysentery, including the Oneida, Catawba, and Creek. Blackberry and raspberry leaves are used as an astringent tea that is effective in treating diarrhea. This is a popular remedy for children, along with alumroot. Blackberry was also used for treating gout, along with Indian root.

Blackberry and blueberry leaves are used as "stabilizing teas for those with blood sugar problems." An elder said that blackberry was also used with viper's bugloss, or blue devil *(Echium vulgare),* for addressing kidney and urinary complaints. The berries are used as a tonic and blood builder today and recognized as powerful antioxidants for their iron, potassium, calcium, manganese, and vitamin C contents.

Black cherry tree (see Wild cherry tree).

**Black cohosh *(Cimicifuga racemosa* or *C. americana).* ** Also known as black snakeroot, black cohosh is used as a relaxant, sedative, and antispasmodic. Its name comes from an Algonquian word meaning "rough." While the flowering wands of the plant are attractive at six feet tall, with a cluster of white flowers, it is the rhizome that is sought for West Medicine. Black cohosh is a member of the Buttercup family. Today it is used in treating diarrhea, as a diuretic for reducing fluid retention, and for treating inflammation. This plant is at risk in its natural environment. Do not use during pregnancy or while nursing.

**Black-eyed Susan *(Rudbeckia hirta* and *R. fulgida).* ** This plant was used for treating urinary complaints and related conditions. As James Duke, Ph.D., has indicated about this state flower of Maryland, it is a strong immune stimulant, similar to echinacea. Orange coneflower *(R. fulgida)* has daisy flowers of yellow to orange with raised cone centers. A hardy perennial, it makes a good garden flower that brightens the landscape.

**Blackgum tree *(Nyssa sylvatica).* ** The Cherokee used the inner bark of the blackgum tree in a formula for ridding the body of worms and other intestinal problems. Also called black tupelo, it was used in several remedies with other tree barks for addressing various problems, including diarrhea and sexually transmitted diseases. The formulas have been lost, but from what the elders could remember about the barks used in these fomulas, astringents and strong antibacterial agents were apparently the active constituents. An elder said that blackgum bark used to be combined with the bark of bush pepper *(Berberis canandensis)* in a tea for treating diarrhea. Blackgum, a member of the Dogwood family, is liked by birds for its juicy fruit.

**Blackroot *(Veronicastrum virginicum).* ** Sometimes called culver's root or bowman's root, blackroot was used by the Cherokee as a purgative and tonic and as an antiseptic for the liver. Mountain folks called blackroot by the same names, but they also call it "physic root" and cautioned that it be prepared only by those who knew how to use it. An elder said blackroot is good as a root tonic to strengthen the "insides for a day's work." In earlier years, gulver root *(Leptandria alba)* was combined with blackroot for "an entire cleansing of the internal systems." Today blackroot is used for treating constipation and liver problems.

Black snakeroot (see Black cohosh and Snakeroot).

Blazing star (see Fairywand and Button snakeroot).

**Bloodroot *(Sanguinaria canadensis).* ** Also known as red root or Indian paint, the reddish sap in the rhizome is used as a special Medicine for treating indigestion. Bloodroot is one of those plants that had a specific use instead of being used as part of a formula. There is an old myth that a piece of dried bloodroot carried in the Medicine bag will keep bad spirits away, but my teachers were not sure how this myth originated.

Bloodroot was combined in a formula with coltsfoot and Solomon's seal for addressing digestive problems and ulcers. Bloodroot contains tannins and phenol compounds that are antibacterial and anti-inflammatory. Today bloodroot is used for treating constipation and to stimulate digestion. This plant is considered at risk in its natural environment. Do not use bloodroot during pregnancy.

Blue cohosh *(Caulophyllum thalictroides)*. Known as papoose root, this small plant is found in the damp woodlands in the mountains of the Southeast. The berries are poisonous, and the plant itself is an irritant to the skin. Earlier Cherokee used blue cohosh as an antispasmodic and as a treatment for rheumatism for the elderly.

Blue devil *(Echium vulgare)*. Sometimes called viper's bugloss or blueweed, a tea was made from this plant and combined with others for treating kidney and urine problems. An elder said, "This is a devil of a plant to work with since it causes severe dermatitis."

Blue-eyed grass *(Sisyrinchium angustifolium)*. A tea of the roots of blue-eyed grass was used for treating diarrhea in children, and the grass was cooked as greens for regularity in elders. Except for the purplish blue flowers, blue-eyed grass looks very much like star grass.

Blue flag *(Iris versicolor)*. The Creek and Cherokee prepared the roots of blue flag by cleaning and boiling them, and then crushing them between stones to make a poultice. The poultice was used on persistent sores, and as a diuretic to purge the body of toxins. In earlier years blue flag was used as a tonic and stimulant called *oo wa su yu,* "liver lily," used to "cleanse the liver of persons who drank too much." Like other iris species, blue flag iris is used as an expectorant for respiratory problems. Today it is used for treating constipation, as a diuretic for addressing fluid retention, for liver problems and inflammation, and to stimulate the bowels. Blue flag should not be mistaken for sweet flag *(Acorus calamus)*.

Boneset *(Eupatorium perfoliatum)*. Boneset was called Indian sage, or "feverwort" by American Indians, for its use in reducing fevers and aches. It was also used for treating arthritis. Boneset is probably a diaphoretic that causes perspiration, which helps break a fever, rather than being a fever-reducing agent. The plant was always intriguing to me because of the white flower heads in a cluster at the top of the plant's stem, and the lance-shaped leaves that grow in opposite pairs that are joined at the base. A cousin, Joe-pye weed *(E. purpureum),* is used to reduce fevers as well. An elder said, "Just keep in mind that it [boneset] is good for almost anything." Boneset is also used with peppermint in a warm tea for alleviating coughs and is used as liver Medicine "when you need it most."

Bouncing bet (see Soapwort).

Bowman's root (see Indian physic).

Branch lettuce *(Saxifraga pensylvanica)*. Several varieties of leafy greens found in the mountains of Appalachia and the Great Smoky Mountains are used in salads. A salad usually includes dandelion leaves and ramps when in bloom. These are also mixed with "greens grown in the garden and cooked in water with collards and pepper to stimulate the physical body and the spirit, especially after the ailments of winter."

Broom sedge (see Beard grass).

Buckthorn tree *(Rhamnus caroliniana* and *R. catharticus)*. Carolina buckthorn *(R. caroliniana)* is a shrub or small tree that is also called Indian cherry or yellow wood. It is a buckthorn without spines that was discovered in South Carolina and is also found in Tennessee. Mountain folks know it as "polecat tree." According to John Lust, alder buckthorn *(Rhamnus fragula)* was used to purge the body when a person was sick with stomach, constipation, or liver problems. *A ga do li,* or "eye tree," as it was called by earlier Cherokee, was used for "cleansing the entire system." Such a cleansing might have taken place before seeking a vision.

There is also a European buckthorn *(R. catharticia)* found in eastern North America, from North Carolina to Nova Scotia. It is used to purge the digestive system or as a mild laxative. Today buckthorn is used as a bark and berry remedy for cleansing and as a laxative. The dye is used for coloring baskets made from the bark. Do not use during pregnancy or while nursing.

Burdock *(Arctium lappa* and *A. minus)*. The roots of great or common burdock are used as a diuretic and as a liver tonic to "clear the body of poisons." The leaves are prepared as a mild laxative, and the seeds are used in a formula as an antibacterial substance. My father said that the word *dock* was Old English for "plant." *Dock* is still in use by some mountain folks.

Burdock, sometimes called burr or sticky plant, was used for treating arthritis. It was considered "good Medicine" when added to alfalfa or buffalo weed for treating colon complaints and internal bleeding. Burdock was used in association with sweat lodge ceremonies to cleanse and detoxify the system. It was also combined with cleavers or bedstraw as a tea for treating gallstones. Today it is used for addressing abdominal pain and diarrhea.

Bull thistle *(Carduus altissimus* or *C. lanceolatus).* The leaves of *tsi tsi* were boiled to make a tea for treating neuralgia "from the inners." This was considered a "soreness or pain that came from within the body," as opposed to rheumatism aches. Very few plants were used specifically for addressing neuralgia.

Bull thistle is not to be confused with milk thistle *(Silybum marianum).* There is also a blessed thistle *(C. benedictus)* used for intestinal, stomach, and liver complaints.

Butterfly weed *(Asclepias tuberosa).* An elder mentioned butterfly weed, or pleurisy root, being used as an antispasmodic, a diuretic, a laxative, and a remedy for indigestion. This plant with colorful orange flowers is found in the dry countryside of Appalachia. It was combined with common phacella, or *u s te s gi,* for easing swollen joints.

Button snakeroot *(Liatris spicata* or *L. regimontis).* Commonly called blazing star, button snakeroot was used as an anti-inflammatory and for "pain of backaches from being sick inside." It was used for treating kidney complaints, as a diuretic, and for addressing painful or difficult menstruation. Another plant called button snakeroot *(Eryngium aquaticum),* or water eryngo, was also used as a plant helper. *Eryngium yuccifolium,* or rattlesnake master, was also called button snakeroot. As with the yellowroots, it's important to know the button snakeroots to use them "in a way of right relationship."

Cabbage *(Brassica oleracea).* Though it is a food, the Cherokee valued cabbage for its medicinal qualities and its ability to heal gastrointestinal problems and ulcers. It was considered a natural antacid and good for treating yeast infections. It was not listed in the formulas, but was mentioned many times as a gift from the Great One to maintain "cleansed insides." Cabbage has anti-inflammatory and antibacterial properties and can be used for addressing "weak livers of folks." The same elder said, "This is another one that someday those researchers will find what earlier Cherokee already knew. This plant is good for many things that ail a body, not just for food." We now know that raw cabbage juice contains two antiulcer compounds that are as effective as antacids in treating ulcers. In recent years pot marigold *(Calendula officinalis)* has been used with cabbage juice for stimulating the immune system.

Calamus root *(Acorus calamus).* Also called sweet flag, this rhizome grows along rivers and in wet areas. It is used for treating stomach pain and gas. In earlier years it was used as a stimulant or tonic. The leaves are used with dandelion and watercress for a "spring salad."

Calamus is a popular water plant used in a formula for healing. One elder said, "The water will be pure where calamus grows." I found out that the Tartars and Mongolians in the eleventh century believed that calamus could purify drinking water, and so they carried it on all their conquest expeditions.

The Cherokee used calamus as a tonic for a "strong stomach before hunting." It was used to relieve heartburn and as a wash for treating sores and burns. Today it is used for digestion problems and for diabetes in a formula with bitter weed. It is effective as a powder or as a poultice for killing lice. Other uses include treatment for headaches, gallbladder problems, swelling, and kidney problems.

Caraway *(Carum carvi)*. Found in the woods and near rocks, caraway was not a native plant in North America. (It is important to distinguish caraway from other poisonous plants in the Carrot family, such as water hemlock.) Caraway seeds have been used as flavoring in breads, but they also can be used for relieving gas pains. The Cherokee used caraway to stimulate digestion in the elderly and for stomach and intestinal health. Today it is used for treating constipation, indigestion, gas, and stomach ulcers.

An elder said that caraway was a very old species of plant that is difficult to transplant. It is still in use today as an antispasmodic and as a cooking spice.

Carolina jessamine *(Gelsemium sempervirens)*. Also called yellow jessamine, in earlier years the roots and rhizome of this plant were dried and used for treating "headaches and nervous conditions by those trained." Caution should be exercised by those using this plant if you have cardiac problems. This plant is not to be confused with yellow flowering jasmine *(Jasminum odoratissimum)*.

Carolina pink *(Spigella marilandica)*. Also known as Indian pink, or *u si la,* Carolina pink has an unusual funnel-like flower that is red on the outside and yellow inside, with the leaves being opposite and connected on the single stem. The roots would be harvested after flowering in the fall and used for treating indigestion. An old formula combined anise, senna, turtlehead, and Carolina pink to cleanse the system of any worms, parasites, or infestations. Sometimes called pinkroot or evening trumpet flower, this plant is a member of the Logania family and native to the Carolinas.

Carrot *(Daucus sativus)*. Carrot plants have roots in various shapes and colors that were used as natural energy bars (especially for those with hypoglycemia), chronic diarrhea bouts, and as a "cleanser" for the intestinal tract. Carrot was included in tonic formulas and was cooked with other plants and fed to infants and children with diarrhea. Raw carrots are used today for developing the strength of ballplayers and competitors. Carrots are high in pectin fiber.

Castor mole bean _(Ricinus communis)_. This plant was mentioned by an elder as a gift from the Iroquois, used to purge the body. It was used in the "black drink" for ceremonial purposes. The seeds were crushed for the oil and used along with anise to rid dogs of worms. The elder said the preparation "was too strong for humans." Another elder said that castor oil was combined in small quantity with giant ragweed _(Ambrosia trifida)_ as a worm formula. Today it is used for treating bowel problems and intestinal worms.

Catnip _(Nepeta cataria)_. Catnip leaves were used for relieving intestinal cramps or infant colic, and possibly for treating gas pains in elders. Catnip is often used with boneset for treating colds and fevers, but also for "fevers caused by an imbalanced system." It was also mixed with other herbs and used as a formula for female Medicine as an antispasmodic or for calming nerves, especially during the menses. It was also combined with maypop, or passionflower _(Passiflora incarnata)_, for addressing internal inflammation, fever, and liver problems. Today catnip is used for treating diarrhea, indigestion, and gas.

Cedar tree _(Thuja occidentalis)_. Called arbor vitae or Eastern white cedar, the leaves of this gift from the Iroquois Indians are prepared as a drink for treating gout. Cedar is a member of the cypress family. There is an Eastern red cedar, or red juniper _(Juniperus virginiana)_, that is used in ceremonies. Do not use cedar during pregnancy.

Celery _(Apium graveolens)_. The plant stalks and seeds of celery were an only remedy for ridding the system of uric acid in the joints "that cause pain of gout." It was also used in an arthritis formula, as well as for lowering blood pressure. Dr. James Duke mentions the anti-inflammatory properties of celery and recommends that adults eat at least four celery stalks daily to lower cholesterol in the blood. Do not use celery therapeutically during pregnancy.

Cherokee rose _(Rosa palustris)_. Cherokee, or wild, rose was mentioned by Mary Chiltoskey for treating diarrhea and to expel worms from children. The roots were boiled for treating diarrhea as a very old remedy. A more recent formula used wild rose for treating inflammation in a mouth gargle with wild cherry bark for healing sore throats. It was also used for treating children with fever and "for cooling, to dispel the cause of the fever's influence." The child would be sprayed by using a wooden straw with a cool water "mix of Cherokee rose" and other plants.

Chickweed _(Stellaria media)_. The Cherokee enjoyed this little plant, found in fields and pastures. A formula of chickweed and corn silk was used to control appetite. The most common use was in an antitussive formula for treating coughs and as a "blood cleanser" for addressing a cut, along with gingerroot. Chickweed is a member of the Pink, or Carnation, family. Today it is used for treating stomach ulcers and obesity.

Chicory (*Cichorium intybus*). Chicory was used for "soreness internally, and with digestive problems." The plant has beautiful blue flowers and is found in the open fields. Chicory is a member of the Aster, or Composite, family. Today it is used for treating constipation and as a diuretic for addressing fluid retention.

Cinquefoil (*Pontentilla simplex*). A tea of cinquefoil, or five-finger, was used for its astringent properties in treating dysentery and other, more serious, internal diseases. The roots and leaves were used to treat inflammation of the digestive tract, especially when there was bleeding and severe diarrhea. Cinquefoil is used today as an antispasmodic and an astringent.

Cleavers (see Bedstraw).

Colic root (*Aletris farinosa*). The rootstock of colic root, or stargrass, was gathered and dried for use as a tonic or tea for indigestion and colic, especially for children who experienced "the pains of gas." It was also called love plant in the East Medicine and was referred to by mountain folks as "blazing star" and "devil's bit." Asafoetida is also called colic root.

Colic weed (see Lion's foot).

Columbine (*Aquilegia vulgaris* or *A. canadensis*). Wild columbine is an astringent and diuretic; the root is used to treat diarrhea. The Creek used wild columbine in a formula as a salve for mouth sores. It was used for addressing a variety of internal ailments, including liver and abdominal complaints, and was used as a sedative. The name comes from the Latin *columba,* which means "dove." The petals and flowers remind us of the shape of a dove. My grandmother Edna Rogers called columbine "jacket." The flowers have long, drooping, colorful petals that attract hummingbirds to the nectar. This member of the Buttercup family was also considered a "love Medicine" by some earlier Indian tribes.

Comfrey (*Symphytum officinale*). A Cherokee formula uses common comfrey, burdock, and yellow dock as a powerful ulcer healer. Called *oo ste e oo ste* in Cherokee, comfrey was combined with dandelion and chicory roots to make a coffeelike drink that was enjoyed by mountain folks and Indians alike during the Depression. Today comfrey is used for treating ulcers of the bowel, stomach, liver, and gallbladder. It is recommend that comfrey not be taken internally because of alkaloids that have been shown to cause cancer when ingested in large quantities. Note the comments made about comfrey in the East Medicine section of the book.

Do not use comfrey during pregnancy or while nursing. Warnings from the U.S. Food and Drug Administration and the American Herb Products Association warns agains taking comfrey internally due to plant alkaloids that can cause liver damage.

Corn (Zea mays). Indian corn, maize, or *se lu* as it is known in Cherokee, is a staple food for the Cherokee, as well as for many Mexican and South American Indian tribes. *Se lu* was used as a diuretic and for treating urinary problems. There was a formula for treating kidney and bladder problems using cornsilk. "A small amount of the silk tuft at the tip of the ear of corn would be put in a mason jar in the sun for up to several hours, then mixed with a cup of boiled water and some mint for urinary problems." The corn silk was also combined with richweed *(Pilea pumila)* for a natural appetite depressant. This remedy was used for overweight children to reduce excessive hunger.

The corn silk are the silky strands surrounding the corn cob. These are actually stigmas and styles that contain the insoluable sugars, potassium, and flavonoids, and (very little) volatile oil. The fresh, cleaned silk was used as a diuretic. It is also a mild antiseptic, which means it is good for calming the urinary tract. It was used with thyme and peppermint, especially for Indian children with active bladders, and for bedwetters among the mountain folks' children. Indian corn was used in Cherokee ceremonies and the special rituals of many other tribes.

Couchgrass (Agropyron repens). It is unclear if use of this grassy weed as a remedy came from American Indians or was brought over from Europe with the mountain folks who settled here. Also called witchgrass, couchgrass was used for treating bladder and kidney stones and as a diuretic. This use was verified by James Duke, Ph.D. Couchgrass was included in a spring tonic with sassafras and chamomile. A tea would be made for gout. Mountain folks used witchgrass with witch hobble *(Viburnum lantanoides)* to "keep the spirits of the witches away." An elder said that couchgrass was used with knotgrass *(Polygonum aviculare)* and several barks and plants as a formula "for the internals, and breathing for the wind," or for bladder, kidney, and intestinal problems, and for the lungs. Couchgrass has a spreading root that is very difficult to get rid of in a yard or garden.

Cowslip (Caltha palustris). Also known as marsh marigold, cowslip was used as an antispasmodic. This is one plant that was used by itself, rather than being used in a formula. For that reason I suspect it was a latecomer to North America. Today it is used to treat physical anxiety and irritability. A different plant called cowslip, primrose *(Primula officinalis)*, was used for treating rheumatism, as well as for dressing wounds and assisting with birthing in earlier years.

Cramproot (see Asafoetida).

Cranberry *(Vaccinium vitis)*. Commonly called mountain cranberry, this plant is not the same as American cranberry *(V. macrocarpon)*. The leaves are a natural antiseptic and diuretic. This herb would be received in trade from our Indian brothers from the north and Canada.

Cranberry juice was used in earlier years as a blood purifier. It is one of the mountain favorites for treating many ailments, including kidney and urinary problems. It is also used as a tonic with other plants for treating asthma. It is one of my grandmother's favorites, along with carrots and whatever was fresh, such as cucumbers, for treating respiratory conditions such as asthma and complaints of gastrointestinal upset. Cranberry prevents bacteria from adhering to the bladder lining. It has preventive anti-infection and anti-inflammatory value when consumed daily because of proanthocyanidins, compounds that prevent *E. coli* bacteria from affecting the urinary tract.

Cucumber *(Cucumis sativus)*. The entire fruit of the cucumber was used for bladder and kidney complaints. It is a natural diuretic, sometimes mixed with carrot or Queen Anne's lace. Today cucumber is used as a diuretic for addressing fluid retention.

Culver's root (see Blackroot).

Daisy fleabane *(Erigeron philadelphicus)*. Daisy fleabane was used for treating gout and kidney problems. It was used in several old formulas as a diuretic. An elder said, "The flowers are like white strings stretching out in a circle with a daisy yellow center. They drive the fleas away." My grandmother Flora Garrett-Watson called this plant "morning bride." She also liked growing daisy fleabane, especially *Erigeron speciosus*, in her flower garden. The purplish flowers have a bright yellow center. This member of the Aster family is a perennial that likes moist, well-drained soil and full sunshine.

Dandelion *(Taraxacum officinale)*. While often considered a pest in the lawns and gardens of today, dandelion has always been a powerful medicinal plant used by American Indians. Also known as yellow flower, the leaves of the dandelion plant were used in a tea as a tonic, and the flowers were used as dye (and wine by the mountain folks). The leaf tea was also a diuretic and was a helper to the liver in that it seemed to enhance the flow of bile. Dandelion stimulates the metabolism and helps in the healing of biliary problems.

An elder remembered dandelion being used for gout and rheumatism. The leaves contain high amounts of vitamins and minerals, particularly as a source of vitamin A. The leaves are used along with other greens as a spring salad. Today dandelion is recognized for treatment of jaundice, gallstones, hepatitis, bile duct inflammation, and liver congestion. It is used to relieve constipation and digestive complaints and as a diuretic for addressing fluid retention, gallbladder and liver disorders, and obesity, and to stimulate bile production. An elder from Arkansas called it "'yellow drifter plant,' 'cause the bristles would push the seeds in the air for the wind to carry it anywhere." Recent studies recognize dandelion as cleansing and strengthening for the liver and gallbladder. Dandelion contains vitamins A and C and potassium. It can be taken long-term.

Devil's bit (see Fairywand).

Devil's shoestring (*Tephrosia virginiana*). Devil's shoestring is also known as goat's rue or rabbit pea. Called *a su ah s gi*, or "fishing plant," by the earlier Cherokee, it was used as a wash to condition and strengthen hair. It was also used by the ballplayers as a rub on arms and legs to "toughen them." A tea was given to a child to make the child strong. It was also used in a formula for treating kidney or urinary problems and to expel intestinal worms, according to Mary Chiltoskey. This was one of those plants considered to be "a man's plant. Creek Medicine men used it with sassafras for weakness." I think the weakness referred to was the bladder. One elder said it was used for "good fishing."

Dock (see Sorrel and Yellowdock).

Dogtooth violet (see Adder's tongue).

Dogwood tree (*Cornus florida*). The flowering dogwood, or *ka nah si ta*, with its unique cream white flowers with notched petals, is a very distinctive tree. It was used by the Cherokee as an appetite stimulant, particularly for the elderly. The inner bark was used for reducing fevers. Uncle Grady remembered dogwood being used for making weaving shuttles and mallet heads by settlers in the mountains. A red dye was used from the roots.

Dutchman's pipe (*Aristolochia macrophylla*). A very old root remedy was used for treating swelling of the feet and legs. Dutchman's pipe is a climbing vine with heart-shaped leaves and a flower that has the shape of a Dutchman's long, swirling pipe. An old formula includes elecampane with dutchman's pipe for treating urinary inflammation.

Dwarf iris (*Iris cristata*). An old formula for treating hepatitis and urinary complaints included dwarf iris and several other plants and barks.

Eastern hemlock (*Tsuga canadensis* and *T. caroliniana*). The inner bark of young Eastern hemlock and Carolina hemlock trees were used to treat kidney ailments and diarrhea. An elder said that hemlock was used in an old formula with other plant diuretics for treating kidney ailments. The inner bark has anti-inflammatory and astringent properties. It is my understanding that the plant was not collected until about 1850 and was finally named in 1881. Today Eastern hemlock is pruned and shaped as an ornamental plant.

Echinacea (see Purple coneflower).

Elder *(Sambucus canadensis)*. The inner bark of American elder was used in several formulas "to kill the pain of something going on inside." It was combined with rabbit tobacco or plantain-leaved everlasting *(Antennaria plantaginifolia)* for bowel and intestinal problems. Spanish needles *(Bidens bipinnata)* was added to make a drink for getting rid of worms in children. Elder is a large shrub or small tree that is common in the eastern half of the United States. Mountain folks have enjoyed elderberry jellies, preserves, and wine since settling here. Elderberry pie, as an elder said, "is the way to die." My grandfather made popguns and whistles from the stems of elder by removing the pith and using his woodworking skills to gift us with toys we all enjoyed.

Evening primrose *(Oenothera biennis)*. The Cherokee found *hu tsi lah ha,* or "flower" helpful in treating gastrointestinal problems and diabetes. High in gamma-linolenic acid (GLA), the oil is used for reducing blood pressure. Evening primrose was used in many formulas for protection and prevention in earlier years. Catawba and Creek Indian remedies combined it with yucca for addressing pain and inflammation, sometimes with meadowsweet.

As one elder said, "There is much more to this plant that will be discovered in the future. It is one of the Great One's special gifts." This is one of those must-have plants in your herbal and flower gardens.

Fairywand *(Chamaelirium luteum)*. Fairywand was also called devil's bit or blazing star. While popular for addressing female health issues, it was used for those elders with poor appetites and those who were "just feeling down." The male flowers are white, while the female flowers are green. Earlier Cherokee used the white flower plant roots for rattlesnake or copperhead bites, along with horehound. The green and white flower plants were used as a diuretic for addressing female health issues and for urinary tract pain. Fairywand was noted by William Bartram during his travels to the mountains of North Carolina. It should not be confused with devil's claw *(Harpagophytum procumbens)*, which is used for back pain.

False aloe *(Agave virginica)*. "A chew of the root is good for diarrhea when alumroot don't work." False aloe was mentioned by Paul Hamel and Mary Chiltoskey as being used for addressing liver complaints and expelling worms.

Fennel *(Foeniculum vulgare)*. Called common or wild fennel, this licorice-tasting plant was traded among the tribes and settlers in earlier American life. The Cherokee used it as an antispasmodic, ingesting the seeds for treating indigestion and cramps. It was used as an appetite depressant along with corn silk to "take a step away from food to make you feel good." It has antibacterial and anti-inflammatory properties but was used mostly with lemon balm for its calming action on the digestive system. It has also been found to contain phytoestrogens, which means that pregnant women should not use it.

Fennel is one of my favorite plant helpers for intestinal upset, as well as for improving the appetite. It is considered a heal-all for colds and bronchial problems. Fennel and peppermint made into a tea, with the addition of thyme, makes a calming and heal-all herbal remedy for general malaise.

Fern, bracken *(Pteridium aquilinum)*. This two-foot fern with large fronds has brown fruiting bodies under the surface of the fronds. It was used along with loblolly pine *(Pinus taeda)* to expel intestinal worms. It was also used to relieve stomach cramps and for treating kidney complaints. This is a member of the Polypodiaceae Fern family, along with maidenhair and Christmas fern.

Fern, female *(Polypodium vulgare)*. The Cherokee called female fern *a ge yu tsa,* or "girl fern." It was used for treating gout, constipation, and liver ailments. The creeping woodstock of female fern, or common polypody, has tannic acid used for "chronic constipation by steeping in hot, not boiling, water." An elder called this plant "feather fern."

Fern, male *(Dryopteris campyloptera)*. A tea called "mountain wood fern" was made of "this fern with several tree barks to expel worms." Earlier Cherokee called it *a tsu tsa,* or "boy fern." The old Cherokee name for the ferns was *u gi da li,* or "feather."

Feverwort (see Boneset).

Five-finger (see Cinquefoil and Ginseng).

Flax *(Linum usitatissimum)*. The entire flax plant is used as an antiseptic and anti-inflammatory. It is a mild laxative or "cleanser" for the system, especially used "with elders that need a cleaning and a picker-upper for their energy and spirit."

Frostweed *(Helianthemum canadense)*. An elder said that a leaf tea of frostweed or frostwort was used for treating kidney problems. This use was also mentioned by Paul Hamel and Mary Chiltoskey. An elder said this plant was a sunflower with crystals that appear on the stem in the late fall, making it look like winter.

Galax (*Galax aphylla*). Galax was mentioned by Paul Hamel and Mary Chiltoskey for treating kidney problems and as a tea for the nerves. The leaves turn a golden red color in the winter. The white flowers with broad, round, shiny leaves are on a long stem, similar to fairywand or black co-hosh. An elder said galax was used "to calm the entire system, especially where ailments include the urinaries and kidneys, and was used with blue devil."

Gall-of-the-earth (*Prenanthes trifolilata*). Gall-of-the-earth was used for the "aching stomachs of children." It was also mentioned by Paul Hamel and Mary Chiltoskey for this use, as well as being used in fresh salad. Other names for gall-of-the-earth included cancer weed and canker root, names that describe other uses for the plant.

Garlic (*Allium sativum*). A member of the Lily family, the Cherokee used garlic for getting rid of parasites and intestinal worms in children. Garlic is a good antispasmodic and is used as a "heal-all" in formulas for treating heart irregularities and respiratory problems, particularly among the elderly. Its value as a helper is to maintain healthy cholesterol levels and good cardiac and circulatory functioning. Today garlic is used for treating constipation, bacterial infections, and diabetes, and some still use it to ward off evil spirits that influence the physical body.

Gentian (*Gentiana lutea*). Also called yellow gentian, this plant has been valued in the mountains as "nature's digestive aide [besides wild ginger]." It was also used with elders to increase appetite. According to Vogel, the Catawba used gentian roots to treat stomach pains.

It is used with goldenseal and ginger to "strengthen and protect the entire digestive system from disease and upset ailments." Mountain gentian (*Gentiana decora*) was also combined in the formula to aid digestion. Bees work to pry open the cluster of flowers for food and pollination.

Ginger (*Zingiber officinale*). The primary use of ginger by the Cherokee is as a carminative or digestive aid. In earlier years it was also used as a stimulant and a tonic. Today it is used as a stimulant and a diuretic. Most people probably know ginger as a culinary herb and a remedy for motion sickness, but it is a powerful medicine in other ways. Ginger was used in several formulas that were referred to as "heal-all." It was used instead of capsicum for system cleansing by the Cherokee in sweats and other ceremonies. It was used in a formula for easing the pain and swelling of arthritis. Today it is used for treating bacterial infections and digestive problems.

This ginger is not to be confused with wild ginger (*Asarum canadense*), sometimes called black snakeroot, colic root, or Indian ginger. *Asarum* gingers were used to treat irregular heartbeat and for general pain relief.

Ginseng *(Panax ginseng).* Various ginseng plants are used by many cultures. Ginseng was a "cure-all" for the Cherokee, especially for stimulating the appetite of the elderly and of tribal members who had severe cold, flu, or infections. Some Medicine men and women would chew the root and blow through a wooden tube on the area of pain. Today it is known as an immune stimulant and adaptogen, to help the body deal with stress. It is not recommended for people with high blood pressure and heart palpitations. Ginseng is recognized for its use as a diuretic in remedying fluid retention, treating diabetes and liver problems, boosting the appetite, enhancing physical performance, and resisting stress. It takes about seven years for ginseng to mature; digging the "sang" too early takes a gift from nature before its time. So many plants have been lost that it is discouraging to go picture hunting for ginseng in the mountains today.

Goat's beard *(Aruncus dioicus).* A tea of goat's beard is made to treat excessive urination. The yellowish white clusters of "strings flowing in the breeze" are seen in May and June in Appalachia. An elder said that he does not see as much of the plant as when he was a small boy. Another plant called goat's beard is also known as meadow salsify *(Tragopogon pratensis);* my grandmother Flora Garrett called that plant "go-to-bed-at-noon" because the flower closes during the day. *Tragopogon dubius* is similarly known as goat's beard.

Goat's rue (see Devil's shoestring).

Goldenrod *(Solidago odora).* Goldenrod tea, made from the leaves of the plant, was used by the Cherokee for treating intestinal gas and for fevers. The flowers were used as a dye by mountain folks. While probably not valuable for reducing fevers, goldenrod has been validated as a carminative for treating intestinal gas. Today it is used for treating bladder stones, exhaustion, and fatigue and as a diuretic to treat fluid retention, kidney and intestinal inflammation, and kidney stones.

Goldenseal *(Hydrastis canadensis).* Goldenseal was also called yellowroot and Indian paint. It grows to about a foot in height and has seven lobed leaves at the apex. It has a green-to-white flower at the top of the leaves with no petals. It was used to treat mouth ulcers and as an astringent.

Goldenseal is considered a "heal-all" plant; it aids circulation, reduces internal bleeding, aids in digestion, is effective on the mucous membranes, and is considered nature's antimicrobial. Mountain folks in Appalachia used a tea from the goldenseal roots as a general tonic. A natural antiseptic and anti-inflammatory, goldenseal is usually combined with plants of similar healing value, such as dandelion as a diuretic and goldenrod for addressing many internal ailments. Today goldenseal is used for improving appetite, relieving constipation and digestive disorders, and as a diuretic. Goldenseal is at risk in its natural environment. Like ginseng, it has been stripped from the mountains as a cash crop, an action that is quickly destroying this beauty of nature and this gift to the world from the Cherokee.

Gooseberry (Ribes rotundifolium). Gooseberry was used for treating bowel complaints and as a tea for nerves. There is little in the herbal literature on this plant. Thanks to Paul Hamel and Mary Chiltoskey, at least this much information has not been lost.

Grape, fox (Vitis labrusca). A tea made from the leaves of the fox grape is used for treating liver problems, as well as for diarrhea. *Vitis vinifera* has been mentioned in the herbal literature for use as an anti-inflammatory and for improved circulation. Grapeseed extract has become popular due to a chemical compound called pycogenol, also found in pine bark. It strengthens blood vessels and can reduce the risk of heart attack. Its use is suggested for treating inflammation, cancer, and varicose veins and for improving circulation.

Harebell, southern (Campanula divaricata). A tea made from the roots of southern harebell was used for treating diarrhea. Most commonly seen at lower elevations in the Eastern mountains, the small blue flower of this plant hangs like a bell.

Campanula glomerata, or clustered bellflower, a hardy plant with purple to violet flower clusters, is a good plant for the home flower garden.

Hawkweed (Hieracium venosum or H. pratense). Known as rabbit's ear, hawkweed was used for addressing bowel complaints. These yellow flowers are common in the Appalachian Mountains and along the roadsides in the Great Smoky Mountains. Other names include "rattlesnake weed," "hawkbit," "adder's tongue," "smoke plantain," and "bloodwort," all names used by mountain folks in North Carolina, Tennessee, and West Virginia for the plant the Cherokee called hawkweed.

Heal-all (Prunella vulgaris). The roots of heal-all were used in a tea for diarrhea; there were several formulas for this use. Heal-all was also called self-heal and woundwort. As the name implies, it was used in many formulas for internal healing. Today it is used for treating diarrhea, hemorrhage, hepatitis, intestinal gas, stomach upset, and related pains.

Heartleaf (Hexastylis virginica). A drink made of heartleaf was used in earlier years to stop internal bleeding.

Hearts-a-bustin' shrub *(Euonymus americanus)*. Also known as strawberry bush, hearts-a-bustin' was used for treating "the problems of spitting blood," urinary problems, and stomachache. The special story of how this shrub earned its name (see chapter 3) gives this plant special significance regarding the connection of plants to our lives, not just as herbal helpers but as helpers of the spirit. Another plant called strawberry bush is wahoo *(E. atropurpureus)*, a shrub or small tree native to the eastern United States.

Hepatica *(Hepatica acutiloba* and *H. nobilis)*. Hepatica was called liverwort and sharp-lobed liverleaf. It was used for the digestive system, as a laxative, and to improve the liver. It was even suggested for treating swollen breasts.

Hepatica is a member of the Buttercup family. It contains an irritant that is poisonous to the central nervous system; the irritant is eliminated by drying the plant. As an astringent, it was considered a good helper in earlier years for gallbladder and liver ailments. Do not use hepatica during pregnancy.

Hog peanut *(Amphicaapa bracteata)*. A tea of hog peanut root was used for treating diarrhea. Hog peanut is a member of the Pea, or Bean, family. It was used as a food as much as for Medicine. The plant was also called American licorice and wild peanut.

Hops *(Humulus lupulus)*. A tea of common hops or hop vine was used for treating kidney and urinary problems and pain. According to an elder, "The entire plant was crushed between two rocks and put into water, heated, and used for the restless physical spirit of a person going through stuff." It is a sedative that can be used as an antispasmodic and for nervous conditions.

Horehound *(Marrubium vulgare)*. The bark of white horehound was used as a tonic. The plant was used a mild laxative and for kidney complaints and was also used as a stimulant. It is a member of the Mint family. An earlier use for horehound was providing strength after an illness. Black horehound *(Ballota nigra)* is the plant used for treating nausea and motion sickness.

Hornbeam (see Ironwood shrub).

Horse balm (see Stone root).

Horse chestnut tree *(Aesculus hippocastanum)*. The inner bark of horse chestnut tree was used to improve bloodflow. The leaves and seeds can be poisonous, but roasting the seeds destroys the poison. This plant is worth looking in to for problems affecting the veins and arteries.

Horseradish *(Amoracia rusticana)*. Horseradish was used as a diuretic and to increase appetite. It was used with ginger to "improve digestion of the elders" and combined with honey for children with colds. An elder said the roots were good for treating infections in the kidney and bladder. Horseradish is a member of the Cruciferae, or Mustard, family.

Horsetail *(Equisetum hyemale* or *E. arvense)*. Horsetail, a plant also known as shave grass, was used as a diuretic; for treating gout it was prepared as a tea with mint. An elder mentioned the use of horsetail in earlier years with broadleaf plantain to stop bleeding. Horsetail was well respected in earlier years as a conditioner for the hair and for dry skin. It is used for bronchitis and pulmonary problems. Earlier Cherokee used horsetail for "keeping the hair young and the kidneys clear by using the fresh plant in a formula with goldenseal."

Huckleberry *(Gaylussacia dumosa* and *G. frondosa)*. Huckleberry, or *ka wa ya* as the Cherokee called it, was used in a formula for diabetes by the southeastern tribes. Sometimes bitter weed and calamus were used as well in an anti-diabetic formula with bilberry or blueberry *(Vaccinium myrtillus,* also called huckleberry). *Gaylussacia frondosa* was used as an astringent and an antidiarrheal.

Indian corn (see Corn).

Indian paint (see Bloodroot).

Indian physic *(Gillenia trifoliata)*. Indian physic, also known as bowman's root, grows along the roadsides in the mountains. It reaches about four feet in height and has narrow white petals. Indian physic was used in earlier years as an emetic to induce vomiting. It is still used for treating chronic diarrhea and as a blood purifier. An elder said that *oo la oo ya te,* or Indian physic, was used in cleansing the liver. Ipecac *(Cephaelis ipecacuanha)* was used in combination with Indian physic to induce vomiting to kill amoebas or intestinal parasites. In earlier years Indian physic and elecampane would have probably been the choice for ridding the body of parasites. Such a formula would have also included a plant such as goldenseal for use with children.

Indian pipe *(Monotropa uniflora)*. This plant was considered "special Medicine" for children. The roots were used for treating convulsions and "fits." It was also used as a North Medicine for treating sore eyes, as a South Medicine for treating polyps and other skin growths, and with a prayer-chant to the direction of the West. This unusual white plant earns the name ghost plant because it lives off other plants. It grows about seven inches high in the dense woods.

Indian root *(Aralia racemosa)*. Also called American spikenard and Hercules' club, Indian root was used as a tea for treating aches internally and was also used externally with willow or dogwood bark. A formula included this root in a tonic for gout and as a stimulant to increase perspiration. The old formulas used it for "blood poisoning," as a poultice for sores, and in a cough remedy. Do not use during pregnancy.

Indian sage (see Boneset).

Indian tobacco (see Lobelia).

Ironwood shrub *(Carpinus caroliniana)*. The bark of ironwood, or American hornbeam, was used as an astringent for "flux," or diarrhea, and urinary problems. Another plant called ironweed, *Vernonia noveboracensis,* was used by the Seneca Indians and Indians in Kentucky for increasing perspiration in traditional sweats and for cooling a fever. An elder referred to hornbeam as "a flyer, 'cause the seeds move through the sky like a dragonfly." There is also a tree called ironwood, or Eastern hophornbeam *(Ostrya virginiana),* that was used as a laxative in earlier years.

Jack-in-the-pulpit *(Arisaema triphyllum)*. The fresh bulb or corm of Jack-in-the-pulpit, also called Indian turnip, was dried to eliminate a caustic substance contained in the fresh bulb and then used for treating stomach problems. It was also mixed with wood ashes and used as a natural insecticide in the planting field, especially around beans and tender tomato plants.

Jack-in-the-pulpit grows in the home garden where the soil is humus-rich and moist. Children and adults both enjoy the unique flower, with its hood in the summer and bright red berries in the early fall. Jack-in-the-pulpit can take several years to bloom, but it really has no insect or disease pests.

Joe-pye weed *(Eupatorium purpureum)*. Joe-pye weed, also called gravel root, was a favorite in earlier years among mountain folks and American Indians for treating urinary tract problems. Joe-pye weed was used as a diuretic, a stimulant, an astringent, and a tonic. The Cherokee Medicine men and women that I worked with mentioned the plant, but they did not use it very much. They did point out the vanilla-like smell and its use as a diuretic and astringent for female menstrual pain and associated problems. Mountain folks called this plant "queen of the meadow." The large clusters of pink to purple flowers stand about twelve feet tall in moist areas.

Juniper tree *(Juniperus communis)*. Common juniper, or dwarf juniper, was used as a diuretic and "to calm the gut." Its use has been almost forgotten by the Cherokee, except for the berries and twigs being used in one formula as a "blood tonic." Juniper contains a volatile oil valid for use as a diuretic and treatment of conditions of the kidney and bladder and for its carminative action in calming indigestion and flatulence. The berries are also used as an antiseptic for the urinary tract and a uterine stimulant. Juniper also has antiviral compounds that are effective in treating flu and herpes. Juniper is a member of the Cypress family.

Kelp *(Laminaria digitata).* Several of nature's gifts were traded between American Indians who lived in the mountains and those who lived by the coast. A special gift from the coastal Indians was kelp and ground shells, health-bringing now, we know, for their calcium and mineral contents. It is uncertain how kelp was used, because it was not mentioned in any of the Cherokee formulas. I suspect it was used to treat rheumatism. Today a derivative from kelp called algin is used in cosmetics and foods. Algin soothes mucous membranes, such as are found in the respiratory tract. Kelp is used as an iodine source and to treat obesity. Kelp and young barley shoots have been added to a formula that was considered sacred but has been lost with time.

Knotweed *(Polygonum aviculare).* Often called knotgrass or birdgrass, this plant was used for treating diarrhea. An astringent, it is especially useful for treating internal bleeding in a formula with yellowroot. This member of the Smartweed, or Buckwheat, family likely got its name from its characteristically knotted stems and leaves. While considered a weed, it does attract beneficial insects that eat aphids and mites. I call this plant "Joi dock" after my niece who, like knotweed, is hardy and has abilities yet to be discovered.

Lady's slipper *(Cypripedium calceolus).* Lady's slipper, also called moccasin flower and known to the Cherokee as *oo ka ou la su lo,* or "nerve root," was used in a formula for treating intestinal worms in children and elders in earlier years. Only trained Medicine people would use this plant, which was also "used as a way to calm the body down and for nerve problems that made people jumpy." Lady's slipper is a mild sedative that is used for treating epilepsy, headaches, and nervousness.

Lamb's quarters *(Chenopodium album).* Lamb's quarters was popular with American Indians and with mountain folks in the Appalachian region. It was nature's "over-the-counter" laxative, using the entire plant at full bloom, the leaves when mature, and the seed in the summer. Lamb's quarters is an edible plant that can be put in salads. It is a member of the Goosefoot family.

Licorice *(Glycyrrhiza lepidota).* Called American licorice, this herb was popular with American Indians for treating digestive problems and gastritis; the formula would include goldenseal. Licorice can raise blood pressure and heart rate. It was used for treating liver conditions related to cirrhosis and chronic hepatitis, as well as gout. In 1980 a group of researchers from Japan visited the Cherokee Reservation to find out more about licorice. The way the Chinese described using the plant was very similar to the Cherokee uses.

Lily, Turk's cap *(Lilium canadense)*. The roots of Turk's cap lily were used for treating dysentery and "bloody flux." The mountain folks called this plant with its beautiful spotted orange petals that were stacked several levels high "superbum." Turk's cap lily is unlike the Carolina lily *(L. michauxii)*, on which the flowers sit atop the stem. Turk's cap lily was combined with St. Andrew's cross *(Hypericum hypericoides)* for treating internal bleeding and bowel complaints. Lilies were traded by the southeastern tribes in earlier years. These gifts from Mother Nature included the pot-of-gold lily *(L. iridollae)* and Michaux's lily *(L.michauxii)*, which were traded with the Catawba and the tribe now called the Lumbee, according to an elder.

Lion's foot *(Prenanthes serpentaria)*. Sometimes called colic weed or snakeroot, the roots of lion's foot were used for treating children and adults with stomachache. This is plant information that would have been lost, but thanks to Paul Hamel and Mary Chiltoskey I was able to verify this use with an elder, who also said the plant was called cancer weed or canker weed by mountain folks.

Lobelia *(Lobelia spicata* and *L. inflata)*. Called pale spike lobelia, this plant was mentioned by Paul Hamel and Mary Chiltoskey as used in a Medicine for treating tremors and arm shakes. Indian tobacco *(L. inflata)* was used when the plant was mature and as the leaves were turning yellow, as an emetic to purge the system. It was also mentioned by an elder from Oklahoma as being used for treating croup and asthma.

Loosestrife *(Lysimachia vulgaris)*. Loosestrife was used for treating kidney problems. Hamel and Chiltoskey listed whorled loosestrife *(Lysimachia quadrifolia)* as a plant that was used for treating kidney complaints. Loosestrife is an anti-inflammatory and an astringent. Purple loosestrife *(Lythrum salicaria)* or various species would be added as an antibiotic for intestinal tract ailments or "mixed with other plant roots and barks for kidney and bowel complaints," according to an elder Medicine man. Whorled loosestrife *(L. quadrifolia)* was sometimes added for bowel and kidney problems, especially for females. Loosestrife can be found along the Blue Ridge Parkway.

Lousewort *(Pedicularis canadensis)*. This plant was used for treating bloody discharge and stomach problems. It was also called wood betony, which should not be confused with another wood betony, *Stachys officinalis,* that is used for expelling worms and for kidney problems.

Maple tree *(Acer rubrum).* Many Indian tribes used the bark of red maple in their formulas for treatment of worms. It is also used in a tonic by some Cherokee. It would be mixed with bark from the mountain maple *(Acer spicatum)* in a formula for ridding the body of intestinal worms. It was said to stimulate the appetite in elders as well. Fraser fir *(Abies fraseri)* is also used in the "worm remedy" with coralbead *(Erythrina herbacea)* using the roots, and the seeds when the plant is in bloom. The formula was used to expel the worms from the intestinal tract. There are several varieties of maple in the Smoky Mountains and along the Blue Ridge Parkway. An elder said, "Maple is Medicine for the spirit." Unfortunately I was not able to learn all the uses of other maples, such as mountain maple and one of my favorites as a youngster roaming the mountains, goosefoot or striped maple *(A. pensylvanicum).* The name goosefoot comes from the web-foot shape of the leaves; the same tree was also called Pennsylvania maple. The Cherokee name for maple is *tsv wa gi.* Maple was one of the council-fire woods used in earlier days.

Maple-leaved viburnum *(Viburnum acerifolium).* Maple-leaved viburnum was used for treating a variety of internal conditions, for easing cramps, and for cleansing the system. It was also reported to be used as a tonic. It was difficult for me to find anyone who used it, but I was able to verify that it was used for treating cramps.

Marsh marigold (see Cowslip).

Maryland sanicle (see Snakeroot, black).

Mayapple *(Podophyllum peltatum).* Called Indian apple and known as mandrake, *oo ne ski u ke* has a large leaf and a single white flower. An elder said, "Don't touch the leaves with your bare hands because they are poisonous, but the fruit is good. What you want are the roots. You learn to use a wood spatulalike piece made of laurel to dig with, then you dry and crush it to make Medicine. It was used in the old days to purge the body of what ails you." The elder said that "women prefer it for their own use and for the children, roasted, and even use it on difficult sores to heal."

Meadow rue *(Thalictrum dioicum* and *T. pubescens).* Also called crowfoot, this small meadow plant was used in earlier years as a natural diuretic and for "cleansing the entire system." Common rue *(Ruta graveolens)* roots and leaves were used for treating worms in children, as well as for treating diarrhea. There are several species of rue in the Buttercup family, which are called by many names in Appalachia; they are used for purposes similar to those described above.

Meadowsweet *(Filipendula ulmaria)*. The roots and flowers of mead-owsweet were dried and used in the winter months in the Smoky and Appalachian Mountains. It was used for treating cough and fevers related to colds and bronchitis. Meadowsweet contains salicylate, the active agent for pain relief in aspirin, as well as being a diuretic.

An elder said, "Remember the meadowsweet flowers. It is a gift from the Great One for healing to look at and to use internally. Maybe we should have called it 'thank-you-for-healing plant,' or just give thanks every time we see it or use it for Medicine." This same elder would say "thank you, Grandmother" every time we saw a large sunflower.

Milk thistle *(Silybum marianum)*. Growing to about six feet with prickly leaves, this bothersome plant is good for treating appetite and digestion. The milk found in the stalk was used in salads and cooking. The fruit of the milk thistle is a source of silymarin, which is a liver-regenerating compound used in the treatment of hepatitis and cirrhosis of the liver. The seeds are used today for cellular repair with degenerative conditions of the liver, along with dandelion and gentian *(Gentiana lutea)*. Milk thistle is used today for treating hepatitis C, boosting liver function, and in an herbal cleanser. Milk thistle helps protect and renew liver cells. Its value in being a helper to the liver, which is one of the body's largest organs with many functions, cannot be overemphasized.

Milkweed *(Asclepias syriaca)*. Also referred to as common milkweed or cottonweed, this plant was used by the southeastern Indians as a laxative and to induce vomiting. It is a unique plant, with its four leaves midway down the stem and small white flowers in a cluster at the top of the stem. Milkweed is sometimes considered a bothersome weed, but it does attract beneficial insects.

Mouse ear *(Gnaphalium uliginosum* or *Hieracium pilosella)*. This was a difficult plant to classify, so both Latin names are given here. Mouse ear is a small plant with upright flower stems that produce runners, like strawberry plants. The flowers, which grow in clusters, are white in color. Called *ga nu la hi,* or "weed," in Cherokee, mouse ear is found in fields and around rocks in the mountains.

The mouse ear plant was valued as an astringent for treating diarrhea. One elder said it was a gift from the Iroquois, who used it as "a throat gargle" and a diuretic. Mouse ear was combined with red mulberry *(Morus ruba)* for treating serious diarrhea and worms. It is a mountain remedy for bronchial problems and fever. Mouse ear is a member of the Aster, or Composite, family.

Mugwort (*Artemisia vulgaris*). Mugwort was also called white sage and wormwood. It was used for treating digestion and to improve the appetite of elders and as a mild sedative and diuretic. Mugwort is found along riverbanks and in fields; it has a greenish flower head along the stems. Mugwort is well known by most American Indians for its use in ceremonial sweats and for treating fevers and respiratory conditions. It is still used in Appalachia as a moth repellent, according to an elder from West Virginia.

Mulberry tree (*Morus rubra, M. alba,* and *M. nigra*). Red and white mulberry are used in a bark tea for treating internal bleeding at the intestinal tract. It is combined with other plants for treating pain, fever, and severe diarrhea. Mulberry was also used for purging intestinal worms and as a laxative by mixing a decoction from the pulverized bark with honey or molasses.

Nettle, stinging (*Urtica dioica*). Stinging nettle was mentioned for treating upset stomach. It was used for elders as a "special Medicine." The oldest formula I could find used the entire plant for treating rheumatism. In more recent years it is used for treating urinary inflammation. An elder said that a prick from a nettle can help with the pains of swollen joints. "The sting takes the pain away, similar to the way mountain folks use a yellow jacket." Today stinging nettle is used in treating osteoarthritis. It is said to inhibit the chemical pathway involving inflammation and thwarts chemical stimulation that causes inflammation. It is also used for treating urinary infections, bladder stones, and irritable bladder problems.

Oak tree (*Quercus alba* and other species). A juice from the inner bark of the oak tree was used for treating hemorrhoids and rectal bleeding and diarrhea. Oak was also valued as a general antiseptic and was used to fight bacterial infections in several formulas, including use for severe diarrhea and kidney and bladder problems. Today it is a popular antiseptic as well as an agent to fight bacterial and viral infections and diarrhea. The corn beater, or *ka no nah,* was made of oak in earlier years. Oak, or *a da ya hi,* was one of the council-fire woods used in earlier years for tribal gatherings. Other names of oak include white, chinkapin, Black Jack, red, chestnut, black, and post oak; all are members of the Beech family.

Oats (*Avena sativa*). The oats and the plant are used as an antispasmodic and to calm the nerves, especially for "those with a nervous stomach." Today it is used as a sedative, to treat gout, and to reduce blood sugar and insulin levels, as well as for lowering cholesterol.

Onion *(Allium cepa* and *A. cernuum)*. The bulb and the green stem of onion and nodding wild onion were used as an antiseptic for the intestinal tract. A poultice would be made for treating arthritic pain. Onions and garlic are used frequently in Cherokee cooking for taste and for Medicine. Nodding wild onion *(Allium cernuum)* is an especially good helper for the diabetic diet.

Papoose root (see Blue cohosh).

Parsley *(Petroselinum sativum)*. Parsley was used as a diuretic by the Cherokee. It was used by the mountain folks for treating kidney inflammation. It was also used for treating colic, gas, diarrhea, and indigestion.

Parsnip *(Pastinaca sativa)*. Parsnip was used in a formula for "the pain of insides." This root vegetable tastes something like a carrot. The roots were used for kidney ailments, but there is no verification of its effectiveness.

Partridgeberry *(Mitchella repens)*. Partridgeberry tea was used as a diuretic and as a blood tonic in earlier years. About partridgeberry an elder said, "It was a sweet that also did some good." It was used for complaints of the bowel, and diarrhea. Partridgeberry is also known as twinberry, checkerberry, and squaw vine. Know that the word *squaw* is offensive to American Indians.

Peach *(Prunus persica)*. Peach kernels were toasted for use in expelling intestinal worms. One elder remembered peach being used in this way, although he could not recall exactly how the kernels were prepared.

Pepper *(Capsicum annuum)*. Pepper, or cayenne, has been popular with the Cherokee since it was first introduced by the French as a trade item, according to elder Cherokee historian Carl Lambert. Pepper is popular for adding flavor to foods, as well as being used for its Medicine properties. As one elder said, "Pepper makes the heart strong for battle or for love. Either can get you killed these days, but the latter is safer and is also good for your heart!" Pepper was used as a circulatory stimulant and as a digestive aid, along with wild ginger.

Pepper bush *(Berberis canadensis)*. Also known as mountain sweet, the bark of pepper bush was used as a tea for treating diarrhea. It was used with yellow-eyed grass *(Xyris caroliniana)* and a mild plant such as mint, for calming. A cousin of the plant species is barberry *(B. vulgaris)*, which has been studied for its effectiveness in reducing blood pressure. Pepper bush was found to contain berberine, an alkaloid that stimulates this action. Pepper bush also stimulates bile excretion, reduces fever, stimulates intestinal peristalsis, and has an antibiotic effect.

Peppermint *(Mentha piperita* and *M. spicata)*. Peppermint and spearmint were used in many Cherokee formulas and were found in many Medicine bags. Peppermint in particular was carried during hunting and journeys as a stimulant and antispasmodic for treating indigestion, settling the nerves, and treating headaches. Peppermint is a "heal-all" plant used by many tribes. The value of the leaves are for aches and pains, gallstones, indigestion, and nausea. The oil is an antimicrobial substance with diuretic effects. It is also a mild sedative. Eastern tribes combine wild or marsh mint *(Mentha aquatica)* with peppermint in a tea for treating diarrhea. These same plants were used in the very old "Sun-drink" formula, which would sometimes be used with St. John's wort and yellowroot in ceremonies, but was also used for treating chronic intestinal upset. The formula was used for purging, to "rid the body of conjuring, influence, and worms." There is much more that has been lost about the Sun drink that somehow connects earlier Cherokee with other southern and Mexican Indian cultures.

Persimmon tree *(Diospyros virginiana)*. The bark of persimmon, or possumwood, was chewed for heartburn, a use that was confirmed by Mary Chiltoskey. Persimmon was used in cases where there was blood in the urine or "dark discharge from the bowels." It was also mentioned by an elder for "problems with gravel and bile, as well as for cleansing the liver." While I was not able to validate any of these uses, there is nothing in the resources reviewed that deny any of these uses. The formula, an "internal tonic Medicine," is an old one that includes tree barks such as walnut, wild black cherry, alder, as well as dandelion, and comfrey in more recent years. The persimmons were dried in the sun, similar to other wild fruits, beans, and corn. Persimmon is a member of the Ebony family.

Pine tree *(Pinus virginiana, P. sylvestries,* and other species). The inner bark of pine was used with balsam fir and alder for expelling intestinal worms and parasites. In earlier years pine was used as a stimulant and tonic, called *no te.* The needles and bark strips were used to make baskets, and the leftover bark would be saved and crushed for use in several formulas "of value for Medicine of the internals." There was mention of broadleaf plantain *(Plantago major)* and rattlesnake plantain *(Goodyera repens)* added to one formula with wild cherry, wild ginger, and twinleaf *(Jeffersonia diphylla)*. Red root *(Lachnanthes caroliniana)* was also used by some Medicine men and women. Pine bark was considered as a sacred West Medicine used in several formulas for healing of the physical and the spirit.

Piney weed *(Hypericum hypericoides* and *H. gentanoides)*. Sometimes called St. Andrew's cross, this plant was mentioned by Paul Hamel and Mary

Chiltoskey as being for "bloody flux" and bowel complaints. As a West Medicine, piney weed was considered to have "special abilities to give strength to ballplayers and runners." The elder said that Jim Thorp, the Indian Olympic distance runner, knew of its strength. Piney weed was used with St. John's wort, ginger, and ginseng.

Pipsissewa *(Chimaphila umbellata* and *C. maculata).* Called pip, this plant was popular with American Indians for treating stomach problems by using the leaves for a tea. It was used as a tonic to increase urine and for treating rheumatism and kidney problems. It is used as "high octane in the kidney formula." Today it is used for treating diarrhea and as a diuretic for relieving fluid retention. An antiseptic, pipsissewa is used in treating urinary ailments.

Pitcher plant *(Sarracenia purpurea).* The leaves and roots of the pitcher plant were used as an astringent and a tonic for the digestive system and for treating kidney problems. Also called Indian cup, an elder said that "you had to be trained on how to prepare and use the insect catching plant." This plant, found in the swamp areas of the eastern Carolinas, is indigenous to the United States.

Poke or pokeweed *(Phytolacca americana).* The root of pokeweed was used as a "blood purifier" by the Cherokee. One Medicine man used the leaves and the roots as a natural antibiotic, particularly in treating the kidneys. It was used for treating cancer, nervousness, fever, swelling, and sores. He said, "Pokeweed has many uses inside the body to get rid of toxins, but it must be the young plant." The plant becomes poisonous with maturity, and it can be extremely toxic if ingested.

Poor robin's plantain *(Erigeron pulchellus).* This plant was used as a diuretic and for kidney complaints. It was also called "frost root," and was mentioned by Paul Hamel and Mary Chiltoskey as an astringent for internal bleeding.

Poplar tree *(Liriodendron tulipifera).* The poplar, or tulip tree, was used in a formula for treating kidney problems. Poplar bark was used in an old formula, with dogwood bark as a stimulant.

Prickly ash *(Zanthoxylum americanum).* As a West Medicine the bark of prickly ash, or toothache tree, was used along with other plants and barks in an internal tonic formula. It was used to "improve circulation in earlier times" as an East Medicine. As a North Medicine it was chewed for toothaches. A salve of bear grease and prickly ash was used as a poultice for wounds and sores in earlier years, especially in treating boils; this was its use as a South Medicine. One elder said that a "pinch" of crushed or powdered willow bark was added for reducing pain. Another plant called prickly ash is devil's walkingstick *(Aralia spinosa)*. Today prickly ash is used to stimulate digestion and for treating intestinal gas.

Pumpkin *(Cucurbita pepo)*. The fruit of the pumpkin was a favorite with the Cherokee for pies and cooking. While traveling out West with the Indian Health Service I learned that the Yuma tribe used pumpkin seeds for wound healing. The Catawba ate the seeds for treating kidney problems. The Cherokee used the seeds as an anthelmintic, an antiparasitic that helps dispel intestinal worms and parasites from the body. The seeds were also used for intestinal and bladder complaints. It is not sure if the Cherokee learned this remedy from the mountain folks, or vice versa. Today pumpkin seeds are used for treating prostate problems and intestinal worms and parasites.

Purge root *(Ilex glabra)*. Called gall berry by some tribes, this evergreen was used as an emetic to induce vomiting. It was used by southeastern tribal Indians in the ceremonial "black drink" in earlier years. While little is known about the ceremony, I suspect the use was similar to the earlier Cherokee ceremonial sweats to purge the body for a "clearing-way" as part of the fasting process. This is a traditional American Indian way to "begin-again" in a physical and spiritual sense. Caution should be used, as the elder said, "to do things a proper way, building up to this ceremony, such as taking fluids to avoid dehydration, knowing what you are taking to avoid body stress with stimulants, and having enough experience to handle the heat temperatures in the sweat lodges." Proper training can lead to a wonderful experience with a cleansing feeling of this form of clearing-way and ceremony.

Purple coneflower *(Echinacea purpurea)*. In earlier years this plant was referred to as purple daisy and purple snakeroot. Today it is still called purple coneflower, but it is better known as echinacea. Purple coneflower's use in formulas was for treating infections and inflammation. It is probably best known as an immune system booster for increasing the production of killer cells to eliminate infectious diseases. Echinacea stimulates the body's defenses to fight bacterial infections. Today it is used for treating colon and liver cancer and urinary tract infections. It is one of the plants in my Medicine bag for using when a cold starts or when I feel any type of infection.

Purple wake-robin (see Trillium).

Purslane *(Portulaca oleracea)*. Called common purslane, this plant is also known by mountain folks as "chickweed." An edible weed, it is used in an old formula for expelling worms and parasites from the body. Purslane was used for "digestive cleansing" in earlier years, as well as for headaches.

It is a good source of magnesium, which may contribute to helping with headaches.

Queen Ann's lace (see Wild carrot).

Rabbit pea (see Devil's shoestring).

Rabbit's ear (see Hawkweed).

Ragweed *(Ambrosia artemisiifolia)*. Common ragweed, or feather tops as it was known by earlier Cherokee, was used for treating intestinal worms and related intestinal problems. It was also used to reduce fever. While there is no verification of the results, it is not used today for those purposes. Ragweed is recognized as a major cause of hay fever.

Ramps *(Allium tricoccum)*. Ramps are gathered in the spring almost as a ritual for many Cherokee. Sometimes called skunk cabbage, ramps were thought to cleanse the system and clear the sinuses for "an awakening of the spirit in the spring and summer and keeps those away that you don't want to be around." It certainly does that very well because of the smell. We enjoy ramps and early collard greens in the spring for a special food that is also a Medicine, cleansing the body of winter toxins.

Raspberry *(Rubus idaeus, R. occidentalis,* and *R. strigosus)*. The leaves of raspberry were used by the Cherokee as an astringent for diarrhea, along with other berry plants. It was also used as an antispasmodic for women, particularly during painful menstruation. It was also used to treat the stomach complaints of children. Today it is used as a diuretic for relieving fluid retention and for treating gallstones, infections and inflammation, kidney stones, and urinary problems.

Red root *(Lachnanthes caroliniana)*. Red root was used as a remedy for treating bowel complaints and blood in the urine and stools. It was used as an astringent in several earlier formulas, including one for sore throats. Red root or New Jersey tea *(Ceanothus americanus)* was used for treating thrush or throat and mouth infections. Another plant called red root, amaranth or smooth pigweed *(Amaranthus hybridus)*, was used for diarrhea and for "cleansing the entire system in earlier times."

Rheumatism root (see Twinleaf).

Rhubarb *(Rheum palmatum)*. The rhubarb plant was used for treating constipation, probably due to its being a slight irritant to the digestive tract, which stimulates movement. An elder said, "You know about rhubarb pie, but the earlier Cherokee used the seven-year-old plants as Medicine. It was used for children and elders to cleanse their systems. They like it because of the pleasant taste, even adding some honey." The elder told me how to sow the seed in the early spring, then how to prepare them for cultivation.

Rosemary (*Rosmarinus officinalis*). Most people know of rosemary as the scented oil used in toiletries and in cooking. Rosemary was also used as a carminative for relieving intestinal gas. The Cherokee used rosemary as an antispasmodic. It is an astringent and an antiseptic, and it is used as an antidepressant and an antispasmodic. Rosemary became part of the "love Medicine" earlier Cherokee used to encourage romance. Today it is used for treating indigestion, intestinal gas, and circulatory problems.

Rue anemone (see Windflower).

Sage (*Salvia officinalis*). Wild sage is an aromatic evergreen that is one of several species of sage in the Mint family. In earlier years it was used as a stimulant or tonic. It is used by American Indians as a smudge, a kind of incense in which the dried sage leaves are lit by fire in a large shell. Sage smudge is used to clear an area of "unwanted spirits that can interfere." Sage is also used as a tea in traditional sweat lodge ceremonies. The Cherokee used it with "sacred tobacco" in ceremonies as well. Sage is used to relieve gas pains and is used externally on sores and wounds. It is considered a sacred plant, a special gift from the Great One for protection and healing. It is also known as red, white, and garden sage. Its popular use today is for treating diarrhea and gastrointestinal problems.

Sarsaparilla (*Smilax sarsaparilla*). A "spring tonic" includes this plant and others to rejuvenate the entire system after a cold winter. Sarsaparilla was considered a blood purifier in earlier years by the Cherokee and mountain folks. The plant contains organic sulfur, magnesium sulfate, iron, calcium oxalate, potassium chloride, and magnesium. Research has also found that it simulates the action of estrogen in women. The roots of another plant known as yellow sarsaparilla, *Menispermum canadensis* or "moonseed" in Appalachia, are used for treating skin conditions and as a laxative, a strength tonic, and a nerve relaxant. Sarsaparilla was called *su yu e yu ste* in Cherokee. Today sarsaparilla is used as a diuretic for addressing fluid retention and kidney problems.

Sassafras (*Sassafras albidum*). A tea made from the root bark of sassafras, known as *ka sta ste*, was used to treat kidney problems and to purify the blood. Today sassafras is used as a diuretic for treating fluid retention, gout, and intestinal complaints; as a tonic; and to promote sweating. It is not recommended for use due to findings that sassafras oil contains a carcinogen, and so carries toxic risk. Of course, this plant has been used by many generations of American Indians and mountain folks as a tonic and as a tea for energy.

Savory (*Satureja hortensis*). Savory, or summer savory, is a member of the Mint family. It was used as a tea for treating cramps, intestinal problems, and indigestion and as an astringent. Yerba buena or Oregon tea *(S. douglasii)* is used for the same purpose in Mexico.

Saw palmetto *(Serenoa serrulata)*. Saw palmetto berries were traded by the Seminole and Catawba Indians; they were used for treating throat and bronchial problems and to reduce mucous discharge in the lungs. Saw palmetto was also used as a mild diuretic. The active constituents of volatile oil and other substances have been found to be effective in reducing the prostate. The palmetto plant had a practical use in earlier years for making brooms, hats, and baskets. There is a Carolina palmetto *(Sabal palmetto)* that is also called Spanish palmetto.

Self-heal (see Heal-all).

Senna *(Cassia* or *Senna marilandica)*. Known as wild senna, or *a su ge te sa se yu sta,* this plant was used in a "warm drink or tea" for treating cramps, along with mint. Another plant was used for more serious intestinal cramping, but the elder could not remember the name. A description of the plant made me think it was possibly nightshade *(Solanum dulcamara)*. He remembered it could be poisonous if too much was taken. Wormwood *(Artemisia biennis)* was also used in the mixture, which has been used for treating cramps in the past, along with peppermint. While senna husk is used today as a mild laxative, the leaves were used in earlier years for purging by southeastern tribes. Today it is used for treating constipation, intestinal worms, and bowel problems.

Serviceberry tree *(Amelanchier arborea)*. Mary Chiltoskey referred to serviceberry as being used with several barks to expel worms from young children. It was also used in a spring energy tonic with sassafras and various berries. Mountain folks called serviceberry "sarvis" or "shadbush."

Seven-bark shrub *(Hydrangea arborescens)*. Seven-bark shrub, or wild hydrangea, is a small shrub found on streambanks. The inner bark was used in earlier years as a stimulant and tonic. It is used as a diuretic and to stimulate appetite for the elderly, as well as for "sour on the stomach." While it would induce vomiting, Mary Chiltoskey also also mentioned that seven-bark shrub stopped children's vomiting as well. It is very strong as a remedy. An elder said that a person should always use a plant formula to calm the system, such as a natural antispasmodic to "heal the upset and to keep from causing more of a problem with the cure." Skullcap *(Scutellaria lateriflora)* would sometimes be used as a nerve sedative, or peppermint would be used to settle the system after cleansing.

Shavegrass (see Horsetail).

Shepherd's purse *(Capsella bursa-pastoris)*. Shepherd's purse was used for treating internal bleeding. Today it is used to treat bloody urine, diarrhea, and as a vasoconstrictor for internal bleeding and to raise blood pressure.

Skullcap *(Scutellaria lateriflora)*. Skullcap was used in severe cases where a strong antispasmodic and sedative was needed for remedying physical conditions. While not used very much today, it is still a well-known plant remedy in Appalachia.

Slippery elm tree *(Ulmus rubra)*. The inner bark of slippery, or red, elm played an important role in a Cherokee Medicine bag. Slippery elm was considered to have special power for the lungs and the gastrointestinal tract. It is a strong demulcent, removing mucus and parasites and worms. It was used with another plant or herb or with oatmeal as a food to cleanse the system in a way that would stop irritation of the colon and small intestines; it was also used as a mild laxative. A small handful (1 ounce) of the ground bark is added to a quart of water. This member of the Elm family was used with licorice for soothing inflammation of the gut, sometimes combined with meadowsweet *(Filipendula ulmaria)*. Today slippery elm is used for treating digestive ailments.

Smartweed *(Polygonum hydropiper)*. Smartweed is used for painful urination or blood in the urine. I was not able to confirm the effectiveness of this use, but I did find that mountain folks use rhubarb root, sticklewort, and smartweed for "the gravel and stones." They said this plant use was learned from the Cherokee.

Snakeroot (see Lion's foot).

Snakeroot, black *(Sanicula smallii* and *S. marilandica)*. Mary Chiltoskey identified the use of pink lady's slipper with black snakeroot for treating stomach cramps and colic. Maryland sanicle *(S. marilandica)* was also called self-heal in the West Virginia mountains. This was a very old formula using lady's slipper as a sedative rather than an antispasmodic. One elder suggested that it was Canadian snakeroot *(Sanicula canadensis)* that was used for cramps and colic.

Snakeroot, sampson *(Psoralea psoralioides)*. A tea of sampson snakeroot was used for treating colic and indigestion in earlier years, but an elder said it was "too strong for general usage today."

Snakeroot, white *(Eupatorium rugosum)*. White snakeroot was used in earlier years for treating kidney and urinary conditions, along with yarrow *(Achillea millefolium)*. There were other plants and tree barks in the formula, which has been lost. Paul Hamel and Mary Chiltoskey mention white snakeroot as a remedy for diarrhea, as well as a stimulant and a tonic.

Soapwort *(Saponaria officinalis)*. Soapwort was used by the Cherokee as a poultice for treating boils and sores, as mentioned by Mary Chiltoskey. One Medicine elder said it was good for treating gout and was used externally as a wash for dermatitis and itching skin. The saponin content of soapwort makes a good antibiotic and expectorant. It is used for treating kidney conditions and gout, as well as used as an antibiotic and expectorant. My grandmother called it "bouncing bet," "that was used as a soapy lather" for washing clothes in earlier years.

Solomon's seal *(Polygonatum biflorum)*. The roots of Solomon's seal are used for countering the effects of poison ivy and other skin irritations. It was also used as a mild laxative and tonic to soothe the intestines. The mountain folks would use it as a remedy for black eyes by crushing the fresh roots and making a poultice.

Sorrel *(Rumex acetosa)*. While little was ever mentioned about common sorrel, one Cherokee-Creek Medicine man did use common sorrel, or dock, as a mild antiseptic and laxative. It was used in a "spring tonic" for adults and children to rid them of worms and parasites. According to John Lust it was used as an astringent, a diuretic, and for treating bladder and kidney problems. Today it is used as an antiseptic, to treat diarrhea, and as a diuretic for relieving fluid retention.

Garden sorrel *(R. acetosella)* is also used for medicinal purposes. However, its use as a juice or tea is not recommended because of possible side effects that could affect the liver, kidney, and heart. The sorrels, or docks, are in the Smartweed, or Buckwheat, family.

Sourwood tree *(Oxydendrum arboreum)*. While the honey from the sourwood tree is well known in the Great Smoky Mountains, the stems were used in earlier years to make pipe stems and arrow shafts. Sourwood is also used in a formula for treating diarrhea and to "calm the intestines." It is also called sorrel tree or lily-of-the-valley tree. It is a member of the Heath family.

Southern wax myrtle (see Bayberry).

Speedwell *(Veronica officinalis)*. The entire plant of speedwell, or veronica, was dried and used as a tonic for the gastrointestinal and urinary tracts, the liver and kidneys, and for treating gout. It was used to purify the blood, as well as being one of those plants that was used when someone in the family "passed over." There are several ceremonial plants used for the "clear way of the spirit to travel to the darkening land, before they come into the light of the Great One and the Universal Circle."

Veronica was also used in earlier years for nervousness and anxiety associated with grief and "feeling down." I am sharing this one to preserve it as a formula that is also used as a tonic for the healing of gout and "other things." Put a teaspoon of the crushed dried leaves in two cups of boiling water and let steep for twelve minutes, then add peppermint and lemon for flavor. Take a cup in the morning and a cup in the evening for seven days and nights. "This is a clearing remedy for when you lose someone or break up a relationship. With each cup, ask for release, clearing, and good Medicine in your own language or way." An old southeastern Carolina remedy of wormwood (Artemisia absinthium) was added to the speedwell for treating bladder and gout problems.

Spiderwort (Tradescantia virginiana). Spiderwort was used for treating kidney complaints and as a laxative, as verified by Paul Hamel and Mary Chiltoskey. A leaf tea was used for treating stomach problems. An elder said that spiderwort was also used in an old cancer formula.

Spleenwort (Asplenium platyneuron). This evergreen fern was used to expel worms in children. Another fern called spleenwort (Comptonia peregrina) is used as a poultice for treating toothaches and diarrhea. It was sometimes called sweet fern and was used in a formula with warm water for expelling worms.

Spreading bladderfern (Cystopteris protrusa). Spreading bladderfern was reported as being used to treat chills. An elder confirmed its use with fennel for treating intestinal and bladder complaints. This is an old remedy that is not much known today.

Stargrass (see Colic root).

Stinging nettle (see Nettle).

Stone root (Collinsonia canadensis). Also called horse balm or richweed, the dried roots and rhizome of stone root is used as a diuretic. The active constiuent is probably the volatile oil with its lemon scent. Stone root was used for treating constipation and gastrointestinal problems in earlier years. This plant was a favorite of some southeastern tribes for dressing cuts and wounds. The stem stands from an underground rhizome; tiny yellowish flowers protrude from the broad leaves and from a distance look like peppers on their stems. Stone root is an old mountain remedy in Kentucky, Virginia, and Tennessee for treating headaches. It is also used as a mild laxative, a diuretic, and a skin wash.

Sunflower (Helianthus annuus). The sunflower seeds are a "digestive treat that helps with constipation." They are also used for general good Medicine. The oil is useful as a dietary supplement, and the seeds are a great energy snack.

Sweet flag (see Calamus root).

Sweet plant (see Anise).

Sweet shrub (*Calycanthus floridus*). While sweet shrub was mentioned by several elders for use with bladder and urinary conditions, it has not been used since earlier years, according to an elder who remembered it back when he was a child in the early 1920s. Paul Hamel and Mary Chiltoskey reported that sweet shrub was used for failing eyesight.

Sycamore tree (*Platanus occidentalis*). The inner bark of American sycamore was used in many formulas for treating internal ailments. Its was considered sacred as much for being the "first tree to have fire and give life" as for being a healing agent.

The story of the sycamore involves the Thunder Beings, who struck a large sycamore on an island across a body of water from where the humans in the beginning of time were living, cold and hungry. It took little Water Spider weaving a web and crossing the body of water to gather a hot coal and carry it back to the humans. Today the fire is started at each ceremony with giving thanks and offering tobacco. The story is much longer, but this glimpse shows that the sycamore has earned a special place in the traditions of the Cherokee. This tree is a member of the Sycamore family.

Tansy (*Tanacetum vulgare*). This was a plant used for "special Medicine," for treating intestinal worms, along with wild carrot, or Queen Anne's lace. Tansy can be poisonous even when used externally, according to John Lust. It was mentioned as being for female Medicine, and Mary Chiltoskey mentioned it as being used to expel worms in children in a formula that included meadow rue and crowfoot with honey. An elder said that swamp rose (*Rosa palustris*) was used as well. Today tansy is used to treat diarrhea and to expel intestinal worms. Do not use tansy during pregnancy and only use it under the supervision of a trained herbalist or naturopath.

Terrapin's foot (*Epigaea repens*). Terrapin's foot is also called trailing arbutus and mayflower. The Cherokee used this plant for treating digestive problems and for the kidneys, along with wintergreen and yellowroot. Terrapin's foot is found in northern Appalachia and is considered a sacred plant by several tribes. The leaves and roots were used for treating indigestion. The mountain folks used it for treating kidney complaints and considered the aroma of the small white to pink flower a "perfume of nature." It is an astringent and a diuretic.

Thyme (*Thymus serpyllum*). Another old remedy of the Cherokee uses this creeping ground plant, with its narrow and oblong leaves and pink to purple flowers that bloom on branch-end heads. Thyme has a lemonlike odor. A Cherokee stew or sauce would not be without thyme or wild thyme.

It was also used as an antiseptic, a diuretic, an expectorant, and an anti-spasmodic. After a meal it would be used as a carminative to alleviate intestinal gas.

All these uses have been validated by pharmacological studies on the active constituents of thyme. Thyme is a natural antibiotic with the anti-viral constituent thymol for fighting unfriendly bacteria while relaxing the muscles and blood vessels. It is also interesting that thyme is used with other aromatic herbs, such as peppermint, rosemary, sage, and savory, to purify water to avoid diarrhea and fever. Today thyme is used for treating indigestion and intestinal gas and for expelling intestinal parasites.

Tickseed (*Coreopsis tinctoria*). Paul Hamel and Mary Chiltoskey mentioned tickseed roots as being used for treating "flux" and for making a red dye. The thread-leaved coreopsis (*C. verticillata*) is a close cousin. It has large, beautiful yellow flowers and is a great plant for home flower gardens.

Tobacco (*Nicotiana rustica*). In earlier years when tobacco was used as a "special Medicine," it would be made into a tea decoction and then sprayed on the area of the body that needed healing by using a wooden tube or reed. There was always a chant or prayer or incantation that would go with the healing ceremony. These chants of giving thanks and seeking healing were very practical and clear in their message to the Great One. This is all sacred Medicine that is not to be shared, but is learned by those chosen to carry on the Medicine Way. Medicine people are very humble and will only say things such as, "I know a little something" or "I learned a little something about that" as a way to not appear boastful.

Tobacco is sacred. The leaves contain nicotine, a toxic alkaloid that is poisonous and can be absorbed through the skin. Like everything else in nature, one must use these substances in moderation and only as a helper.

Trailing arbutus (see Terrapin's foot).

Trillium (*Trillium erectum*). Also known as Indian balm, bethroot, or purple wake-robin, trillium is used as an astringent for stopping bleeding or "runny or bloody flux or diarrhea." Trillium, a member of the Lily family, is at risk of extinction in its natural environment. Do not use trillium during pregnancy.

Trout lily (see Adder's tongue).

Trumpet vine (*Ipomea pandurata*). A natural diuretic, trumpet vine was used for treating kidney complaints and as a mild laxative. It was also mentioned as wild potato vine, used for treating urine and bowel complaints. In earlier years a wash was made to "soak potato eyes before planting, to keep the insects away." Trumpet vine is also called morning glory and wild rhubarb in Appalachia.

Turtlehead (*Chelone glabra*). The plant was used to increase the appetite of the elderly and those recovering from illness and was used in formulas for reducing fever and to rid children of worms and parasites. The leaves are used as a mild laxative and in a formula for expelling intestinal worms. It is also called pink turtlehead, even though the plant can have white flowers. The name comes from the small turtlelike snout that protrudes from the flower cap. The plant is also known as snakehead, old woman's cap, and shell flower in Appalachia.

Twayblade (*Liparis loeselii*). A tea of the twayblade roots was used in an old formula for treating kidney and urinary problems. It was combined with the plant called ladies' tresses for treating urinary problems. The plant has broad shiny green leaves with one stalk and "little gourdlike flowers."

Twinleaf (*Jeffersonia diphylla*). Also called yellowroot and rheumatisum root, twinleaf is used for urinary problems related to "the milky urine and gravel that causes lots of pain." It was sometimes used with vervain (*Verbena hastata*) for bowel complaints that are chronic. It was also used with blue weed (*Echium vulgare*).

Vervain (*Verbena officinalis*). This member of the vervain family is considered a "wild weed"; it is used in a formula for treating kidney and liver problems. It is also known as Indian hyssop.

Viper bugloss (see Blue devil).

Virginia creeper (*Parthencissus quinquefolia*). Called American ivy, Virginia creeper was used in a formula with red alder and ash tree bark for treating liver problems and was sometimes mentioned as being used with wood betony. Paul Hamel and Mary Chiltoskey mentioned its use for treating yellow jaundice. This clinging vine is distinguished from poison ivy by the fact that it has five leaves and is not poisonous.

Virgin's bower (*Clematis virginiana*). The roots of virgin's bower were used with milkweed for treating kidney, nerves, and stomach disorders. This very old remedy enjoyed great popularity in the early 1930s and '40s. Virgin's bower was also known as devil's thread and devil's hair.

Walnut tree (*Juglans nigra*). The inner bark of walnut tree, or *se di* in Cherokee, was used for treating persons with parasites in earlier years. I suspect that the tree's content of potassium iodine as a strong antiseptic is probably the reason for the plant's effectiveness. Walnut was used in earlier formulas for treating nerves, skin conditions, sores, bleeding, diarrhea, inflammation, ringworm, dandruff, and even blood-sugar level. Black walnut is still used for expelling tapeworms and parasites and their larvae from the body. Today black walnut is valued for its antifungal properties and is used both internally and externally. As an elder said, "Maybe someday others will recognize what earlier Cherokee knew about the gift of this bark as a natural helper and healing agent." Black walnut is a member of the Walnut family.

Watercress (Nasturtium officinale). As a food and Medicine, watercress was used for addressing internal pain and inflammation. Water plantain (*Alisma subcordatum*) was mentioned by an elder as being used with "cresses" for internal cleansing and bowel complaints. Watercress leaves are chopped and put into salads, coming into season at the same time as ramps and other wild greens. A "spring tonic" that includes watercress is still popular in the mountains. Do not use watercress medicinally during pregnancy.

Watermelon (Citrullus vulgaris). Watermelon seeds would be used for treating kidney problems, as mentioned by Mary Chiltoskey. While use of the seeds as Medicine has been forgotten, some elders do remember watermelon remedies that were considered sacred Medicine.

Wax myrtle (see Bayberry).

White mustard (Sinapis alba). While not a native plant to Turtle Island, or North America, the small seeds of white mustard were recognized as being good for relieving acid indigestion. The oil of mustard was also used in ointments for external relief of minor aches by mountain folks. The Cherokee have always recognized the value of accepting new remedies from other tribes, as well as from the Europeans.

White sage (see Mugwort and Sage).

Wild carrot (Daucus carota). Also called Queen Anne's lace, wild carrot was used in a formula, sometimes with ginseng, to "straighten them right up, when they are sickly due to the weather." It was used for treating colds, especially with children. The large cluster of white flowers in umbels are easily recognized in large fields and along the roadsides. One elder remembered wild carrot being used in an old formula for expelling intestinal worms.

Wild chamomile (Matricaria chamomilla or recutita). Wild chamomile was used as an antispasmodic, to heal inflamed stomach and intestines, and for calming. German chamomile (*Matricaria recutita*) has been researched extensively for its anti-inflammatory, antioxidant, antibacterial, and other healing properties. Chamomile is effective for treating cough and bronchitis, fevers and colds, skin inflammation, mouth infections, wounds, and burns.

Wild cherry tree *(Prunus serotina)*. The "inner scrapings of the bark" of wild cherry tree was used for treating bladder and urinary problems. Wild cherry bark and berries are often mixed with cranberries in healing formulas. Wild cherry, a member of the Rose family, is also called black cherry.

Wild comfrey *(Cynoglossum virginianum)*. The roots of wild comfrey were used for treating cancer, itch, and milky urine. The elders I worked with remembered its use for treating urinary problems. Cancer formulas were sacred.

Wild garlic *(Allium vineale)*. Wild garlic was used in formulas for expelling intestinal worms and parasites. It was also used in formulas for cleansing the entire system. Garlic contains antiviral and antibacterial properties. Do not use while nursing. Common garlic *(A. sativum)* is used as an anticlotting agent and for treating colds.

Wild geranium *(Geranium maculatum)*. Wild geranium is probably better known in the mountains as alumroot, crowfoot, or cranesbill. It is used as an astringent for treating diarrhea, especially with children and elders. It was used in earlier years with agrimony in a formula for gastrointestinal problems. A native geranium known as Carolina cranesbill *(G. carolinianum)* can be found along the Blue Ridge Parkway.

An elder who could speak very little English said the seedpods will "pop open to spread the seeds into the air." This elder, William Hornbuckle, smiled as he showed me how the pod would explode. He would make it explode, and then laugh, over and over again. I will always remember those events when learning as much about nature as about the plant uses themselves. Of course, those elders will always be very special to me. William Hornbuckle taught me much about the wonders of life in the mountains as he perceived them, and through his cunning sense of "knowing" about plants.

Wild horehound *(Eupatorium pilorum)*. Wild horehound was known in Appalachia as a bitter tonic. Earlier Cherokee used it as a drink for sweats and to induce perspiration to cleanse the system, as well as for treating constipation. One elder remembered the plant being used as a stimulant and tonic, as well as for treating women's breast complaints when used as an East Medicine. This plant is different from white horehound *(Marrubium vulgare)*, used as a flavoring in cough drops.

Wild hydrangia (see Seven-bark shrub).

Wild hyssop *(Verbena hastata)*. Also called blue, or wild, vervain and ironweed, wild hyssop was used as an emetic to induce vomiting. Earlier Cherokee called it *te stu yu te na* and used it as a West Medicine for treating cramps, colds, sore eyes, skin itch, kidney problems, parasites, and diarrhea. An elder Medicine man from the Lumbee tribe mentioned that several of the coastal tribes used wormwood *(Artemisia absinthium)* with wild hyssop for gallbladder and bile problems, sometimes along with wild mercury. Blue, or wild, vervain is often found with Joe-pye weed. Vervain *(V. officinalis)* is also called wild hyssop.

Wild mercury *(Acalypha virginica)*. The roots of wild mercury were used for treating gallbladder and kidney ailments. While mentioned by several elders and in some of the old formulas, it seems this plant use has been lost. However, it was popular at one time in what an elder called "mountain Medicine."

Wild oats *(Uvularia sessilifolia)*. Called bellflowers, or *tsu hi tsu gi* by the Cherokee, wild oats were used for treating "stones," urinary problems, and diarrhea, and as a tonic. It is also called sessile bellwort due to the shape of the leaves with their single drooping flower.

Wild plum *(Prunus americana)*. Wild plum was used in earlier years as a bark tea for treating kidney and bladder complaints. It was used with wild indigo for treating colitis. Thanks to Paul Hamel and Mary Chiltoskey, this use would have been lost if they had not recorded it.

Wild potato *(Convolvulus pandurata)*. Also known as wild jalap, wild potato was mentioned by an elder as being used to "settle a nervous stomach, but also used in an earlier formula for urine problems." Wild lettuce was used with this plant as an antispasmodic. William Bartram reported wild potato's use during his travels. Wild potato is not to be confused with mayapple, which is also called jalap. (Jalap is the name of a village in Mexico.) Also called trumpet vine *(Ipomoea pandurata)*, wild potato is a member of the Morning Glory family.

Wild strawberry *(Fragaria vesca* or *F. virginiana)*. A tea made of the roots of wild strawberry was used for treating kidney and bladder problems, dysentery, and for calming the nerves. In addition to being a special Medicine in Cherokee myth, the wild strawberry fruit was used for internal system cleansing, along with blackberries and raspberries as "wild berries that help calm the young spirit in youth." A tea of the leaves is used to "strengthen the gastrointestinal tract." It was also used for treating gout, liver ailments, and arthritis for the elderly. In the West Medicine, strawberry was always referred to as wild strawberry, as though there was a mystic power in the plant for young people and romance. Wild strawberry is a member of the Rose family.

Wild yam *(Dioscorea villosa)*. This plant and fruit was used in a formula to relieve the pains of childbirth for Indian women. In one old formula yellowroot was used with it. Wild yam was also used for treating rheumatism. The plant has a steroidlike substance that makes the plant effective when the root is boiled or crushed and prepared as a poultice. My grandmother said wild yam was used for treating gallbladder problems and for colic. Today it is used to treat the adrenal glands and to address inflammation in the colon, dysentery, gallstones, and stomach and muscle cramps.

Willow tree *(Salix nigra, S. exigua, and S. discolor)*. The bark of willow or black willow is used for treating pain in a formula that also includes licorice. Today a combination with meadowsweet *(Filipendula ulmaria)* provides acetylsalicylic acid, a natural form of aspirin. The pussy willow and sandbar willow are also popular in the Northwest.

Windflower *(Thalictrum thalictroides)*. Also called rue anemone, the roots were used as a tea for treating diarrhea and as an emetic. Several of the elders mentioned this plant, but few have used it "since the olden days."

Winter cress *(Barbarea vulgaris)*. Also called bitter cress, winter cress greens are eaten to cleanse the system. It is added to collards, cabbage, dandelion, watercress, and other "wild greens" as a "good cleanser and purifier of the system and the blood, and a good tonic."

Wintergreen shrub *(Gaultheria procumbens)*. This small shrub is also called teaberry or mountain birch. The roots were chewed in earlier years for treating chronic indigestion and dysentery. One elder said that wintergreen prefers growing around pine trees. Wintergreen is also used for its good taste.

Witchgrass (see Couchgrass).

Witch hazel *(Hamamelis virginiana)*. As a small tree or shrub, witch hazel was used in a formula for treating diarrhea, along with several other tree barks. It is a member of the Witch Hazel family, along with sweetgum. Witch hazel is found along the streams in Appalachia.

Wood betony *(Stachys officinalis)*. Betony, or wood betony, was used to expel intestinal worms and to treat kidney problems. The plant is used for treating diarrhea, but not with pregnant women due to the stimulating effect on the uterus. Another plant called wood betony, which is also known as lousewort, is included in the West Medicine. Today betony is used for treating heartburn, kidney problems, and stomach pains.

Woodbine *(Lonicera japonica)*. Also called honeysuckle, this long vine with narrow, heart-shaped leaves and trumpet-shaped flowers was used for treating gout. It was also used for treating the kidney and liver, for mouth sores, sore throat, and bronchitis, and as a diuretic.

Wormseed (Chenopodium ambrosioides). Also known as Mexican root or Jerusalem oak, this plant was used for children with "weak stomachs" and to rid their intestines of parasites. A small amount of the juice was added to peppermint tea, along with licorice. Another plant called wormseed (*Erysimum cheiranthoides*) is used by the British for treating coughs.

Wormwood (see Mugwort).

Woundwort (see Heal-all).

Yaupon shrub (Ilex vomitoria). Yaupon shrub was used in a mixture called "Indian black drink," a purging drink for certain ceremonies. As a tonic it is slightly narcotic. In the coastal area of North Carolina a plant called wormseed, or gall berry (*I. glaba*), was used by the southeastern Indians in the ceremonial "black drink," a piece of information shared by one of the elders.

Yarrow (Achillea millefolium). Called common yarrow, this plant is used as a tonic to stimulate the intestinal system and to increase urine flow. The small white cluster of flowers and fernlike leaves are found in Appalachia. Earlier Cherokee used the leaves for treating diarrhea, fevers, internal bleeding, and insomnia. Yarrow is also used in the mountains with dandelion leaves for treating gout and backache. It was used in earlier years for blood sugar problems or diabetes. There is also a "sneezeweed yarrow" (*Achillea ptarmica*), a plant with a sharp and pungent smell that causes sneezing. Yarrow was used to increase the appetite of elders. Do not use during pregnancy.

Yellow dock (Rumex crispus). Also called curly or curled dock, yellow dock was used for treating digestive and stomach problems, as well as chronic constipation. Today it is also used for relieving fluid retention. It is used by the elders to increase their appetite, especially after an illness.

Yellow-eyed grass (Xyris caroliniana). This plant was used in earlier years for treating diarrhea in children. This was mentioned by Mary Chiltoskey, and an elder mentioned yellow-eyed grass as used with sourwood (*Oxydendrum arboreum*) for treating diarrhea in adults or with little vine (*Clematis virginiana*), which was used in the Green Corn Ceremony in earlier years with the Cherokee. A blue-eyed grass (*Sisyrinchium angustifolium*) blooms at Mile High, or Spirit Mountain, on the Blue Ridge Parkway near Cherokee, North Carolina.

Yellowroot (Xanthorhiza simplicissima). Cherokee Indians still recognize this plant by the yellow crystalline alkaloid, now known as berberine, which gives the roots their yellow appearance. The healing agents of this alkoloid are the reason the plant was used for treating sore throat, ulcerations in the mouth, and stomach problems. The root was chewed in earlier years for a fresh taste in the mouth or used to make a mouthwash.

Found along the streams in the southeastern mountains, yellowroot grows from a rhizome; the single stems have a cluster of bright green leaves at the end of the stem. The flowers, at the base of the leaves and stem, droop in clusters of purple flowers that bloom in April and May. Yellowroot is one of my favorite plants in my Medicine bag for taking care of hoarseness when I'm teaching and giving presentations. Twinleaf and goldenseal are also commonly known as yellowroot.

Many uses of plants by southeastern Indians for West Medicine have been lost over the years. In case any readers know how or what these plants were used for as West Medicine I would appreciate hearing about it. The plants that were used in earlier years for West Medicine include obedient plant *(Physostegia virginiana)*, tall ironweed *(Vernonia gigantea)*, rose pink or meadow beauty *(Sabatia angularis)*, heart-leafed aster *(Aster cordifolius)*, nodding pogonia *(Triphora trianthophora)*, pine-sap *(Monotropa hypopithys)*, grass pink *(Calopogon tuberosus)*, cardinal flower *(Lobelia cardinalis)*, trumpet honeysuckle *(Lonicera sempervirens)*, Indian paintbrush *(Castilleja coccinea)*, mountain myrtle *(Leiophyllum buxifolium)*, flame azalea *(Rhododendron calendulaceum)*, Indian pink *(Spigelia marilandica)*, sweet shrub *(Calycanthus floridus)*, puttyroot *(Aplectum hyemale)*, bristly locust *(Robinia hispida)*, bleeding heart *(Dicentra eximia)*, mountain laurel *(Kalmia latifolia)*, Indian cucumber root *(Medeola virginiana)*, little brown jug *(Hexastylis arifolia)*, whorled pogonia *(Isotria verticillata)*, showy orchid *(Galearis spectabilis)*, pinxter flower *(Rhododendron periclymenoides)*, cross vine *(Bignonia capreolata)*, North American pawpaw *(Asimina triloba)*, gay wings *(Polygala paucifolia)*, and creeping phlox *(Phlox stolonifera)*.

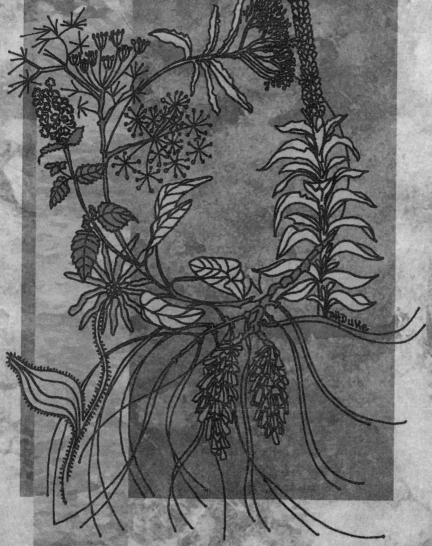

NORTH

7

Plant Medicines of the North

North Medicine is about a sense of freedom and a connection to the stars and the greater Universal Circle. The focus is on the respiratory system, the nervous system, the ear, nose, throat, and mouth, as well as on allaying those influences that interfere with our balance and breathing.

The Medicine plants and tree barks were used to bring back balance for the person who was affected by the wind or by breathing, lung weakness, and other respiratory issues. As one elder described it, "North is the direction of calm, the coolness in the early morning on the mountain." Continuing, the elder said, "It is about going on the mountain, either in person or in your mind. There is a peace, a calm state, as you experience freedom. It is a time to give thanks to the Great One for this day, a special day to be alive, to hear the birds sing, to watch how life becomes busy about survival, and it is about learning and sharing. You have to be free of thoughts that interfere to be able to learn and teach the Medicine."

The North Direction is about early morning and dew on the leaves of the trees, seeing for miles from the top of a mountain and hearing the creations of nature awakening to a new day. It is about our senses making us acutely aware of everything around us and in our circle of being. The connection between the animal world and humans was considered so special that earlier Cherokee believed that the animals taught the hunters how to "be in the 'right way' with the animals, with giving thanks and having ceremony before hunting for skillful and successful hunting." The same sensitivity and awareness of the early morning was the acuteness and skill of a hunter tracking and protecting Mother Earth in the pursuit of food for survival. There is much to learn from the North Medicine about harmony and balance.

The color of the North is sky or dark blue or purple. The vision of the sky and stars in the late afternoon is the image used to describe the North. There is a story of two young Cherokee trying to capture a star as it sat near the top of a mountain. As the story goes, one of them did manage to sneak up and grab the star, which was like a large cotton ball that could not be held. As they looked at the one youth's arm, there was a sparkle. Suddenly the young boy started rising from the ground until he arose in the sky, never to be heard from again. Today we look up at the stars in the sky to see the North Star, the young Cherokee looking down on his village brightly so all can see him early in the evening as they leave the planting fields.

Other than the hawk circling in the sky, the deer is the animal that probably best represents the North Direction. To the earlier Cherokee the deer was considered sacred as a cunning and sensitive animal in the forest. It seemed to have an awareness and connection to the Universal Circle that hunters would learn to follow in learning to be excellent at their skill. The deer, or *a wi*, was honored and prized for its soft skin. The deerskin was treated and used in a sacred way, as a wrap for crystals and "to keep special things as part of our Medicine bundle." Everything about the deer was treated with sacred respect so that even the venison hunters were specially trained in just the right way to take the life of a deer, similar to the eagle hunters.

North Medicine includes Medicine formulas and prayer-chants that relate to the calm and quiet of the North, with soft songs and drumming in the distance. The flutes share a quiet melody with animal sounds made with instruments and vocals. In the same way that Cherokee Medicine is related to the Four Directions, so are the "spirit" connections to animals, birds, and natural substances such as plants and trees. The focus in the North was more on calmness, to relieve tension, and on prevention rather than treatment. North Medicine focused on protecting and clearing the "wind" for us to survive with a "good Medicine breath of life."

The following is a listing of plants and their uses as North Medicine.

Adam and Eve root *(Aplectrum hyemale).* This member of the Orchid family is also called puttyroot. It is used as North Medicine for addressing bronchial and pulmonary problems. This bulb is found in moist woods; the flowers are in a purplish spike. The name "Adam and Eve root" is reflective of the two bulbs—one small and one larger—connected at the single leaf and stem. The flowers, which bloom in the spring, are purplish mixed with yellow, brown, and white.

Alder tree *(Alnus serrulata* **and** *A rugosa).* The young leaves of common, or hazel, alder were "soaked or crushed with willow bark in a formula that included ginger and sassafras for fevers." The tannins in the alder bark were used in a formula for sore throats. The inner bark was used for treating colds, coughs, eye conditions, thrush, and fungal infections in the mouth. According to an elder, "it was mixed with balsam fir in equal parts in a formula." Alder is a member of the Birch family of trees.

Alexanders *(Angelica atropurpurea).* Also called angelica, the roots of this plant were used in cold formulas for treating fevers and sore throats. I met a Cherokee elder in Arkansas who recalled his grandfather using this plant and knew how to mix the formula. The flavor of the plant is similar to celery and parsley leaf used in cooking soups and fish dishes. The seeds are used as a seasoning, and the roots are eaten like parsnips. Alexanders is also an old remedy for asthma.

Allspice (see Spicewood).

American spikenard (see Indian root).

Anemone *(Anemone lancifolia, A. nemorosa,* **and** *A. blanda).* An elder mentioned the "wind flower," or wood anemone, a May-blooming plant that grows to about six inches tall and bears three leaves and a white flower with five petals. It is used for treating headaches and "dizzy spells." An elder remembered it combined with tulip tree and cardinal flower for addressing colds, croup, fever, and headaches.

These members of the Buttercup, or Crowfoot, family are found in moist woods. My father called this plant "crowfoot"; my grandmother Flora Watson, who grew up in the Great Smoky Mountains, used the plant for treating stomachaches, gout, and asthma. The plant is also called pasqueflower. My father said that early Irish settlers used wood anemone

(A. lancifolia) and thimbleweed *(A. virginiana)* "like the Cherokee, for summer colds and fever." Grecian windflower *(A. blanda)* is a species commonly found in home flower gardens. Rue anemone *(A. thalictroides)* was a root starch similar to potato that was dug in the mountains. These small plants have pink to white flowers.

Angelica *(Angelica archangelica).* The leaves and roots of angelica, or masterwort, are used in a formula for addressing respiratory complaints and the sinuses as an expectorant and a stimulant. Angelica was also combined with dogwood in traditional sweats and ceremonies. Calamus root was usually included in the formula, along with butternut bark *(Juglans cinerea).*

Angelica was used for treating asthma symptoms, hay fever, and headaches. One elder called angelica "powder puff." The white flowers, in compound umbels, have a honeylike aroma and stand up to five feet tall. Angelica reminded earlier Indians of the "powder puff used by fancy White women." Today angelica is used for addressing backache, leg and circulation complaints, and menstrual and menopausal symptoms. It is also used for loss of appetite and gastrointestinal complaints and is an effective diuretic.

Anise *(Pimpinella anisum).* Anise was called *u ga na s dah,* or "sweet plant," by the Cherokee, because the seeds taste sweet. While this plant is native to the Mediterranean, it is used in a Cherokee formula for treating asthma, severe colds, and stubborn coughs and as an expectorant. Sometimes it was combined with hophornbeam for treating toothaches. It is also used with alumroot for treating inflammation and sores in the mouth. Today it is used for the same conditions, and it is also used externally for muscle spasms and scabies and to repel insects.

Anise contains an essential oil that is effective as a cough remedy and as an expectorant. Do not use anise during pregnancy.

Apple tree *(Malus sylvestris).* The inner bark of wild, or common, apple was used as "wind Medicine" for addressing throat and voice problems. As an elder put it, "For earlier Indian runners and hunters, it was important to have energy and endurance." The apples "were small, not like the golden delicious apples of today." Apple juice has been a choice fruit juice to give children for energy, along with blackberries and raspberries, especially for children who were sick with colds. An apple-bark tea is still used for "voice problems."

According to the Audubon Society, there really was a Johnny Appleseed who traveled for almost fifty years sharing the seeds of apples from Pennsylvania to Illinois. The sweet crab apple *(M. coronaria)* is found in southern Appalachia. The southern crab apple *(M. angustifolia)* is a popular sweet fruit for small animals. Apple *(M. domestica)* is the apple used for applesauce; this variety has a pectin that is useful today for addressing constipation. Apple is a member of the Rose family.

Arnica (*Arnica montana* and other species). Arnica is called *a ga do li,* or "yellow eyes," in Cherokee. It was used to calm the nerves and as a mild sedative. It was also called mountain tobacco and was used by some in Appalachia for treating colds, fever, cough, and bronchitis. An elder said the Catawba used arnica for back pain. Today it is used for joint and muscle aches and pains and is used topically for bacterial infections and inflammation. Use is not recommended for pregnant women, as the plant was once used for stimulating uterine contractions. A question has been raised about reports that it is not safe for use on open wounds and with children, due to potential heart and kidney effects. Arnica should not be used internally due to the toxic effects of lactones.

Arrowhead *(Sagittaria latifolia).* A leaf tea was used for fevers in babies and young children. An elder said that the lanceolate leaves were thought to make his arrow "go straighter and true to its mark" if he kept some of these leaves with his sacred tobacco.

Arrowroot *(Arum maculatum).* Also known as arum, or *ga tli da* in Cherokee, arrowroot is combined with the rootstock of wood betony and used for treating bronchitis and asthma symptoms. Sometimes red spruce *(Picea rubens)* was added for treating more severe colds. Arrowroot is a member of the Olive family.

Arum (see Arrowroot).

Asafoetida *(Ferula foetida).* The gummy resin from the roots of asafoetida was used in a formula for treating severe cough, asthma, and bronchitis. It was also mixed with peppermint or a flavor such as horehound for use as a sedative.

Ash tree *(Fraxinus americana).* White ash is called *tsu ga no nah* by the Cherokee. It was used in a formula for a topical remedy for rattlesnake and copperhead bites in earlier years. Another use was as a bark drink for "strengthening the wind of the runners." The tree is sometimes called biltmore ash, and the wood is used to make baseball bats.

The various species of ash brought over from Europe were a gift to America of a valuable cold and fever remedy. Mountain folks used ash for treating gout, arthritis, and bladder conditions and as a mild laxative. An elder called ash "a reliable analgesic for rheumatism and arthritis from the old country." There is a Carolina ash *(F. caroliniana)* found along the eastern coastal region that was used similarly by Native tribes. Ash is a member of the Olive family.

Balm, melissa *(Melissa officinalis)*. This member of the Mint family is also called lemon, or bee, balm. The leaves were used "to calm the spirit and the nerves of the wind." It is valued as an antidepressant and a calming agent for the nervous system. For stronger action one can combine melissa with lavender and/or valerian. For even stronger action one could use melissa and peppermint in combination with skullcap. This remedy should be prepared by someone trained in herbal medicine. Melissa has antibacterial and antiviral properties and is used as an antispasmodic.

Balm-of-Gilead (see Balsam fir tree).

Balsam fir tree *(Abies balsamea)*. Also known as Balm-of-Gilead, the inner bark was used with other barks in a formula for treating colds. The leaves were smoked as an inhalant for addressing pulmonary problems. While there were no elders who could remember smoking the leaves, one remembered using them as part of a "sweat for colds and feeling bad." The needles of balsam fir last longer than most other trees that are used as Christmas trees. Earlier Cherokee used the needles for ceremonies, especially for the Friends-making Ceremony where the needles are bundled and held in the hand during a dance. Douglas fir *(Pseudotsuga menziesii)* and Fraser fir *(Abies fraseri)* needles and cones were used for gifting and in traditional sweat lodge ceremonies. The scotch pine *(Pinus sylvestris)* was used in a similar way by western tribes. Balsam was combined with goldenseal for treating colds and diarrhea. Balsam fir is a member of the Pine family.

Baneberry *(Actae pachypoda, A. ruba,* and *A. spicata)*. The roots of baneberry, a plant called "herb Christopher" by my English friend Simon, was used as an emetic and a cold remedy. It is considered poisonous in some uses but was popular in earlier years to "cleanse the system and to get rid of body worms and toxins after the sickness of winter [colds and flu]." Baneberry was also known as button snakeroot, which is also a common name for blazing star *(Liatris spicata)*. White baneberry *(A. alba)* is a variety of white cohosh.

Baneberry was used in an old North Medicine formula with wild geranium and alumroot for treating thrush and sore throat. An elder reminded me that thrush is also something that horses get on their hooves from "being in a wet stall." These conversations remind me of all there is to learn from our elders' experiences.

Basswood tree *(Tilia americana)*. The leaves of *wa ou li si,* or bee tree, are used for treating colds, coughs, and sore throats. American basswood is a species commonly used as a diuretic, a mild sedative, and an expectorant. Basswood is a member of the Basswood, or Linden, family.

Bayberry shrub *(Myrica cerifera).* This shrub was known as southern wax myrtle and southern bayberry. It is an evergreen shrub or small tree with lanceolate leaves that are easily identified year-round. It was used in a cough and cold formula. The active compounds validate its value as a stimulant and an astringent. The name wax myrtle comes from the substance that surrounds the black seeds, which protects the seeds up to several years in the soil, until germination. Mountain folks place the fruit in boiling water to extract the waxy substance for making candles. The shrub is popular in the eastern and northern regions, where it is known as waxberry and candleberry. Bayberry is a member of the Bayberry, or Wax Myrtle, family.

Bearberry shrub *(Arctostaphylos uva-ursi).* As one Cherokee-Creek elder remembered, a "smoke with bearberry is a mixture to take the edge off the bitter tobacco and to relax the spirit. We learned this from our brothers in the West, who traded bearberry for Cherokee tobacco." Bearberry is a member of the Heath family, with wintergreen, mountain laurel, and cranberry. It has unique, small, pitcherlike flowers with berries combined. Sometimes bearberry was combined with celery seeds and used as an antiseptic and for treating urinary tract infections. Today it is used for conditions of fluid retention and for septic care of the urinary tract. Bearberry has been called by several names, including foxberry, bear's grape, crowberry, hogberry, and uva-ursi. Do not use bearberry during pregnancy.

Bee tree (see Basswood).

Bilberry shrub *(Vaccinium myrtillis).* Called *ka wa ya,* or "huckleberry," bilberry makes a juice akin to cranberry juice. The bilberry juice is used as a mouthwash. It is an astringent and is valued as an eyewash. The dried leaves and berries are used as an astringent for treating inflammation of the mouth and pharynx.

Bilberry is sometimes combined with cranberry for antibacterial properties and is a "special Medicine for the gums and teeth for inflammation. Use hawthorn and you can get a cleaning like you'd get at the White man's dentist." Today bilberry is used for treating cataracts, diabetic eye problems, glaucoma, macular degeneration, and poor night vision, as well as varicose veins and poor circulation. Bilberry is a member of the Heath family.

Birch tree *(Betula alba* and *B. lenta).* Indian Medicine men and women recognized the astringent abilities of white and sweet birch bark. The inner bark of mountain birch, or *a ti sah gi,* was used as a stimulant and in a formula for treating colds and respiratory problems. In the early 1900s sweet birch oil was popular as a form of methyl salicylate. Black, or cherry, birch *(B. lenta)* used for oil of wintergreen and salicylic acid or aspirin compound. It was also tapped like maple for the sap, which was used to make birch beer. Today birch bark is used for treating headaches and for pain relief. It is a member of the Birch family.

Bird's foot violet *(Viola pedata)*. Bird's foot violet was used for treating pulmonary conditions and coughs in earlier years. There were other species of violets used in a cold formula, but this is the one I was able to verify as used by American Indians and mountains folks alike. Others used included Canada violet *(V. canadensis)*, common blue violet *(V. papillionacea)*, halberd-leaved violet *(V. hastata)*, sweet white violet *(V. blanda)*, longspurred violet *(V. rostrata)*, smooth yellow violet *(V. pensylvanica)*, and round-leaved violet *(V. rotundifolia)*.

Bittersweet *(Celastrus scandens)*. The roots of American bittersweet were chewed for allaying coughs. There is another plant called bittersweet nightshade *(Solanum dulcamara)* that has been used for treating venereal disease. It was also used by mountain folks for treating bronchitis.

Blackberry *(Rubus villosus* and *R. hispidus)*. Several of the species of blackberry plant were used in tonics for treating sore throat, including dewberry *(R. hispidus,* sometimes called swamp berry) as an astringent for colds. Blackberry was also used with wild geranium for treating thrush or fungal inflammation in the mouth. An elder called it *oo se na tu.*

Black cherry (see Wild cherry tree).

Black cohosh *(Cimicifuga racemosa)*. The value of this plant as a North Medicine was as a sedative to "relax the nerves and to settle the heart and spirit." It is also known as black snakeroot, used in earlier times as a popular snakebite remedy. Do not use black cohosh during pregnancy or while nursing.

Black-eyed Susan *(Rudbeckia hirta* or *R. fulgida)*. Called *a ga do li, gah ne ge i* ("black eye") in Cherokee, black-eyed Susan was mixed with yellow dock and yarrow and used in liquid form for treating earache. It was known by mountain folks as "deer-eye daisy." The Cherokee name of *a wi a ka ta* was mentioned by Mary Chiltoskey.

Blackgum tree *(Nyssa sylvatica)*. A small twig from the blackgum tree would be used to clean teeth and to "prevent disease of the mouth and gums, with a gargle of alumroot." Marigold *(Calendula officinalis)* was added when there was inflammation of the mucous membranes of the mouth and throat, sometimes with chamomile for its anti-inflammatory properties. Blackgum is also called black tupelo. It is a member of the Dogwood family.

Black mustard *(Brassica nigra)*. The entire black mustard plant was used for treating asthma, fever, croup, and nervous conditions. An elder said the seeds were used for treating colds, with the leaves being used for headache and toothache. This is the same mustard whose seeds are used as a food spice. Mustard is still used as a remedy for rheumatism in Appalachia, and to relax the intestines. It has an antibiotic effect due to its sulfur content.

Black snakeroot *(Aristolochia serpentaria)*. Also known as Virginia snakeroot, the roots of this plant were chewed and then sprayed or blown on a person with a fever. Black snakeroot is mixed with several other plants and barks in a tea for treating fever.

Blazing star *(Liatris spicata)*. Blazing star was also known as button snakeroot and devil's bit. It was used as a gargle for sore throats. It was also used as a diuretic, as well as an expectorant for respiratory problems. According to Mary Chiltoskey, it was used for backaches. Baneberry *(Actae pachypoda)* is also called button snakeroot.

Blessed thistle *(Cnicus benedictus)*. Blessed thistle was combined with willow or dogwood bark for use in treating respiratory inflammation and fever. Arnold Krochmal, Ph.D., mentions use of this plant by Indians as an infusion for contraception. Some mountain folks say it is used for elders with "fevers from digestive problems of chronic inflammation." In earlier years it was used for treating digestive problems and digestive tract inflammation, as well as being used as an astringent.

Bloodroot *(Sanguinaria canadensis)*. Bloodroot, sometimes called red root, or *tsi tsi* in Cherokee, was used as an expectorant. The large basal leaves from a bud on the rootstock, and the white flower, make bloodroot distinctive in the shaded and rich soils of the mountains.

I was instructed to be very careful to use bloodroot only in very small amounts. Bloodroot was used in small doses in a formula for treating cough and lung problems. Today it is used as an expectorant. Do not use bloodroot during pregnancy.

Bluebells *(Mertensia virginica)*. Little is written in the herbal literature about bluebells' use or effectiveness. Virginia bluebells was combined with several other plants for treating difficult respiratory complaints. Mountain folks still use the entire plant in making a remedy for respiratory complaints. Also known as Virginia cowslip, the plant has beautiful blue flowers that hang downward with trumpet-shaped bells. It is a great plant for the home flower garden. Bluebells is a member of the Forget-me-not, or Borage, family.

Blue flag *(Iris versicolor)*. Called snake lily, or *i na dah,* blue flag was used for treating earaches and as an eyewash. It was used with yarrow for eardrops and was sometimes "mixed with puffball for ear infections." It was also combined with echinacea and skunk cabbage for treating sores in the mouth. Crested dwarf iris *(I. cristata)* and southern blue flag *(I. virginica)* were also used with the earache remedy, which also included garlic. Today blue flag is used more for treating bruises, constipation, fluid retention, inflammation, liver disease, and sores and to stimulate the bowel.

Boneset *(Eupatorium perfoliatum)*. Boneset is also called feverwort and Indian sage. It was used for treating colds, flu, and sore throats, as also mentioned by Mary Chiltoskey. It is a member of the Aster, or Composite, family, with the unique lanceolate leaves that join on opposite sides of the stem. Today boneset is used as an expectorant and a sedative for treating bronchitis, fever, and respiratory problems.

Burdock *(Arctium lappa* and *A. minus)*. Great burdock and common burdock are used for treating coughs and asthma by making a tea from the roots. Mullein is added to the tea; mullein is also smoked to relieve coughs. Crushed burdock seeds were used as anti-inflammatory and antibacterial agents in treating fevers. Arnold and Connie Krochmal confirmed the use of common burdock in treating lung disease. A member of the Aster, or Composite, family, the burrs of the burdock plant were called "stick buttons" by mountain folks. Do not mistake burdock for common cocklebur *(Xanthium strumarium),* which grows in wet soils and was considered poisonous to livestock.

Butterfly weed (see Baneberry and Blazing star).

Butternut tree *(Juglans cinerea)*. Butternut was used for treating toothaches, as remembered by several elders. This member of the Walnut family was also used in the place of or with rhubarb as a mild laxative. The inner bark of the root and leaves were used, rather than the hard nut fruit. The nuts were eaten by wildlife, and the nut oil was used in a very old ceremony. The nut shells were used as a dye. Butternut wood was used for making boxes for "keeping special things."

Button snakeroot (see Blazing star).

Calamus root *(Acorus calamus)*. Also called sweet flag, the roots of calamus are used for treating colds and are mixed in a cough formula with nodding onion and wild cherry bark. It was used to stimulate "a sweat or perspiration for a fever." Arnold and Connie Krochmal reported that American maidenhair *(Adiantum pedatum)* was used with sweet flag to loosen phlegm and to soothe the mucous membranes in the throat. Sweet flag is used with maidenhair *(Adiantum capillus-veneris)* in a cough and respiratory formula.

Canker root *(Coptis trifolia)*. This plant is probably better known as goldthread. The small, three-leaf plant growing from yellow rhizomes resembles a strawberry plant. It is valued for treating canker sores and irritations in the mouth, as well as sore throats. It used to be mixed with alumroot, or wild geranium, as a gargle for treating mouth sores. Creeping sourgrass *(Oxalis corniculata)* was added for treating sores in the mouth and would be chewed for nausea as well. An elder said that the Penobscot Indians used it for indigestion and as an eyewash. The crushed rhizome contains the alkaloid berberine, which is a mild sedative. Goldthread is not to be confused with golden thread, or dodder *(Cuscuta megalocarpa)*, which is a parasitic plant used for treating insect stings and as a laxative. Goldthread was also called yellowroot by the southern tribes.

Carolina hemlock (see Hemlock).

Carolina horse nettle *(Solanum carolinense)*. Also known as bull nettle, Carolina horse nettle was used as a strong sedative and for treating severe asthma and bronchial conditions. This plant is a member of the Nightshade family, along with jimson weed and similar plants with prickly spines.

Carolina jasmine *(Gelsemium sempervirens)*. Carolina jasmine, sometimes called yellow jessamine, has a sweet aroma and bright yellow flowers on an evergreen vine. It was used by the eastern Indians as a sedative and painkiller in earlier years. It is a member of the Loganiaceae family.

Carolina poplar tree *(Populus deltoides)*. This tree was sometimes called southern cottonwood. This hardwood is a large tree used for everything from making matches to boxes. It was included in an earlier formula for "clearing the head"; other Medicine uses are unclear.

Carolina silverbell *(Halesia carolina)*. Carolina silverbell was called "opossum wood" by the mountain folks of the Great Smoky Mountains. The inner bark was used in a cold formula "when your mind and nose became as stuffed as the fog in the mountains." Mountain folks "used it to clear the sinuses."

Catnip *(Nepeta cataria)*. This plant familiar to the Cherokee and the mountain folks was popular as a mild central nervous system stimulant and as an antispasmodic. It contains several acids, volatile oils, and tannin, as well as nepetalactone isomers that are similar to compounds found in valerian that are effective for addressing insomnia and using as a sedative. This member of the Mint family is a favorite with children and infant "restlessness problems, especially when sick."

Catnip has many uses today, including addressing bronchitis, colds, fever, headache, and restlessness and inducing perspiration. Studies by the U.S. Forest Service have confirmed that catnip does repel some insects. The studies also found that a very small percent of the essential oil repels mosquitoes, compared to the repellent DEET, which is ineffective at low concentrations. This might be an alternative to some repellent products on the market today, given the safety concerns connected with many. The Cherokee used certain natural products to discourage insects from eating young plants in the spring planting season.

Celery *(Apium graveolens)*. The roots, leaves, and seeds of celery are used as a sedative. Celery today is used for treating many conditions, including bronchitis, asthma, cough, fever, headache, nervous conditions, and tension, as well as being a good high-fiber vegetable. Do not use celery in a medicinal way during pregnancy.

Chamomile *(Matricaria chamomilla or recutita)*. Also known as wild chamomile, this plant used for calming and insomnia is a more recent plant introduction to North America. The Cherokee recognized the value of chamomile for calming the nerves and valued the natural oils for treating allergies. Today chamomile is used for treating eye irritations, insomnia, migraine, menstrual disorders, and throat discomfort.

Chaparral *(Larrea tridentata)*. While used by western tribes, chaparral was traded with the southern tribes. It was known as creosote bush resin, a remedy for coughs. An elder said that eastern tribal members who moved to Arkansas and Oklahoma during the forced relocation of the Cherokee in the 1830s learned of chaparral's value along the Trail of Tears. When some returned to the Carolinas they brought back several chaparral plants and other similar plants for use as Medicine.

Chaparral has antibiotic, antiseptic, and anti-inflammatory properties. The resinous substance was used in a poultice by mountain folks for treating arthritis pain. While today it is used for treating acne and for slowing the skin's aging process, chaparral has been reported to cause liver damage. Another elder from Oklahoma said chaparral was used to protect the skin from the sun's harmful radiation, a use learned from our Mexican Indian brothers and sisters who were aware of its value for fighting skin cancer.

Chestnut tree *(Castanea dentata)*. The bark of American chestnut was used as a mild sedative, especially for treating severe coughs and chest congestion. Arnold and Connie Krochmal mention its use in treating worms and dysentery as well as whooping cough, or pertussis. It was also mentioned as part of a formula with blue cohosh *(Caulophyllum thalictroides)* for relaxing the system and treating sore throat and severe coughing. While no longer commonly found in the mountains, the chestnuts are still remembered as an item of trade with other tribes. Chestnut is a member of the Beech family.

Chickasaw plum *(Prunus angustifolia)*. Wild plum was used for treating fever. It was more popular in Georgia, where it was also used for treating head lice.

Chickweed *(Stellaria media)*. Chickweed was included in cold formulas and was used for treating fevers and related symptoms. A chickweed poultice was used on eye infections "and bruises." An expectorant, chickweed is used today to treat cough, fever, and sore throat. Chickweed is a member of the Pink, or Carnation, family.

Chicory *(Cichorium intybus)*. A chicory poultice was used in earlier years for treating sore eyes. Called "blue dandelion" by some mountain folks, chicory was used earlier as a nerve-tonifying tea and as a flavoring agent with coffee. Chicory has a soothing effect on the lungs.

Chinkapin tree *(Castanea pumila)*. Similar to chestnut, Allegheny chinkapin was used as a strong astringent. An elder mentioned it as being in a formula for "the effects of serious colds, especially for children." The leaves contain tannin and flavonoids, but there is little in the herbal literature to verify this. Chinkapin is a member of the Beech family.

Cinquefoil *(Potentilla simplex)*. Cinquefoil, or five-finger, was used as a gargle for treating thrush and other fungal inflammations and sores in the mouth. A plant cousin to cinquefoil is five-finger grass *(P. reptans)*, which has been found to contain tannins and flavonoids and is effective as an astringent.

Potentilla erecta, a plant found in damp areas, is used in a similar way as alumroot for treating inflammation of the gums, mouth, and throat. Several varieties of cinquefoil were used for treating fevers, inflammation of the mucous membranes of the mouth, and toothache. Cinquefoil is a member of the Rose family.

Coltsfoot *(Tussilago farfara)*. The yellow flower head of coltsfoot looks somewhat like a dandelion flower. It has heart-shaped leaves that are used as an expectorant. The flowers and leaves were used in cough syrups and as a tea or smoke for treating asthma and bronchial problems. The yellow flowers were used as an antispasmodic.

Coltsfoot has been shown to cause cancer if taken in large doses, probably due to toxic pyrrolizidine alkaloids in the plant. The plant has been banned for human consumption in the United States and Canada. This single hairy-stemmed plant is a member of the Aster, or Composite, family.

Corn *(Zea mays)*. The leaves of Indian corn, maize, or *se lu,* were used in a very old formula with rabbit tobacco and mullein for treating fever and colds. The active compounds are saponin, essential oil, and tannins. Corn kernals can be used as a stimulant for cardiac muscles and to increase blood pressure. An elder said that a "corn mush combining crushed up carrots and other vegetables" would be fed to the very ill in earlier years "to give them strength."

Cotton (*Gossypium* species). Natural fibers brought to America by the Europeans quickly found their way to the mountains. The fibers were absorbent and could be used to hold an ointment. As an elder said, "It was a newfound thing, this cotton, but the seed oil was used for asthma." Cotton was also mixed with yellow dock and yarrow and used in an earlier formula for treating earaches.

Couchgrass *(Agropyron repens)*. Also known as witchgrass, couchgrass is a remedy for respiratory complaints and coughs, including inflammation and bronchitis. An elder mentioned this is one of the favorites of an elder Medicine man who had passed on to the otherworld. It is also known by the name of triticum.

Cowslip *(Primula veris* or *P. officinalis)*. This favorite "root remedy" of the mountain folks in earlier years was "learned from the Indians." It was used for treating coughs "that were dry and had tickles." American cowslip is used for treating anxiety and insomnia, but there are side effects, such as diarrhea and nausea. While chewing the leaves was the way to take it, cowslip can irritate the digestive tract. Today the flowers are used by some as a mild sedative for children and elders. Another plant called cowslip is marsh marigold *(Caltha palustris)*, a member of the Buttercup family. Cowslip is also called primrose, not to be confused with evening primrose *(Oenothera biennis)*.

Cucumber magnolia (see Magnolia tree).

Daisy fleabane *(Erigeron philadelphicus)*. Daisy fleabane was used for treating coughs, colds, and fever. A formula used this plant with balsam fir and willow bark for people who had difficulty getting over the common cold or had a recurring low-grade fever. It was combined with wild yam and senega snakeroot for "a sore and quiet throat." An elder mentioned the combination with frost root for treating eyesight difficulties and use of this formula with urinary ailments.

The earliest record of fleabane is John Bartram's, who in 1751 mentioned its use for treating snakebites. The large white daisy flower of fleabane stands out. It is as a member of the Aster family.

Dandelion *(Taraxacum officinale)*. The leaves and roots of dandelion, "yellow flower" or *hu tsi la ha,* were used in a tea to calm the nerves. Sometimes dandelion was combined with licorice or mint leaves to ease the bitter taste. Dandelion is a member of the Aster family, along with thistle.

Devil's bit (see Blazing star and Fairywand).

Devil's shoestring *(Desmodium perplexum)*. The roots of devil's shoestring would be "used as a chew for sore gums." A wash or bath would be used to comfort a person experiencing cramps, especially for ballplayers. An elder mentioned that Creek Medicine used this plant with sassafras for treating colds.

Dogwood tree *(Cornus florida)*. The root and inner bark of *ka nah si di,* or flowering dogwood, are used to treat pain and aching muscles and headaches related to colds. It is also used in a formula as a wash for mouth sores, along with wild cherry and spicewood. Dogwood is a member of the Dogwood family. Its beautiful white flowers "are a sign of early spring with early planting of corn in the mountains."

Eastern red cedar tree *(Juniper virginiana)*. This small evergreen is also called red juniper. It is used for treating bronchitis. The nuts, leaves, and twigs were used in a boiling mixture as an inhalant and in sweat lodge ceremonies. It was used in other ceremonies as well, and for the aroma, which would "protect the house from the spirits not friendly." It is also used to "warm the spirit" by gifting the cedar shavings to a sacred fire.

An elder mentioned using Eastern red cedar with borage *(Borago officinalis)* for treating respiratory complaints. This hardy evergreen was chosen for making furniture and small boxes and was used as a finish wood in log cabins for the perfume of the wood and leaves. My father remembered cedar wood pencils in school. Cedar is a member of the Cypress family.

Echinacea (see Purple coneflower).

Elder *(Sambucus canadensis* and *S. nigra)*. Common or American elder is a large shrub or small tree that is used for treating headache and mucous congestion in the lungs and bronchial system. Sometimes willow bark is used, along with goldenrod as an anti-inflammatory. It is also combined with ground ivy for treating colds and hives. The ripe fruit and flowers are used with goldenseal and fennel for treating colds and fever. The flowers are used for treating fever and the chills; in earlier years a traditional sweat lodge would be undertaken as well "to sweat out the fever." It is a member of the Honeysuckle family.

Elecampane *(Inula helenium)*. Called wild sunflower, the roots are used with elecampane in a formula for treating coughs and lung problems. The daisylike flowers and roots are also combined with slippery elm and wild cherry. Elecampane is an astringent and an antiseptic and is regarded as a cure-all plant. Today it is used for treating asthma, bronchitis, cough, and indigestion and to stimulate the appetite. It has a bitter taste, so licorice or honey is added for sweetening. Elecampane is a member of the Aster family.

Evening primrose *(Oenothera biennis)*. Evening primrose was used for treating coughs and colds, as well as for mild depression or "feeling low." An astringent and an internal stimulant, today there are many uses for primrose oil, including being used as a treatment for asthma, cough, nerve pain, and nervousness. *Primula veris*, a plant also known as primrose, is reported by James Duke, Ph.D., as effective for treating bronchitis, cough, and laryngitis.

Due to the presence of the unsaturated fatty acid GLA, the oil from evening primrose seeds has been valued for a variety of conditions, including regulating hormonal activity and calming hyperactive children. Mountain folks used the oil in cosmetics to soften the skin and to relieve chapped or cracked skin and hands during the cold winters and the dry heat of summers. Evening primrose is a member of the Evening Primrose family.

Eyebright *(Euphrasia officinalis)*. Eyebright made its way into the American Indian Medicine bag after being used since the Middle Ages for irritated eyes and hay fever triggered by grass and tree pollens. It was combined with buckthorn and mullein in a formula for congestion, cough, and colds. Eyebright is an astringent, expectorant, and decongestant, as well as an anti-inflammatory. Today it is used for treating inflammation of the eyelids, conjunctivitis, eye fatigue, and styes. An elder said that eyebright is not as effective as other plants that were used by earlier Cherokee Medicine men and women. Eyebright is a member of the Figwort, or Snapdragon, family.

Fairywand *(Chamaelirium luteum)*. Called by common names such as devil's bit, rattlesnake root, and false unicorn root, fairywand was used as a "root chaw" for treating coughs. The unique rosette that grows from the basal leaves at ground level are easy to identify. The male flowers are white and the female flowers are green. Arnold and Connie Krochmal report that the crushed roots were used for treating uterine pain and depression. Use of fairywand is not recommended if you are pregnant. Fairywand is a member of the Lily family.

False Solomon's seal (see Solomon's seal, false).

Fennel *(Foeniculum vulgare)*. Common, or wild, fennel was used as an expectorant for respiratory conditions but was probably better known as an antispasmodic and stimulant. It was used in a formula for treating fever and coughs and as a "special Medicine" for the "sickly or weak or those who need wind." It is a member of the Carrot, or Parsley, family.

Fern, bladder *(Cystopteris protrusa)*. Bladder fern was used in a cold tea for treating fever and chills, according to Mary Chiltoskey. One elder said, "It was just one [plant] that was used in a fever remedy that really worked, if you used it early on."

Fern, brakeroot *(Polypodium vulgare)*. Brakeroot fern was used for treating coughs and respiratory problems; it was combined with honey locust *(Gleditsia triacanthos)* for addressing more serious respiratory complaints.

Fern, crested field *(Dryopteris cristata)*. The roots of crested field fern were used for reducing phlegm in the chest and for fevers.

Fern, Christmas *(Polystichum acrostichoides)*. Sometimes called southern cottonwood, the roots of Christmas fern were used for treating fever, bronchitis, and rheumatism. It was used with Balm-of-Gilead for treating toothache.

Fern, male (see Wood fern).

Feverfew *(Chrysanthemum* or *Tanacetum parthenium)*. The flowers of feverfew are similar to chamomile, although feverfew is a much taller (two to three feet), upright plant. Feverfew's strong odor helps to purify the air around the home, and it is used for alleviating asthma and allergies. Feverfew is also used for reducing fevers and nervousness. It "helps those with low spirits" and with muscle tension. The leaves are used for treating colds and indigestion. Arnold and Connie Krochmal noted the use of feverfew with children, who were given the leaves to chew for cold and fever.

Feverfew seems to have been used less by earlier Cherokee than willow bark or dogwood tree bark for treating pain. However, it was used as an anti-inflammatory and for relaxing the blood vessels. Today feverfew is used for treating asthma, fever, migraines, and toothache. It should not be used during pregnancy or while breastfeeding, according to an elder who works with female Medicine.

Fever tree *(Pinckneya pubens)*. Also called Georgia bark, fever tree was a gift from another tribe. As the name suggests, it was used to treat fever. Fever tree is a member of the Madder family, which was used by several southern Indian tribes from lower Georgia and upper Florida. It was sometimes called Indian fever bark and Indian fever root, but little is known about its use today.

Fireweed (*Epilobium angustifolium*). From the Evening Primrose family, fireweed is a native plant of Turtle Island. American Indians used it as an antispasmodic and to treat asthma. The leaves were used as a demulcent to soothe the mucous membranes. This member of the Evening Primrose family has been researched as a willow herb species. The findings show that it is an antimicrobial and an astringent. As an antimicrobial it is helpful in treating staph infections and fungal problems.

Five-finger (see Cinquefoil and Ginseng).

Foxglove, false (*Aureolaria flava*). False foxglove was used for treating asthmalike conditions and dysentery. It has been suggested for treating apoplexy and muscular weakness due to vessel constriction. Foxglove (*Digitalis purpurea*) is known as a heart stimulant and is also used for treating fever and asthma.

Fraser fir tree (*Abies fraseri*). The inner bark of Fraser fir, also called big tree or she balsam, was used as a stimulant and for treating fluids in the lungs. Sometimes Fraser fir is referred to as spruce. Both are members of the Pine family.

Georgia bark (see Fever tree).

Ginseng (*Panax quinquefolius*). Ginseng, *o ta le ga le* to the Cherokee, is also called sang or five-finger plant. It was used to help with the "wind sickness," or dizziness caused by inner ear problems, as well as headaches, vertigo, and general malaise. A tea made of ginseng and wild geranium was used as a mouthwash for treating thrush or sores in the mouth. Sometimes the leaves of *Trollius laxus,* spreading globe flower, were combined with ginseng to make a mouthwash.

Dwarf ginseng (*Panax trifolium*) was reported by Paul Hamel and Mary Chiltoskey as being used for treating cough, along with other uses. Today ginseng is used as a sedative and sleep aid for treating depression and mood swings, as well as for improving mental concentration. Ginseng is at risk of extinction in its natural environment due to "sang hunters," who can get top dollar for this plant on the overseas market. Ginseng is a member of the Ginseng family.

Globe flower (*Trollius laxus*). Paul Hamel and Mary Chiltoskey mentioned using the globe flower's leaves and stems for treating thrush, caused by fungus in the mouth. The fresh plant was used in the formula, which is an old remedy. Research on another species of globe flower has shown that the plant loses most of its active properties in drying. Globe flower was used by Europeans for treating scurvy in earlier years. It is an irritant to the gastrointestinal tract.

Goldenrod *(Solidago odora)*. The roots of goldenrod would be made into a tea for use in a tonic as a stimulant agent for "balancing the nerves, particularly for young people before ceremonial dances and competition." It was also used in a formula for wellness of the throat. Goldenrod, sometimes called sneezeweed, is a member of the Aster family. It was used with common ragweed *(Ambrosia artemisiifolia)* in a formula for serious colds. Today it is used for treating exhaustion and fatigue and sore throats.

Goldenseal *(Hydrastis canadensis)*. Also known as Indian paint or yellowroot, goldenseal was popular with the Cherokee for many uses. In the North Medicine it was used for treating a sore mouth and as part of an eyewash formula. It is used as an astringent and for antimicrobial properties to clear phlegm. The root is also combined with mullein flowers for treating earaches and ringing in the ears. Goldenseal is not to be confused with *Xanthorhiza simplicissima*, also known as yellowroot. Goldenseal is in my Medicine bag for treating sinus problems, along with yellowroot *(Xanthorhiza simplicissima)* for sore throats. Today it is a very popular plant and flower remedy used for treating eye conditions, mouth sores, and inflammation.

Gooseberry *(Ribes rotundifolium)*. A tea was made from gooseberry leaves for calming the nerves and settling the stomach. It was combined with giant ragweed *(Ambrosia trifida)* for treating colic.

Gravelroot *(Eupatorium purpureum)*. Called sweet Joe-pye weed or Indian gravelroot, gravelroot was added to an old formula with juniper *(Junipers communis)* and calcium salts for treating urinary problems. Gravelroot was used as a tonic and stimulant by mountains folks to induce sweating and to break a fever. It was used in earlier years as a soothing agent, along with juniper, an antiseptic, for taking care of respiratory problems. Another plant called gravelroot, meadowsweet *(Filipendula ulmaria)*, is listed as a West Medicine, but it was also used by earlier tribes for toothaches, headaches, and colds. Gravelroot is a member of the Aster, or Composite, family.

Ground ivy *(Glecoma hederaceae)*. An ivy tea was used in a formula for colds and as a remedy for treating hives in young children. Ivy, a member of the Mint family, has been naturalized in America. It is considered effective for clearing phlegm and is used with bayberry bark as an astringent for treating sinusitis, an expectorant for bronchitis, and a natural antiviral substance. It was also used for treating headaches and toothaches.

Hazel elder (see Elder).

Hedge mustard *(Sisymbrium officinale)*. A poultice of hedge mustard was made for treating croup. An elder said the plant was used mainly for children with colds, along with wild cherry and other mild plants for treating sore throat. Blue-eyed grass *(Sisyrinchium angustifolium)* is included in the formula with hedge mustard for treating colds and sore throat.

Heal-all *(Prunella vulgaris).* Heal-all, commonly known as self-heal and woundwort, was a favorite plant helper of several Cherokee Medicine people for treating sore throats, in the company of wild geranium. Growing in fields and streams, heal-all has small purple flowers found in the axils of the leaves. It is also identifiable by the sweet aroma. It is used to relieve gas and colic. As an elder said, "The small purplish flowers have a hairy tongue that hangs down from the cluster with a cover over it." Heal-all is used with black snakeroot and goldenrod for treating sore throats. The Cherokee added wild ginger to the formula, as well as Spanish needles *(Bidens bipinnata)* for sore throats. Heal-all is a member of the Mint family.

Hearts-a-bustin' *(Euonymus americanus).* Also called strawberry bush, this beautiful plant with the red crimson flowers and berries was used as an astringent and antiseptic in earlier years. It was also known as "heart's-a-bustin' with love." It is still used in a formula as an expectorant.

Heather *(Calluna vulgaris).* Heather was probably introduced to the Cherokee by the early Scots who came to America. Indians in West Virginia used heather as a tea to suppress coughs. It is also used as a sedative to help with sleeplessness. It is an antiseptic and expectorant. There is little in the herbal literature about heather, but it was used as a diuretic and an antimicrobial to help with kidney problems, urinary tract and prostate complaints, and gout. An elder referred to heather as "a woman's plant for healing of wounds and calming the spirit of young females." It was also used in earlier years for treating gastrointestinal and other internal complaints in old North and West Medicine formulas.

Heather is a member of the Heath family. An old Cherokee myth tells of early Medicine men and women who would use a heather stick "to cause it to rain." Heather is the name of my niece, who is sensitive and beautiful, like the plant.

Hemlock *(Tsuga caroliniana).* Hemlock was called Eastern, or Carolina, hemlock. The inner bark was used in a formula for treating colds, and the needles were placed on hot rocks in a traditional sweat when sickness was being purged. Hemlock was also used in a fever formula and as a source of tannin for an astringent. It is a member of the Pine family.

Hepatica *(Hepatica acutiloba).* Called liverleaf or liverwort, the hepatica roots were chewed for supressing coughs, treating bronchitis, and reducing fever. It was used by mountain folks in Appalachia for treating liver complaints, a use that was brought to America from Europe. The brown and greenish leaves in a tri-joined pattern are camouflaged in the fall leaves, except for the small white flowers that protrude from the ground. It is used as a mouthwash and to relieve pain and inflammation. My father called this plant "mouse ear."

Hickory tree *(Carya tomentosa)*. Called mockernut hickory or white hickory, hickory bark was chewed for sores in the mouth and for colds. Hickory is valued for making furniture, baskets, and baseball bats. The nuts were a favorite fruit used in mash, breads, soups, and other foods. Hickory is a member of the Walnut family, with butternut and Eastern black walnut. Carolina hickory *(C. australis)* is found in the Smoky Mountains.

Holly tree *(Ilex opaca)*. The leaves of American holly were used for treating chronic bronchitis. The bitter berries are popular with birds in the winter. Holly was also used for winter decoration due to the bright leaves and red berries. As an elder said about the holly, "The Great One intended for the birds to have plenty of fresh fruit for their survival and so they could sing all year-round." This plant is included in the Holly family, with yaupon.

Hophornbeam tree *(Ostrya virginiana)*. Also called ironwood, a piece of the hophornbeam bark would be held in the mouth with a piece of willow bark as treatment for a toothache. According to Mary Chiltoskey, hophornbeam was used in a hot tea with cucumber as another toothache remedy. Hophornbeam is a member of the Birch family.

Hops *(Humulus lupulus)*. Common hops, or hops vine, is probably best known for its role as a key ingredient in beer. The Cherokee and tribes over most of Turtle Island use hops as a sedative. Hops are fairly common along roadsides and fields. The vine can reach thirty feet long with opposite three- to five-toothed lobes. The small flowers are greenish yellow for male and pale green for female, with a greenish pink fruit cone that contains the hops bitters. Hops is well known as a calming and sleep-inducing plant to calm nervous energy, tension, and restlessness. Today it is used as a sedative and to ease pain.

Horehound *(Marrubium vulgare)*. With all its popularity as a candy, horehound is an effective expectorant, a substance that helps to loosen phlegm in the lungs. Also known as white horehound, it is used in a formula for treating coughs, hoarseness, and colds. It is a member of the Mint family.

Horse balm *(Collinsonia canadensis)*. Mountain folks called horse balm "richweed" and "stone root." As an astringent it was used in a formula for treating chronic bronchitis. It is also used as a gargle for hoarseness with peppermint.

Horse chestnut tree *(Aesculus hippocastanum)*. Horse chestnut, or *ti li, so qui li,* was included in a formula by the Cherokee for treating bronchitis and respiratory problems. It is a member of the Buckeye, or Horse Chestnut, family. Today it is used for treating fever and circulatory problems, including phlebitis and varicose veins.

Horsemint *(Monarda punctata* and *M. fistulosa)*. This member of the Mint family was used for treating fever and colds as well as headaches. It was used to "calm the system, like its cousin bee balm that was also used for nausea and people who were sick and ready to throw up." This plant is native to the eastern United States and was used by several eastern tribes for aiding digestion and reducing congestion. It is also known as wild bergamot *(M. fistulosa),* good for home gardens.

Horseradish *(Armoracia rusticana)*. Horseradish was used as a gargle for sore throats, and to treat colds and bronchitis. It was also used to prevent contracting colds in the winter months. It was used for diseases of the tongue and mouth, according to Mary Chiltoskey. An elder said the root cuttings were a gift from the settlers in much earlier years. Horseradish is used as a stimulant; it is often combined with agrimony for treating inflammation.

Horseweed *(Erigeron canadensis)*. Also called bittersweet or fleabane, horseweed leaves were used for treating sore throats and respiratory complaints. Arnold and Connie Krochmal noted that Indians used the tops of the leaves and the blooms in sweat lodges by placing them on the hot rocks. This plant is native to the eastern United States. As a stimulant, it is not recommended for pregnant women. The entire plant was used in earlier years for treating rheumatism and "sore back muscles from playing Indian ball." Horseweed is a member of the Nightshade family.

Huckleberry (see Bilberry).

Hyssop *(Hyssopus officinalis)*. A member of the Mint family, the hyssop flowertops are used for treating respiratory problems, as an expectorant to reduce phlegm, and for treating allergies, along with flaxseed. It is also used for treating coughs, hoarseness, and sore throat, sometimes mixed with horehound. A formula included wild cherry and anise to "relax a cough." As an expectorant hyssop relaxes the blood vessels.

Hyssop was used in many formulas and remedies as an astringent, an antiseptic, and an antibacterial. Today it is used for treating anxiety, asthma, bronchitis, colds, and sore throats. This plant should not be confused with Indian hyssop or vervain.

Indian cucumber *(Echinocystis lobata)*. Also known as wild cucumber or balsam apple, Indian cucumber was used for treating chills and fever. It is a unique plant in that it has three leaves at the top that have yellowish flowers that hang under the leaves, while a bare stem goes to another group of about eight leaves several inches below it. An elder said, "The leaves become streaked with the blood of Cherokees lost in battle in the fall. The black berries remind us of the sacredness of life."

Indian hemp *(Apocynum cannabinum)*. Also called "dropsy weed" by mountain folks and "wind weed" by earlier Cherokee, Indian hemp was used to treat breathing difficulties and asthma. This is not to be confused with hemp *(Cannabis sativa)*, which is the narcotic commonly known as marijuana.It is combined with a fern *(Pteridium aquilinum)* and cow parsnip *(Heracleum lanatum)* for treating headaches, a remedy also used by mountain folks. Indian hemp was also used to make baskets and fibers that were spun for other uses. Only use Indian hemp under the supervision of a person having expertise is the use of this plant, because it is an intestinal irritant that can increase heart contractions and lower blood pressure. Indian hemp is a member of the Dogbane family.

Indian hyssop (see Vervain).

Indian physic *(Gillenia trifoliata)*. Indian physic was used for treating asthma and colds. This is not to be confused with American hemp, which was also called Indian physic and was used as a laxative.

Indian pipe *(Monotropa uniflora)*. Earlier Indians used the juice of Indian pipe with water as an eyewash. The earlier Cherokee also used Indian pipe as a mild sedative and antispasmodic. Mountain folks referred to it as "ghost plant" because it lives from the roots of other plants. Pinesap *(Monotropa hypopithys)* is a similar plant that is cream and brown in color and is from the Wintergreen family. Indian pipe is a member of the Indian Pipe family.

Indian root *(Aralia racemosa)*. American spikenard, or Indian root, was called *yah wi ya hi* by the Cherokee. It was used for treating coughs and colds. It is sometimes called manroot, used as a food and for treating backaches. An elder said it was used for "the pains of the old ones, with sage and rabbit tobacco." An elder said that this plant, used by western and Plains Indians, is now at danger of extinction in its natural habitat. Do not use Indian root during pregnancy.

Indian tobacco *(Lobelia inflata)*. The lobeline in this plant is used as an anti-tobacco therapy. An expectorant sometimes called pukeweed, it is used as an upper respiratory stimulant for treating asthma. Indian tobacco is indigenous to North America; it is usually found in fields and meadows. It is also called wild tobacco and vomit root. Indian tobacco is a member of the Lobelia, or Bellflower, family. Another species found in

Appalachia is the great lobelia *(Lobelia siphilitica),* which "was used to cure the bad disease [venereal disease] in those earlier years when White man first came here." Mullein was also called Indian tobacco.

Jack-in-the-pulpit *(Arisaema triphyllum).* Called Indian turnip, Jack-in-the-pulpit was used as an expectorant for treating colds. The distinctive "covered funnel with three leaves standing guard has very small flowers inside the pulpit." Jack-in-the-pulpit was also used as a root poultice for treating headaches according to Mary Chiltoskey. The plant has needlelike calcium oxalate crystals that are extremely irritating and toxic. They will dissipate after exposure to dry heat. The Cherokee and the Catawba used Jack-in-the-pulpit and pitcher plant, both found in the damp woodland and bogs, for sacred purposes. Jack-in-the-pulpit was a protected plant and tribe members were encouraged not to use it except in ceremony. Jack-in-the-pulpit is a member of the Arum, or Calla, family, along with skunk cabbage.

Jasmine *(Jasminum officinale).* The flowers of yellow jasmine were used to "calm the nerves of those that would jump around a lot." Jasmine is a climbing vine and bush that blooms in early summer and into the fall with flowers that are still used in aromatherapy preparations. Jasmine flower tea calms the nerves. It was used in earlier years as a snakebite remedy, as well as "to soothe the skin." Earlier Cherokee used jasmine as a love Medicine.

Jimson weed *(Datura stramonium).* Called crazy weed or locoweed, jimson weed was used as an antispasmodic and for treating asthma. The U.S. Food and Drug Administration declared it to be poisonous; it has the effect of causing rapid heartbeat. Arnold and Connie Krochmal mention its being smoked as a treatment for shortness of breath. Today jimson weed is used for treating asthma and difficult coughs. It is a hallucinogen with potential toxicity and contains alkaloids that reduce ciliary action, an action that is needed as a bronchial expectorant. Jimson weed is a member of the Nightshade family, with wild tobacco.

Joe-pye weed (see Smokeweed).

Jumpseed *(Tovara virginiana).* Jumpseed was used as a leaf tea for treating whooping cough in earlier years. A formula of wild black cherry, wild senna, and the honey locust *(Gleditsia triacanthos)* was used for treating colds and flu. Much knowledge about the use of this plant has been lost, but it was always considered a North Medicine.

Knotweed *(Polygonum aviculare).* Also known as knotgrass or birdgrass, the roots of this plant were used in a formula for treating bronchitis and colds, as well as with alumroot for inflammation and sores in the mouth.

This plant is an astringent as well as being effective for addressing respiratory inflammation and pulmonary complaints. It is a diuretic and can be used to stop or reduce bleeding. Knotweed was used by earlier Cherokee for treating bronchitis and with alumroot or wild geranium for treating inflammation of the gums and sores in the mouth.

Lady's slipper (*Cypripedium calceolus*). This special plant, also called moccasin flower or *o ka u la su lo,* was cherished as a sacred plant by the Cherokee and other eastern tribes. The root was used as a sedative, treating anxiety, nervousness, and especially insomnia. The Cherokee value lady's slipper as an antispasmodic in possibly one or two formulas as well. Arnold and Connie Krochmal refer to it as "yellow lady's slipper," used for headache, jangling nerves, to promote sleep, and to allay pain. A pink lady's slipper *(C. acaule)* can also be found in the Smoky Mountains and Appalachia.

Today lady's slipper is used as a mild sedative and a treatment for epilepsy, headache, muscle spasms, and nervous condition. Lady's slipper is a member of the Orchid family, with puttyroot, or Adam and Eve root. There is concern that this plant is at risk of extinction in its natural environment.

Laurel tree (*Kalmia latifolia*). Mountain laurel bark was used in several formulas for North Medicine for pain relief, including as a poultice for an aching jaw. The laurel wood was used for carving utensils and as a "talking stick" that was used in groups, where only the person holding the stick would be permitted to talk. An elder said, "There are several stories about the rabbit getting caught in the twisted laurel and the prickly bramble of raspberry bushes. It seems that the rabbit was always doing the wrong thing at the wrong time and getting caught in something such as the laurel branches." An eastern cousin, white wicky *(K. cuneata)* also has white flowers but is about half the size of the mountain laurel. Mountain laurel is a member of the Heath family.

Lavender (*Lavandula vera* or *L. officinalis*). Lavender flowers are used as a sedative and a tonic to relax the nerves, as well as for reducing allergies. It is also used for "dull pain that doesn't seem to go away." It is an antiseptic and antispasmodic. According to John Lust lavender was also used as a potion to revive a person who had fainted. An earlier formula used lavender with feverfew and peppermint in a tea as a sedative and an anti-inflammatory to help with constricted blood vessels. Today it is used with tea tree *(Melaleuca alternifolia)* for treating fever and blisters.

Licorice (*Glycyrrhiza lepidota*). A substance in licorice called glycyrrhizin is said to be about fifty times sweeter than sugar and safe for diabetics. The Cherokee use wild licorice for soothing coughs in a cough formula with horehound. Today licorice is used for treating cold sores, the common cold, coughs, and mouth sores. Licorice can raise the blood pressure and the heart rate. It is a member of the Pea, or Bean, family.

Linden (see Basswood).

Liverleaf (see Hepatica).

Locust tree *(Robinia pseudoacacia).* Also known as black locust, the locust tree bears clusters of white flowers in the spring. A piece of the inner bark was placed on an aching tooth for pain relief in earlier years. Locust was popular with the Cherokee as a sacred wood for the ceremonial fire. In earlier years it was used with hickory for making bows, arrows, and other utensils for hunting and fishing. It is a member of the Legume family.

Lousewort *(Pedicularis canadensis).* Also called wood betony, lousewort was used in a cough formula and was a gargle for treating sore throat and colds. It is a member of the Figwort, or Snapdragon, family. The leaves remind me of a fern; the plant has a flower head that blooms in early spring with yellow and brown flowers. Another plant called lousewort *(Delphinium staphisagria)* is used for anxiety and nervous conditions.

Lungwort *(Pulmonaia officinalis* or *P. maculata).* Lungwort was known in the mountains as bluebells and Virginia cowslip. It was used as a remedy for severe coughing and bronchitis. The flowers look like small bells. Mountain folks called lungwort "Jerusalem cowslip" or "spotted comfrey" and used it externally for treating wounds and internally for diarrhea. The bright violet to reddish flowers make this plant a good choice for a wildflower garden. Today lungwort is used for treating bronchitis, cough, and hoarseness. It is a member of the Borage family.

Magnolia tree *(Magnolia acuminata, M. fraseri,* and *M. tripetala).* *Magnolia acuminata* was also called cucumbertree. It was used for treating toothaches, along with hophornbean. It was also used in a formula for "cleansing and the yellow look from poisons of the liver." Paul Hamel and Mary Chiltoskey mentioned its use in treating severe diarrhea with irritation that causes bleeding. Magnolia is also used as an expectorant. Another member of the Magnolia family, the yellow poplar was a very tall tree used for making "long canoes"; mountain folks used it for making furniture and musical instruments.

Maidenhair *(Adiantum capillus-veneris).* Southern maidenhair is used by crushing the rhizome and making a tea of the leaves for treating colds, cough, and hoarseness. This common fern has small leaflets that are arranged alternately on the black stem. An elder said the leaves were dried and mixed with mullein in a "smoke" for asthma. It is used as a stimulant to soothe the mucous membranes in a formula with hyssop and hore-hound. Another plant called maidenhair, or spleenwort, is also used in a cough remedy by mountain folks. Do not use maidenhair during pregnancy.

Mandrake (see Spleenwort).

Manroot *(Ipomoea pandurata)*. Manroot was used for treating asthma and severe pulmonary complaints. An elder said this was a gift from the "eastern tribes in the Carolinas, where they [the manroot] are plentiful as a cousin to the morning glory." Manroot was also known as trumpet vine or wild potato vine.

Maple tree *(Acer rubrum)*. Red maple bark was used in a formula for clearing the eyes and for sore eyes. It was thought to have a special ability to help hunters see long distances. Mountain maple *(Acer spicatum)* was used in the formula for eye infections. The Maple family also in-cludes the silver and sugar maple, used for making sugar and syrup. Arnold and Connie Krochmal noted the use of mountain maple to stimu-late appetite.

Marsh mallow *(Althaea officinalis)*. Marsh mallow was used in a cough formula with wild cherry and other tree barks for swollen mucous mem-branes. It soothes inflamed tissues and is an anti-inflammatory. The mu-cilaginous compound polysacharides is the agent that soothes mucous membranes and eases sore throats. The same compound is also found in plantain and linden, or basswood. Marsh mallow is used with hyssop as an antispasmodic and expectorant. The leaves are preferred for bron-chial healing, while the flowers are used in a cough formula.

Mallow *(Malva moschata)* was often used with marsh mallow to coat irritated membranes in the throat and for soothing coughs. An old Lumbee and coastal tribal remedy used bladderwrack *(Fucus vesiculosus)* and calen-dula flowers *(Calendula officinalis)*.

Several elders said that marsh mallow was introduced from the "set-tlers," the mountain folks, and were not one of the "old" formulas. How-ever, a combination with this plant and marigold *(Calendula officinalis)* was used for treating inflammation of the mucous membranes of the mouth. Today marsh mallow is used to soothe coughs and throat irrita-tions. Marsh mallow is a member of the Mallow family.

Masterwort (see Angelica).

Milkweed *(Euphorbia maculata)*. Also called "milk purslane" by the moun-tain folks, the milkweed root was used for treating toothaches. Another species of milkweed, *Asclepias syriaca,* or common milkweed, is used as an expectorant and to treat asthma. The four-leaved milkweed *(Asclepias* *quadrifolia)* grows in the Smoky Mountains and is used as a North Medicine. Milkweed is a member of the Milkweed family, with butterfly weed.

Mint *(Mentha arvenis).* Also known as field mint, mint was used as a tea and a stimulant for reducing fever. Mint was mixed with calamus root, dogwood bark, yarrow, and chestnut seeds crushed with flaxseed as a toothache remedy. The leaves of downy wood mint *(Blephilia ciliata)* was used with other mints as a poultice for treating headache, according to Mary Chiltoskey. Mint is a member of the Mint family.

Mistletoe *(Phoradendron flavescens).* Mistletoe was used by the Cherokee in a protected formula to calm the body and as an antispasmodic. Mistletoe is high in nutritive ingredients, including calcium, magnesium, potassium, and sodium. The quality of the plant that was protected by the formula was as a catalyst or stimulant when used with other plants. Mistletoe was used for treating nerve conditions, convulsions, and heart conditions by several tribes. Today it is used for treating depression, epilepsy, headaches, insomnia, tension, and heart conditions.

Mockernut hickory (see Hickory tree).

Motherwort *(Leonurus cardiaca).* Motherwort was used to calm nervous conditions, along with wild lettuce *(Lactuca canadensis),* which is a sedative. Motherwort was considered "too strong for general use in a cold formula, but mixed with wild lettuce it helped to calm an anxious person." Today it is used for treating heart conditions with palpitations.

Mountain dittany *(Cunila origanoides).* A tea of mountain dittany was used for treating colds, fevers, and headaches. The name *dittany* seems to have been around with mountain folks for a long time, "brought over from the old country." Mountain dittany was used for treating scalp complaints.

Mountain laurel (see Laurel tree).

Mountain mint *(Pycanthemum flexuosum* **and** *P. virginianum).* Mountain mint was used for treating fevers and colds. There is also a field mint *(Mentha arvenis)* that is sometimes called mountain mint.

Mountain tobacco (see Arnica).

Mouse ear *(Gnaphalium uliginosum* **or** *Hieracium pilosella).* Mouse ear was mentioned by an elder as used in a formula for treating colds and coughs. The herbal literature indicates that mouse ear has tannins and flavonoids that make it useful as a diuretic and as a treatment for asthma. The aerial parts of the plant were used for making remedies, including the flowers "to put some color in your face when you are sick for a long time from the winter cold and needing a spring lift."

Mullein *(Verbascum thapsus)*. Great mullein, also called Indian tobacco, or *su la e u ste* by the Cherokee, is used as a leaf or flower tea for treating colds, bronchitis, and asthma. The oil in the flowers were squeezed and used for earaches "when children would get the Oconaluftee [river water] in their ears." (The Oconaluftee is a river in the Smoky Mountains and on the Cherokee Indian Reservation in North Carolina.) Mullein was also used as a mild sedative and an anti-inflammatory. It is a member of the Figwort, or Snapdragon, family.

In earlier years mullein leaves would be used as inner soles in moccasins for comfort, the soft flannel-like leaves making a nice cushion. Panic grass *(Panicum sp.)* was also used for inner soles.

Mullein is used today as an expectorant and a treatment for asthma, bronchitis, and cough, and to stimulate earwax production. Another plant with wooly leaves that enjoys the bright sun is lamb's ears *(Stachys byzantina)*, which makes a good home flower garden plant. It has soft green and dense leaves. The nettle-leaved mullein *(V. chaixii)* with its white flower spikes is used in landscaping.

Nettle, stinging *(Urtica dioica)*. Stinging nettle plant was used by many generations of mountain folks and American Indians for treating asthma, allergies, and bronchitis. A very old formula uses this plant to prick the sore spots related to sinuses and the chest, as well as in a leaf tea for allergies. I have been in sweat lodges in which the use of stinging nettle leaves swelled mucous membranes until perspiration released some of the pent-up fluids associated with bronchial conditions. The plant was used by Indians as an astringent on the scalp, especially with the elders. As confirmed by Arnold and Connie Krochmal, it was also believed to be a sedative.

Stinging nettle is a member of the Nettle family. Another nettle called horse nettle *(Solanum carolinense)*, a plant with spines and purplish flowers, is a member of the Nightshade family. It is is used today as an expectorant and for treating asthma, cough, rheumatism, and many other conditions. Today there are many good references describing nettle's specific uses.

Nodding wild onion *(Allium cernuum)*. This wild onion was used in earlier cold formulas, as well as for treating fevers, nervous conditions, and sore throats. While unable to verify its use with liver ailments, it has been an internal cleanser used by American Indians and mountain folks as well. The combination of onion *(A. cepa)* with honey is good for treating coughs and hoarseness. As members of the Lily family, onion and garlic have antiviral properties.

Oak tree *(Quercus velutina* and *Q. prinus)*. The inner bark of oak tree was used in a formula for treating fevers, bronchitis, and coughs. As Mary

Chiltoskey said, the mortar, or *ka no na* in Cherokee, was used to beat the bark into a mush with other barks for a cold formula. Chestnut or rock chestnut oak was combined with red maple *(Acer rubrum)* or mountain maple *(A. spicatum)* and balsam fir to make an eyewash. A poultice of the same formula included American elm and wahoo tree bark for "sore eyes and to cool the head."

The mountain folks would make up "eyeberry" using raspberry and blackberry roots for sore eyes, then add purple trillium for swelling of the face. Sometimes it is used with maypop, or passionflower, for earaches. Oak was also used in tanning leather due to its high tannin content.

Today oak is used for treating many conditions, including bacterial and viral infections, bleeding gums, eye and mouth inflammation, laryngitis, mouth and throat inflammation, and tonsillitis.

Oats *(Avena sativa)*. An elder told me that "the old ones referred to oats as a nerve tonic that nature provided for the picking." Today we know of oat's ability to lower cholesterol and to calm acute and chronic anxiety. The oat straw is used for treating itch and was enjoyed by earlier Cherokee as a footbath after long hunting trips. As a North Medicine it was a nerve tonic and an "oat meal" for calming.

Orchid *(Habenaria ciliaris)*. Called yellow fringed orchid, this plant was used as a tea for treating headaches. Another Orchid family member, purple fringed orchid *(Habenaria psycodes)* has a cluster of flowers that protrude upward on a stalk about fifteen inches tall.

Pale beardtongue *(Penstemon pallidus)*. The leaves of pale beardtongue are barely seen in a field, and the flowers protrude upward on a stem about three feet tall. The white flowers have lips. The root of pale beardtongue was used as a "chaw" for easing the hurt of a painful tooth. *Penstemon canescens* is used in a similar way.

Pansy *(Viola tricolor)*. A member of the Violet family, pansy was used by the Cherokee as an expectorant and to loosen phlegm. It is a demulcent, a substance that soothes mucous membranes in the respiratory tract. It contains rutin, a natural substance used for treating glaucoma. The common blue violet *(V. papilionacea)* was included with pansy in a formula for treating respiratory complaints and bronchitis. According to James Duke, Ph.D., wild pansy can contain up to 23 percent rutin, a substance that lowers vessel pressure in the eye.

Parsnip *(Pastinaca sativa)*. The parsnip root was used in several formulas for pain relief. It was also used in earlier years for treating colds and "internal complaints"; however, the formula for its internal use has been lost. It may have been used in the same way the herbal literature suggests that parsley roots and hogweed were used for reducing fever. A conversation with an elder leads me to believe this may be so.

Passionflower (*Passiflora incarnata*). Called "maypop" by mountain folks, passionflower was used as a mild sedative for those with nervous behaviors in a formula that included hops, valerian, and hawthorn. Passionflower is an effective calming remedy with peppermint. This member of the Passifloraceae family has a very unusual purple flower with a fringe above the petals. Today it is used for its calming effects.

Pea, butterfly (*Clitoria mariana*). Butterfly pea was mentioned by a Medicine man who recommended it as a gargle for sore mouth and "weak gums." It was mixed in a formula with wild geranium (*Geranium maculatum*).

Pearly everlasting (*Anaphalis margaritacea*). Pearly everlasting was a popular plant used by American Indians in earlier years for treating colds, throat problems, and chronic coughing. This is one of the few plants of which the leaves were chewed or smoked for Medicine. Animals understand the value of this plant, which has antiseptic oils. Pearly everlasting is a member of the Aster, or Composite, family.

Pennyroyal (*Hedeoma pulegoides* and *H. hispida*). The pennyroyal leaves were used for relieving the pain of toothaches, a use that was verified by Mary Chiltoskey. The leaves would be crushed and made into a poultice to place on the head for pain relief, and a calming tea was used that included willow bark and peppermint. Pennyroyal was also used for treating "chest ailments and headaches." A mixture with goldenseal was used as a wash for "sore eyes."

Pennyroyal is often used to increase perspiration for getting rid of colds. The fever formula would either include pennyroyal or catnip. Pennyroyal has been used commercially as an insect repellent. It is a member of the Mint family.

Pennyworth (*Obolaria virginica*). Pennyworth is used in a a cold formula, as well as for cough control with wild black cherry. It was used with small children for treating colic.

Pepper (*Capsicum frutescens*). The plant and seeds of pepper or cayenne are used for treating colds and fevers. The pepper berries were used as a stimulant.

Peppermint (*Mentha piperita*). Peppermint was one of the gifts from Europeans that the Cherokee learned to enjoy and used early on for the nice smell. A member of the Mint family, peppermint is used for calming. The value of the leaves in earlier years was for treating earaches, fever, and pains. It was also used as a breath freshener. Peppermint is antiviral and acts as a mild sedative.

Periwinkle *(Vinca minor).* A member of the Dogbane, or Indian hemp, family, periwinkle was used by eastern Indians as an astringent and for calming the nerves. It was used for treating sore throats but was not used internally for circulatory complaints by the Cherokee. One elder said it was used to stop a nosebleed, and periwinkle was also used by mountain folks to stop bleeding.

An elder Cherokee who spoke very little English shared many old formulas with me that were used by the Cherokee in Arkansas, which is home to some very traditional Indian people. They remembered a "sun drink" that was actually used preventively and to ensure wellness. The drink used periwinkle's pink flowers and marigold flowers. The purpose of the drink was to prevent colds, fever, and sore throat for runners, or "deer riders," who ran long distances to take messages to the various clans of the larger tribe.

Some traditional Cherokee feel that our connection with some Mexican Indians is stronger than we know. The "sun drink" was an ancient remedy that used the sunflower as the key ingredient, as the Cherokee do. We consider the flowers of this special plant as "healing that comes from the Sun as an 'apportioner' looking over us as we work in the planting fields," in the words of one Cherokee elder.

Persimmon tree *(Diospyros virginiana).* As Mary Chiltoskey mentioned, the bark of persimmon tree was used for treating toothaches. The mountain folks also used it as a remedy for throat and tonsil problems. An infusion would include persimmon, alder, walnut, and wild cherry. One elder said that it was used for "thrush and sores in the mouth" related to fungus. Persimmon was called common persimmon or possumwood. The sweet fruit contains tannin, which is an astringent. It was used in pudding and breads. Persimmon is a member of the Ebony family.

Pine tree *(Pinus virginiana, P. strobus,* and other species). There are many species in the Pine family, including shortleaf *(P. echinata),* longleaf *(P. palustris),* spruce, pitch, eastern white, Scotch, and Virginia pine. "Scrub pine," white pine *(P. strobus),* was commonly used in a cough formula with slippery elm. It was also used with witch hazel and spicewood for reducing fever, according to Mary Chiltoskey. Pine bark and needles were used in a tea with apple for the ballplayers, in order that they "have good wind for running."

Pine bark is considered a sacred Medicine for "wind and healing of the spirit." It is used today as an expectorant for treating congestion and coughs.

Plantain, rattlesnake *(Goodyera pubescens).* A wash of plantain and willow bark would be used for relieving toothaches and "aching gums." I suspect that the astringent and antiseptic abilities of the plantain, along with salicin or natural aspirin, provided pain relief. An elder said, "a chew blend of plantain leaf and Spanish needles" was used for treating sore throats. Rattlesnake plantain is a member of the Plantain family.

Pleurisy root (Asclepias tuberosa). Also called butterfly weed, chigger weed, or witch weed, pleurisy root has been used as a carminative, a stimulant, a diuretic, and an expectorant. It was commonly used for treating respiratory problems in earlier years. Several of the southeastern Indian tribes would chew on the dried or boiled root as a remedy for bronchitis and fevers and to promote perspiration. A member of the Milkweed family, pleurisy root is used with cayenne at the first signs of a cold.

Poke or Pokeweed (Phytolacca americana). Poke leaves were combined with lemon balm and used in a tea to reduce phlegm and to "calm the chest when you have a deep cold and cough."

Poplar tree (Liriodendron tulipifera). Also known as tulip poplar, the Cherokee called poplar *tsi yu,* "big tree." This very tall tree was introduced to Europe by early Virginia colonists. The inner bark was valued in a cough formula with wild black cherry. A Medicine elder referred to it as the "ancestor tree," probably because it is native to this part of America. The elder called it white tree, and he said his grandfather used the bark with dogwood bark for "anything that ails you, including fever and colds."

Today poplar is recognized for its use in treating common cold and rheumatism. Tulip poplar was a good hardwood for making canoes in earlier years.

Puffball (Lycoperdon pyriforme). While puffball is not used today, it was part of a formula "used for infections and irritations in the ear." The mature spores of the fungus are used as a powdered or dust substance that was blown into the ear or used as a wash. An elder said it was used for treating nosebleeds, along with plantain leaf. It was suggested by one elder as used for "skin problems," but its exact application was unclear.

Puffball, blue (Myxos). This slime mold, or myxomycetes, is in the kingdom of Protoctista and was used to treat ear and other infections. The mold is a part of the "Great One's Universal Circle with animals, bacteria, fungi, and plants." Puffball was used in the inner ear for treating infections.

Purple coneflower (Echinacea purpurea). Commonly called echinacea today, purple coneflower is used for treating fevers and mouth and ear infections and as an anti-inflammatory. It was used in earlier years with dogwood bark and yarrow for treating toothaches and headaches caused by infection and inflammation. Like ginseng, purple coneflower seems to be less abundant in its natural environment in recent years. Its popularity today for treating colds and as an antibiotic has also caused it to be taken in great quantities from its natural habitat.

Purslane *(Portulaca oleracea).* The inner bark of purslane would be crushed between two rocks, and the juice would be mixed with warm water for treating earaches. One Medicine man added balsam fir and pine to the formula and used it for treating mild depression. Purslane is a member of the Purslane family.

Puttyroot (see Adam and Eve root).

Queen Anne's lace *(Daucus carota).* A special children's formula of Queen Anne's lace used for treating hoarseness and colds includes horehound and wild cherry. The white flowers are in fairly large umbels; they bloom in the summer and into the fall. Also known as wild carrot, Queen Anne's lace is a member of the Carrot, or Parsley, family. Do not use Queen Anne's lace during pregnancy.

Rabbit tobacco *(Gnaphalium obtusifolium).* Also called "sweet everlasting" or "cudweed" by mountain folks, rabbit tobacco was used in a bath to calm the nerves; the leaves were smoked for relieving asthma; a tea was prepared for taking care of colds; and the young twigs were chewed for relieving sore mouth and throat. A formula added pine bark and mullein for respiratory problems. Rabbit tobacco was also known by mountain folks as "catfoot," "golden motherwort," and "white balsam."

Ramps *(Allium tricoccum).* The juice of ramps was added to warm water for treating earache. Ramps were eaten for relieving colds and were combined with nodding onions for treating croup and as a spring tonic. As one elder said, "You didn't have to worry about getting a cold or passing a cold on. If you ate ramps nobody would get within ten feet of you, 'cause of the smell." Ramps were called "wild leek" by mountain folks.

Raspberry *(Rubus odoratus).* Called *yun oo gi sti* by the Cherokee, the root of this member of the Rose family was chewed for relieving coughs. It was used as a poultice and wash for sore eyes along with huckleberry. Raspberry has a red fruit that is popular in Appalachia for making jams. Black raspberry *(R. occidentalis)* is also found in the mountains.

Today raspberry is recognized as effective in treating canker sores, cough, infections, inflamed tonsils, inflammation, and sore throats. Studies demonstrate that parts of raspberry plant are rich in niacin, potassium, and iron. It may even help to inhibit cancer cell growth, raspberry being an excellent source of ellagin acid. Blackberry can be added to a raspberry-based remedy for powerful antioxidants that encourage good health.

Redbud *(Cercis canadensis).* The inner bark of eastern redbud, a member of the Legume family, is used in a formula for treating severe coughs, particularly with children. The pink flowers cover the tree in the spring, which makes it a beautiful tree in a yard. The woods of the Great Smoky Mountains are very beautiful when the redbud blooms in spring.

Red clover *(Trifolium pratense).* Also called wild clover, red clover was used in a formula for treating bronchitis, sore throats, coughs, and colds, as well as for calming the nerves. It is a member of the Pea, or Bean, family. The formulas also included angelica, elecampane, trillium, white pine, white oak, and false Solomon's seal for a "powerful remedy" for treating bronchial problems and as an expectorant. An elder said one of the favorite cold formulas included red clover, angelica, pine or spruce, and rattlesnake plantain *(Goodyera pubescens)* "with a added bit of peppermint and yellow fringed orchid for the headaches of colds. It was also used for toothaches." This use was verified by Paul Hamel and Mary Chiltoskey. An elder of the Lumbee tribe remembered a remedy for purification and ceremony with red clover and yellow dock.

Red clover should not be used during pregnancy or while taking blood thinners. The plant's phytoestrogens are a helper to postmenopausal women.

Red root *(Lachnanthes caroliniana).* Red root was used as an astringent for treating sore mouth and gums and sore throat. It was combined in a formula with poor robin's plantain for treating colds. New Jersey tea *(Ceanothus americanus),* a plant in the Buckthorn family that was used for treating toothaches, was also called red root. Red root was used as a tea substitute in earlier years by mountain folks.

Rhododendron *(Rhododendron maximum* and *R. catawbiense).* The Catawba, or purple, rhododendron leaves were used as a wrap tied around the head for relieving headaches. A tea of willow bark and peppermint or mint would be used internally.

My Uncle Grady referred to rhododendron as "laurel"; in fact, the two plants are often seen together. The home of the Cherokee, next to the Great Smoky Mountains, has a beautiful array (and display, in flowering season) of rhododendron, or great laurel *(R. maximum),* and mountain laurel *(Kalmia latifolia),* a member of the Heath family. He and my father enjoyed telling of their adventures in the mountains. They would always make reference to the beautiful Catawba rhododendron with its show of pink to purple blossom that they would gather for their mother and special young ladies. It is my understanding that the word *rhododendron* is Latin for "rose tree."

Earlier Cherokee prized this beautiful showy plant long before White men set foot in the mountains of North America. There is a story about how the blooms represent the tears of warriors lost in preserving and protecting the tribe from intruders. The Great Smoky Mountains National Park and the Blue Ridge Parkway are teeming with these beautiful gifts of the Great One. The wood is still popular for use in ceremonies and dances at the Fall Festival in Cherokee, North Carolina.

Rue *(Ruta graveolens).* Rue was used by American Indians for cough suppression. It was smoked with tobacco as a sedative and to treat neuralgia by Indians and earlier settlers in Appalachia. Today rue is used for relieving eyestrain. Common rue leaves can cause poisoning if handled fresh.

Sage *(Salvia officinalis).* A tea made of sage leaves was used for treating asthma and colds, as well as for "sores in the mouth." It was used in earlier years for treating inflammation in the mouth and throat. This member of the Mint family was also used for night sweats as a "power plant of special value, given by the Great One." John Lust mentions it being used for treating nervous conditions, vertigo, and with mild depression. Purple sage *(S. purpurea)* was included in a formula "said to be a helper to the elders for good memory," according to a Natchez-Cherokee elder. Today sage is used in treating gingivitis and sore throat.

Sassafras tree *(Sassafras albidum).* Sassafras, or *ka na s da tsi,* was used for treating bronchitis. An elder called it *ka sta ste* and said it was used "in the olden days for pain in the lungs." It was used by the Cherokee as a poultice for sore eyes and for respiratory complaints. It was also used in a drink, along with pine bark, to "give the runners in the old days 'strong wind' so they could flow like the wind." Today it is used to promote sweating and to enhance physical performance. Sassafras contains safrole, which has been shown to cause cancer. It is not recommended for use due to findings regarding this potential carcinogen. It is a member of the Laurel family.

Saw palmetto *(Serenoa serrulata).* Southeastern tribes knew the value of the leaves, roots, and seeds of saw palmetto for relieving intestinal complaints. The dried berries were used as a sedative. It was prepared as a root drink for treating respiratory infections and to "improve the wind in ball players." John Lust mentions it as a tonic for strength. Earlier use was as a diuretic and for its antiseptic properties. Saw palmetto is a member of the Palmetto family.

Senega snakeroot *(Polygala senega).* Senega snakeroot was used in much earlier years as a remedy for poisonous snakebites. More recently it has been used for treating pleurisy and croup. This member of the Milkwort family was included in a formula by the Cherokee and the Seneca Indians for treating pneumonia and pulmonary infections. Today it is considered effective as an expectorant for reducing upper respiratory phlegm.

**Sensitive plant *(Cassia* or *Senna nictitans).* ** Sensitive plant was used with wild senna *(Senna marilandica)* for "weak ballplayers who would pass out." It was also used for children who experienced fainting spells. One elder mentioned its use in a formula for respiratory conditions, particularly with children. The name can be confused with sensitive fern *(Onoclea sensibilis),* which is a tall evergreen fern.

**Shepherd's purse *(Capsella bursa-pastoris).* ** As an elder put it, "In my Medicine bag is the plant sheperd's bag for nosebleed and to clear my chest of that sticky mucus." Shepherd's purse is a member of the Mustard, or Cruciferae, family. Arnold and Connie Krochmal confirmed that the plant was used by Appalachian mountain folks by putting the juice on cotton to plug the nostrils during nosebleed.

**Skullcap *(Scutellaria lateriflora).* ** Skullcap was favored by the Cherokee as a sedative. The entire plant was used in a formula for treating difficult respiratory conditions and bronchitis. It relaxes and promotes healing of "frazzled nerves." Another combination used wood betony *(Stachys officinalis)* with skullcap, especially for relieving tension, stress, and headaches.

A member of the Mint family, skullcap is found in damp areas and near swamps. Today skullcap is used for treating seizures, chronic spasms, stroke, and movement disorders. Be sure to purchase the product from a reputable dealer to avoid adulteration of the alkaloids from germander, or wood sage *(Teucrium canadense).*

**Skunk cabbage *(Symplocarpus foetidus).* ** This member of the Arum, or Calla, family was used for treating respiratory, cough, and bronchial problems. It was also used for treating nervous conditions. Today it is used for treating asthma, bronchitis, nervousness, tightness in the chest, severe cough, and headaches with irritability. The unpleasant smell is a natural defense of the plant to drive away certain insects while attracting others, such as flies.

**Slippery elm tree *(Ulmus rubra).* ** The inner bark of slippery elm was valued for its astringent ability in treating coughs and colds and as a poultice. It was also a Creek remedy for toothache. Today slippery elm is considered at risk of extinction in its natural environment. Slippery elm is a member of the Elm family of trees.

**Smallflower *(Ranunculus abortivus).* ** Also called smallflower buttercup, smallflower was used as a sedative and for treating sore throat and mouth sores. One elder used this plant, but there were others he preferred to collect and dry for the same purposes, including goldenrod and ragweed.

Smokeweed (Eupatorium maculatum). The smokeweed stem was used to spray a liquid substance directly on the body. An elder said the plant stem made a good tube for "blowing the Medicine directly on the wound, like a spray can or bottle does today." The leaves were used with pain plant, a plant that is not known to me, for treating rheumatism, and were smoked with mullein for relieving lung conditions, "but not like tobacco."

Sneezeweed (Helenium amarum and H. tenuifolium). An elder said that "Bitterweed [sneezeweed] should not be confused with other plants, such as goldenrod, that are also called sneezeweed." It was used for "helping with the mucus in the nasal passages." It was also used as a "special plant for fishing." Sneezeweed is also used in a formula for treating colds and sinus complaints.

Soapwort (Saponaria officinalis). Also called bouncing bet, the leaves were used in washing clothes by the eastern tribes. It was used externally as a wash for itchy skin and as a poultice with burdock and dock. The primary use for this member of the Pink, or Carnation, family was as an expectorant for respiratory problems and bronchitis. Today it is used to expel mucus from the lungs. My father and Uncle Grady knew the plant as wild sweet William, a helper for cough and cold remedies.

Solomon's seal (Polygonatum biflorum). A tea of Solomon's seal root was used as a tonic for colds. The plant is different from false Solomon's seal; you can identify Solomon's seal by the small flowers that hang down from the axils of the leaves. It was also used to increase perspiration in sweat lodge ceremonies.

Solomon's seal, false (Smilacina racemosa). A member of the Lily family, the flowers grow in a cluster upright from the rootstock. False Solomon's seal was used as a wash for sore eyes. There were many uses of this plant by American Indians as a tonic. Arnold Krochmal mentions it as "fat solomon plume" (Smilacina amplexicaulis). Mountain folks used it as "a smoke to relieve a fainting person."

Sourwood tree (Oxydendrum arboreum). Commonly known as lily-of-the-valley, sourwood was used in a tea for calming the nerves. It was mentioned by a Medicine elder as being used as a tonic. The leaves were used for reducing fevers in a drink for elders.

Speedwell (Veronica officinalis). This member of the Figwort, or Snapdragon, family was used as an expectorant for treating respiratory problems and migraine headaches and as a gargle for sore mouth. It was used for treating chills and cough, and the juice was used as a warm wash for earache. An old remedy, speedwell was used by mountain folks for bronchitis.

Spicewood *(Lindera benzoin)*. Known as allspice, this plant was used for treating colds and coughs. An elder said it was a plant of choice for "Cherokee mothers whose children had the croup." It was valued as a spring tonic. Spicewood was combined with wild cherry and horehound in a formula for the "winter months of colds."

Spleenwort *(Aspenium platyneuron)*. Called mandrake, this evergreen fern was used with other plants in a formula as an eyewash. Another plant called mandrake *(Mandragora officinarum)* was used for treating skin conditions and warts.

Spotted cranesbill or cranesbill (see Alumroot).

Spruce tree *(Picea rubens)*. Eastern red spruce was used in a cold formula. The Smoky Mountains has virgin spruce fir in the National Park. Spruce is a member of the Pine family. *Picea excelsa* was used as an expectorant and tea for treating coughs and bronchitis, as well as a vapor that included wintergreen.

St. John's wort *(Hypericum perforatum)*. While popular today for calming and treating mild depression, St. John's wort has been used by American Indians for respiratory complaints. It is an anti-inflammatory substance used against bacteria. A helper to the nervous system, a formula includes vervain flowers and leaves, with dogwood and pine for pain relief.

Strawberry, wild *(Fragaria virginiana)*. Virginia, or wild, strawberry was used as a leaf tea to calm the nerves as a North Medicine. Strawberry was combined with other plants in a drink that was refreshing and relaxing after long hunting trips.

Sumac shrub *(Rhus copallina)*. Sumac, or dwarf sumac, is native to the eastern United States. It was used for treating nausea; the taste of the berries were known to "settle the system." Poison sumac *(R. verix)* was used as a "special Medicine" formula for treating fever and asthma. It was combined by "only those trained in how to prepare the Medicine, 'cause it is a poisonous plant." It is a member of the Cashew family.

Sunflower *(Helianthus annuus)*. The large black and yellow flowers of common sunflower are considered sacred by many American Indians. It is one of the first flowers in the old myths to be a gift from the Sun, a peacemaker plant. Sunflower protects the "planting fields and looks over the new shoots coming into this world to be food and helpers." The entire plant was used for treating bronchitis and respiratory conditions. Sunflower is a member of the Aster, or Composite, family.

Sweet everlasting (see Rabbit tobacco).

Sweetgum tree *(Liquidambar styraciflua)*. A tea made of the bark of sweetgum tree was used for calming the nerves.The inner bark, leaves, and rosin were used for "gum and tooth pain." Sweetgum was an important timber tree for production, second to oak for hardwood. The sweetgum, or *se la le,* was obtained by peeling the bark and scraping the resin substance, which would be chewed. Sweetgum is a member of the Witch Hazel family.

Sweet plant (see Anise).

Sycamore maple *(Acer pseudo-plantanus)*. Sycamore maple was used as an eyewash and to treat sore eyes. The inner bark is still used today for treating colds. *Acer* species were used as a "bark wash" for the eyes. Sycamore was also used as an astringent in several formulas. It is a member of the Maple family.

Thimbleweed *(Anemone virginica)*. A tea from the thimbleweed roots was used with other plants in a formula to relieve severe coughing. It is a member of the Buttercup, or Crowfoot, family. Golden glow *(Rudbeckia laciniata)* is another plant that has the common name of thimbleweed.

Thistle, sowthistle *(Sonchus arvensis)*. Sowthistle was used as a tea to calm the nerves or to "settle a person down who has took to the angers." Common sowthistle *(S. oleraceus)* is an old remedy used by mountain folks for calming. The plant attracts beneficial insects.

Thunder plant *(Sempervivum tectorum)*. Also called houseleek, a small amount of the juice of thunder plant was squeezed from the leaves and used in a warm wash for earaches, according to Mary Chiltoskey. Thunder plant is a member of the Saxifrage family.

Thyme *(Thymus vulgaris)*. This plant was traditionally used for treating coughs and spasms. It is an antitussive, which relieves coughing; it is also an antispasmodic, an expectorant, and an antiseptic. Today thyme is used for treating coughs and headaches. It is also good as an antibacterial agent for treating bronchitis. Thyme is one of those special heal-all herbals in my Medicine bag for the healing of mucous membranes, especially when I've contracted a virus. Add one of the mint teas for flavor and calming to relieve some of the restlessness.

Tickseed *(Desmodium nudiflorum)*. The roots of tickseed were used for treating sores and fungus in the mouth and gingivitis. Combined with wild geranium and alumroot, it made a good wash and gargle.Tick-trefoil *(D. canadense)* is also called devil's thistle or tick clover for its burrlike pods that stick to a person or animals. Tickseed is a member of the Pea, or Bean, family.

Tobacco *(Nicotiana rustica)*. Tobacco was used to treat dizziness and fainting. Sacred tobacco *(N. tabacum)* was a favorite for the Cherokee for ceremonial use, along with Indian tobacco *(Lobelia inflata)* in earlier years. Some referred to tobacco rustica as "wild tobacco." Tobacco was used for the external treatment of insect bites and snakebites. It was also used for treating fevers, chills, cramps, nervous conditions, and pain in formulas from earlier years. However, caution is suggested because the leaves contain a toxic alkaloid, nicotine, that can be absorbed through the skin. Tobacco is a member of the Nightshade family.

Tomato *(Lycopersicon esculentum)*. It may seem ironic that tomato was considered a Medicine in earlier years. Several foods were used as Medicine, including cabbage, celery, and carrots. Add tomatoes and nodding onions to a warm soup and you have a very old Cherokee formula for treating colds and fever. This is another plant in which the elders have said researchers will find other healing agents in the future. While a part of the world thought tomato was poisonous in much earlier years, American Indians created some wonderful dishes with them.

Toothache tree *(Zanthoxylum americanum)*. Commonly called prickly ash, a twig of this tree was chewed for relieving the pain of toothache in earlier years. A formula of calamus root, licorice, spleenwort, and skunk cabbage was also used for treating toothaches and inflammation. It was also combined with marginal shield fern *(Dryoperis marginalis)* and rattlesnake master *(Eryngium yuccifolium)* in a formula as a toothache remedy. Toothache tree is a member of the Rue, or Citrus, family.

Toothwort *(Cardamine diphylla)*. The root of toothwort would be crushed between two rocks and applied as a poultice for treating headache. The root would be chewed for treating colds and prepared as a tea for treating sore throats. The bark of hazel alder *(Alnus rugosa)* would be added for treating for toothaches and inflammation.

Trailing-arbutus *(Epigaea repens)*. A formula of this plant with others (now lost) was used for addressing lung complaints. An elder said this plant was a gift from the Catawba and the Creek in the south of Georgia, and "some tribe I cannot remember about a creek [Pee Dee] that would get it from the wetlands." The elder was referring to the Pee Dee River in North Carolina. The Cherokee would trade with the Catawba and other tribes who lived along the river and called trailing-arbutus by the name of "terrapin's foot." Trailing-arbutus is plentiful in the Sandhills areas of the Carolinas.

Twinleaf *(Jeffersonia diphylla)*. Also called butterfly plant, twinleaf was used as an expectorant and as a gargle for treating sore throat by the Cherokee and mountain folks in Appalachia. Sometimes called yellowroot, it is not to be confused with goldenseal or with *Xanthorhiza simplicissima*, both of which are also called yellowroot. An old formula mixes twinleaf with blue cohosh, mayapple, and barberry for "difficult problems of breath," but the mixtures were not identified.

Unicorn root *(Aletris farinosa)*. Paul Hamel and Mary Chiltoskey mentioned the use of this plant for treating colic, cough, fever, and lung ailments. An elder familiar with this plant said it was used as a tonic, but that it did have some narcotic effects as a sedative. Unicorn root was used with peach, wild plum, and wild cherry for a cough syrup in earlier years. It is also known as love plant, blazing star, devil's bit, and colic root. Cherokee elders refer to this plant as "true unicorn root," as compard to false unicorn root *(Chamaelirium luteum)*, another plant that is in danger of extinction in its natural habitat.

Valerian *(Valeriana officinalis)*. In earlier years valerian was commonly known as all-heal. It was used for calming the nervous system and was used for children who experienced unusual excitability problems. This plant was most often used by itself, not in formulas, as a tranquilizer and antispasmodic. The plant was not considered as a "strong Medicine" for the nerves.

The herb's sedative effect is due to the volatile oil in the plant and other compounds known as valepotriates. Valerian acts as a sedative by depressing activity in the central nervous system. It helps to relieve anxiety by reducing excess activity in the brain and spinal cord, and it improves sleep quality. Externally it was used for eyestrain.

Today valerian is used to treat restlessness, muscle spasms, tension, and sleep disorders. A small percent of the population will respond to Valerian as a stimulant. In that case, use chamomile with passionflower, skullcap, or hops. Some folks still get valerian confused with Valium, a prescription drug that can have serious side effects. Valerian is safe in proper dosages.

Vervain *(Verbena officinalis)*. Also known as Indian hyssop, vervain was used for treating fever, along with pine, balsam fir, and dogwood, in a very old formula for reducing fever and chills. My Uncle Grady pointed out plants that were used during the Civil War for treating respiratory and stomach complaints as well as fever.

According to John Lust vervain was used for congestion in the throat and chest. It was valued as a "special remedy for those who felt low a lot of the time," as well as used for the "pains of the back and head." Today it is used for many purposes that include bronchitis, the common cold, eye diseases, insomnia, and to help expel mucus from the lungs and quell severe coughs. Do not use vervain during pregnancy.

Violet *(Viola odorata)*. A member of the Violet family, the leaves and flowers of sweet or garden violet are used as an expectorant to loosen phlegm in the chest and relieve pulmonary problems. It has been mentioned in earlier formulas of the Cherokee for "wind in the chest." The common little violet has been naturalized here in America; it is likely a native of Europe.

Violet is used for calming, insomnia, and nervous conditions and as an anti-inflammatory and expectorant. Violet was combined with American maidenhair *(Adiantum pedatum)* as a "smoke for asthma and fever." Earlier southeastern tribes used it with dogwood for treating pain and headaches, bronchitis, and "deep coughs." An elder referred to violet as *ou ste,* or "little plant with a big punch." The same elder said, "This little plant is good for cooking when you want something for a sweet tooth."

Virginia cowslip (see Lungwort).

Wahoo tree *(Euonymus atropurpureus)*. Eastern wahoo is said to be named from a Creek Indian word. The Creeks and other southeastern tribes used it for reducing fevers. It was also used by mountain people in Appalachia for treating head lice. The crushed bark was prepared to a "fine powder and was used on the scalp for dandruff and its irritation, sometimes with stinging nettle." Eastern wahoo *(Euonymus atropurpureus)* was used for reducing fevers and in Appalachia for head lice. Today it is used for chills, fainting, seizures, and weakness. The seeds are considered poisonous and should not taken internally. Wahoo is a member of the Bittersweet family.

Walnut tree *(Juglans nigra)*. The bark of black walnut, white walnut, or walnut would be chewed for relieving a toothache. Walnut is also used for colds and fevers. This is a popular tree in the Smoky Mountains and Appalachia for furniture making and for use as gunstock, as well as for carving. Walnut was also used for preparing black dye, along with black sumac, butternut, and sourwood. Walnut was considered as one of the sacred woods for carving items used in ceremonies, along with cherry and buckeye. There is also a butternut or white walnut *(Juglans cineria)* used as a laxative to encourage movement in the intestines. Walnut is a member of the Walnut family.

Watercress *(Nasturtium officinale)*. This member of the Mustard, or Cruciferae, family is found near the water and in low, damp places in the woods. It is used for treating colds, nervous conditions, stomach ailments, and hives. Earlier Indians used it in a formula for colds, cough, and bronchitis. The leaves were placed over open hot coals and breathed into the lungs; it was also prepared as a "sipping tea," as well as being chopped and eaten as a salad. My mother would chop and soak the large leaves in warm water before mixing in other wild greens for a salad.

White clover *(Trifolium repens)*. This plant was dried and used in the winter months for reducing fevers. While white clover was specifically mentioned for fevers, red clover *(T. practense)* was used as a mild sedative in the North Medicine.

White hickory (see Hickory tree).

Wild apple (see Apple tree).

Wild carrot (see Queen Anne's lace).

Wild chamomile (see Chamomile).

Wild cherry tree *(Prunus serotina)*. The bark of wild black cherry, or *ta ya, gah na ge,* is probably best known as an ingredient in cough remedies or for relief of pains and muscular soreness. Wild cherry was also used in jellies and jams and was added to wines in earlier years. A native of North America, American Indians have used wild cherry inner bark, or *te te ya,* for many formulas. Sometimes wild plum *(Prunus americana)* was combined with wild cherry to make a cough syrup.

Wild cherry was also used as a tonic to loosen phlegm in the chest and as an astringent for the mucous membranes. Wild cherry is used in cold remedies for treating cough, bronchitis, tuberculosis, and fevers. The volatile oil is used for asthma as a stimulant for aiding appetite and digestion. It is also used to calm the nerves or as a mild sedative to "quiet the nerves of an ill or irritable child."

Wild cherry is a member of the Rose family. Cherry wood is still popular for carvings, along with walnut and buckeye. Today it is used for treating colds, cough, and respiratory conditions.

Wild clover (see Red clover).

Wild geranium *(Geranium maculatum)*. Also known as alumroot or American cranesbill, wild geranium was used for treating sore throats. It was used in a mouthwash for sore throats and thrush in earlier years. For more severe sores in the mouth, it was combined with red root *(Lachinanthes caroliniana)*. It is used as an astringent today for treating lip and mouth inflammation, sores, and sore throat. Alumroot *(Heuchera americana)* is also used for sores in the mouth and sore throat.

Wild horehound *(Eupatorium pilosum)*. Wild horehound was used for treating colds and respiratory complaints, as well as constipation and breast complaints. Another southern tribe, the Lumbee, used rabbit tobacco, pine, and goldenrod for treating colds. The natural horehound flavoring used in candies and drops is white horehound *(Marrubium vulgare)*, which is also used for treating colds.

Wild hyssop *(Verbena hastata)*. In earlier years wild hyssop, also called blue vervain, was used for treating coughs, colds, flu, and fever. It is still included in a formula for treating colds and fever that also includes vervain *(V. officinalis)*, a plant that is also known as wild hyssop. Wild hyssop was combined with white vervain *(V. urticifolia)* by mountain folks and used for treating rashes and hives.

Wild indigo *(Baptisia tinctoria)*. Wild indigo has been used as a tonic and antiseptic for cold sores and colds. This member of the Pea, or Bean, Family was also used as a toothache remedy and in a cold formula in North Medicine. Blue indigo *(B. indigofera)* was used as a blue dye.

Wild lettuce *(Lactuca villosa)*. Wild lettuce was used as a natural relaxant and was mixed with passionflower "for stronger nerve action" when used as a sedative. The leaves were gathered when the flowers had completed their blooming; the flowers were then dried and used "for general pains." An elder said, "Wild lettuce had to be used when nothing stronger was available for persons with deep cuts or wounds, to kinda' sedate the person."

Wild licorice *(Glycyrrhiza lepidota)*. This plant is still a favorite for use in formulas for treating asthma, cough, and sore throats. The European variety, *G. glabra,* is cultivated in the United States and other countries. It is a common variety used as a flavoring and sweetener in products such as toothpaste, beverages, and candies. It is also used in throat lozenges and to treat cold sores, cough, and the common cold. My grandfather had a tobacco blend with licorice in it, and it was used in gum, toothpastes, and lozenges. The concern with concentrated use of licorice is with the heart and high blood pressure problems.

Wild plum (see Chickasaw plum).

Wild sunflower (see Elecampane).

Willow tree *(Salix alba)*. The white willow is usually used with the inner bark of balsam and wild cherry. It is used as an expectorant and to reduce fevers. It is also an anti-inflammatory and antiseptic, as well as an astringent. The Cherokee used it in a formula to reduce congestion by burning the leaves in a "sweat" or as a hot tea. Researchers isolated salicin in about 1830; it has been synthesized as acetylsalicylic acid, or commercially produced as aspirin. Another member of the Willow family is black willow, or pussy willow *(Salix nigra)*, which contains tannins used as astringent and the glycoside salicin for pain. Today willow is recognized for reducing fever, inflammation, and pain.

Wild flower (see Anemone).

Wintergreen shrub *(Chimaphila maculata)*. This evergreen shrub grows to about a foot high; it has dark and shiny green lancelike leaves. The flowers atop the leaves are whitish brown with violet-colored spots inside. The leaves are used in a formula for nervous conditions. Krochmal called wintergreen spotted wintergreen, as the cream-colored flowers have small spots of violet on them. He also noted its use for treating nervous disorders and ulcers. Wintergreen *(Gaultheria procumbens)* was mentioned for use with chronic colds, gum inflammation, and other problems. The wintergreen oil can be toxic and should not be used internally from the plants without having someone specialized in its use administering it. Today wintergreen is used for joint pain and muscle strain.

Witch hazel shrub *(Hamamelis virginiana)*. The leaves, twigs, and bark of this shrub or small tree are used in a tea for fever and sore throats. This member of the Witch Hazel family is a mild astringent. In earlier years it was combined with chestnut bark and hops as a poultice for treating earache.

Wood anemone (see Anemone).

Wood betony *(Stachys officinalis)*. Betony, or wood betony, was used with arrowroot and other barks in a formula for bronchitis and asthma problems. It is used as a sedative "to calm the nerves of someone too caught up in things." It is sometimes mentioned with vervain, peppermint, and skullcap as a "strong calming of the body and spirit." The plant has beautiful whorls of red-purple flowers that "stand and wave in the field." It is a member of the Figwort, or Snapdragon, family, which also includes paintbrush, foxglove, eyebright, mullein, and speedwell. There is also another wood betony *(Betonica officinale)* used as a sedative and for bronchitis.

Wood fern *(Dryopteris filix* or *D. marginalis)*. The plant was steeped in hot water to prepare a tea that would be cooled, then held in the mouth for soothing toothache. It contains tannin, which is effective as an astringent.

Yarrow *(Achillea millefolium)*. Yarrow is dried and used as needed for pain and headaches. It was used as a tonic and as a stimulant for treating colds. A poultice would be made for skin sores and rashes. It is also used for ear problems with chamomile or mayweed as called by mountain folks in a wash. Yarrow is used in a formula with blue flag for ear drops. It was also used with agrimony and sage leaves to stop a nosebleed. The earlier Cherokee used crowfoot *(Ranunculus abortivus)* for the same purpose.

Yellow dock *(Rumex crispus).* The leaves of dock, curly or curled dock are used for treating sore throat and in a tonic formula. It was used for treating colds in earlier years. It is in the Smartweed, or Buckwheat, family.

Yellow jessamine (see Carolina jasmine).

Yellowroot (see Goldenseal).

Yellowroot *(Xanthorhiza simplicissima).* A poultice was made from the roots for soothing sore eyes. An elder mentioned its use for calming nerves. I learned as a young boy to chew on the stem or just steep it in some peppermint tea for a sore throat or hoarseness. The plant was also used as a yellow dye.

It seems to me that less of the North Medicine plants and their uses have been lost through time. However, there are several for which I have not been able to verify earlier use as North Medicine. They are as follows: pinxter flower *(Rhododendron periclymenoides),* waterleaf *(Hydrophyllum virginianum),* prostrate bluets *(Houstonia serpyllifolia),* purple bluets *(Houstonia purpurea),* chicory *(Cichorium intybus),* swamp thistle *(Cirsium muticum),* purple gerardia *(Agalinis purpurea),* spiderwort *(Tradescantia subaspera),* tall bellflower *(Campanula americana),* southern harebell *(Campanula divaricata),* mistflower *(Eupatorium coelestinum),* closed gentian *(Gentiana linearis),* monkshood *(Aconitum uncinatum),* and great lobelia *(Lobelia siphilitica).*

APPENDIX

Medicine Formulas of Plant and Natural Helpers

EAST MEDICINE

East Medicine includes ceremonial formulas, formulas for the circulatory system, some nervous-system and endocrine-system formulas as related to females, formulas for the reproductive system of women and men, and formulas for the wellness of children, adults, and elders.

Tribal ceremonial rites included the ingestion of sacred formulas to give the tribe strength and power for survival and as a "clearing-way" for journeys, wars, and "little wars," or games of competition. These sacred formulas were kept secret within the tribes. There are also sacred formulas for disease and illness that were used by only those trained in the Medicine ways, such as for conjuring or influencing a situation or outcome. These were also kept secret by those trained within the Medicine.

Symptomologies related to female and male sexuality and reproduction were usually not discussed openly among the Cherokee Medicine people. Certain ailments were handled by Medicine women and men who were trained in the uses specific plants related to these conditions. For example, there were specialists who dealt with prostate concerns, as there were specialists trained in the reproductive issues faced by women, including cramping, "hot flashes," profuse bleeding, or abnormal menstrual flow. Usually Medicine women dealt with female conditions and Medicine men with male difficulties. Plants that have diuretic, astringent, or stimulant properties were popular for women's Medicine bags. Such plants include black cohosh, ginseng, comfrey, and others listed below. Strawberries, blackberries, and red raspberries were used a lot for female conditions. Greens and leaves rich in vitamin C and minerals such as potassium were also employed for woman's reproductive health. As an elder woman put it, "Women in that time knew what to do because they learned it from their grandmothers. You didn't have to get an appointment, because these Medicine women lived with you." Special Medicines were used for conditions commonly experienced by women during menstruation. Plant helpers used for profuse bleeding included carrot, cayenne, lemon, raspberry, shepherd's purse, and thyme. Plant helpers used for delayed menstruation included balms, angelica, and fennel, and some foods such as cucumber and beets. For menstrual pain and cramping women used strawberry, peppermint, chamomile, and catnip.

Another important characteristic of East Medicine is its relationship to heart health. Tea made from the inner bark of the wild cherry tree was used to calm the heart. Hawthorn berries used as a heart tonic was introduced by Europeans. The earlier Cherokee used young asparagus shoots as a diuretic to help with edema. They also used rosemary in the formula, along with wild onions. (The essential oils found in onion and garlic may help to lower serum cholesterol levels.)

Early Cherokee knew that the obvious symptoms that we today associate with high or low blood pressure were indeed related to heart health. The symptoms the Cherokee treated with heart-helping herbs included headaches with tightness in the chest, tingling and numbness, excessive perspiration, and cramping with palpitations. Ginger tea was used as a helper for symptoms of low blood pressure. The formula for circulatory-system health used by earlier Cherokee included peppermint, passionflower, ginger, and a mild diuretic. In some remedies, motherwort and garlic were used, along with horse chestnut and pine bark.

Cherokee Medicine of the East also included formulas that were used as general tonics. A traditional Cherokee tonic was watercress leaves in peppermint tea for stimulating the digestive and nervous systems, with anise and/or angelica. Sometimes carrot was used, along with raspberry leaves for women during pregnancy.

East Medicine also focuses on detoxification, or "clearing." The strategy for detoxifying usually involved drinking lots of water and ingesting natural laxatives to irrigate the entire system. In earlier times such a clearing was usually undertaken in preparation for a traditional sweat lodge ceremony. Certain teas or cold drinks would be provided in the sweat lodge or as part of a "vision quest." These were sacred drinks prepared by the Medicine priest. Sage was a common tea for such ceremonies.

Detoxifying teas also included fennel, yarrow, and cayenne. The connection between cleansing and protection seems to go back a very long way. Some earlier Cherokee were almost obsessed with water cleansing and herbal washes and "going to the river." Internal and external cleanliness was important in ceremonial preparation.

When a baby is born into this world, a blessing and a clearing-way are performed to ask for strength, health, and a bright mind to carry on the tribal traditions and life. Gifts of tobacco, sage, and cedar were made to the fire, with prayers to the Great One for clearing and protection. Then there would be prayers to the Four Directions and a thank-you to the Great One. A similar ceremony with the peace pipe reminded participants that we are all connected in the circle of life. These ceremonies were East Medicine.

Today we can have a similar "way," making our own ceremonies in simple things we do, especially with plants. As an example, we can give thanks to the Great One when we are in nature for the plants and all the other gifts of life. We can take a deep breath as we give thanks for this gift of life and healing. We can leave enough plants for regeneration of the circle of plant life. (The traditional means of ensuring regeneration was to make sure there were always at least four plants in an outgrowth before taking any, and that at least four plants were left behind.) We should always remind ourselves that we are here to be the protector of every plant species and ensure the survival of all that come after us, as our ancestors did. As a Cherokee elder and friend, William Hornbuckle, said, "We have been gifted by the special healing plants for food and Medicine. It is our way to protect, preserve, and replant the gift of life for those who come after us." I was fortunate to learn the uses of many plants from this Cherokee elder, thanks to Ann Bradley, who introduced me to him. She continues to encourange Cherokee youth to learn about plants and cultural traditions, as William encouranged her.

The following list gives the herbs used to treat specific situations or conditions. If any of these situations pertain to you, you might want to consider getting to know one or two of the herbs listed here and carrying those herbs in your personal Medicine bundle. Always check with and learn from people trained in herbal or naturopathic medicine, as well as with your physician, before using plants or plant products for healing.

Anemia ("weak blood")
Dandelion, gentian, ginseng, nettle, saw palmetto, and watercress

Birthing and labor (internal remedies)
Balsam fir, blackgum, buckeye tree, bugbane, Carolina hemlock, cinquefoil, dutchman's pipe, greenbrier, golden puffball or dusk snuff, goat's beard, goldenseal, heal-all, hickory, horse balm, horseweed, Indian root, Indian tobacco, lady's slipper, leafcup, melissa balm, moon root, mountain dittany, poke or pokeweed, purple coneflower, ragwort, raspberry, skullcap, sweet flag, sycamore, trillium or Indian balm, stone root, walking fern or walking leaf, wallflower, watercress, wild ginger, and wild cherry

Blood purifiers
Agrimony, alder tree, birch, burdock, button's snakeroot, catnip, comfrey, elderberry, garlic, ginseng, goat dandelion, goldenseal, Indian root, milkweed, prickly ash, and wild cherry

Breast health, sore nipples, and flow of milk
Black cohosh, borage, evening primrose, fox grape, hearts-a-bustin', nettle, oak, partridgeberry, poke or pokeweed, rosemary, saw palmetto, skullcap, stone root, walking fern or walking leaf, and water dragon or lizard's tail

Cervical care
Burdock, echinacea, ginger, goldenseal, Indian root, Indian tobacco, melissa balm, milk thistle, red clover, watercress, willow, yellow dock, and yellowroot

Cleansing (internal, for toxins in the blood)
Black elder, cayenne, chaparral, comfrey, garlic, dandelion, evening primrose, heal-all, Indian root, Indian tobacco, nettle, pansy, peppermint, wormwood, and yellowroot

Cleansing (external "wash" for females)
Heal-all, Indian root, wallflower, and watercress

Circulation
Cayenne, chamomile, elderberry, ginseng, hawthorn, holly, Indian poke, and mistletoe

Depression (female)
Borage, ginseng, lavender, mistletoe, oats, St. John's wort, stargrass, Venus looking glass, and vervain

Fatigue
Comfrey, dandelion, and ginseng

"Female problems"
Wild ginger, dutchman's pipe, and valerian were combined for females who experienced irregular heart rate and anxiety during their menstrual cycles and during menopause. While not verified, this formula may have been used in earlier years during birthing labor. Wahoo, virgin's bower, Indian arrowroot, and black haw were combined in a special formula for "female nervousness around those problems"; sycamore, Carolina hemlock, and golden ragwort were combined, possibly with black haw, for various female complaints around menstruation and birthing. Sampson and black snakeroot were considered "cure-alls" for female conditions; red clover was combined with ginseng and evening primrose in a formula; Indian root and Indian tobacco were used as a "cure-all" with ceremony, especially for births; hop vine was included in a special drink for women having "womb problems." Heal-all was used as well, but the formula and its use is now forgotten or kept sacred; elecampane was considered good Medicine for all female complaints; chasteberry, or vitex, is a good modern-day "squaw root."

Green Corn Ceremony Medicine
Beargrass, broom sedge, comfrey, mint, pumpkin, spring amaranth, virgin's bower, wild lettuce, and others

Heart (arrhythmia, or "nervous heart")
Cayenne, chamomile, fennel, ginger, hawthorn, Indian poke, larkspur, lavender, lemon balm, lily-of-the-valley, maidenhair fern, mountain mint, mullein, rue, sassafras, senna, shepherd's purse, rue, stargrass, valerian, and wahoo

Heart (angina or pain)
Alfalfa, bilberry, cayenne, columbine, dandelion, elcampane, garlic, ginger, ginseng, hawthorn, lily-of-the-valley, mountain mint, mistletoe, motherwort, ragwort, rhododendron, stargrass, stone root, willow, wood betony, and yarrow

High blood pressure
Anise, black cohosh, burdock, caraway, cayenne, chamomile, fennel, garlic, ginger, kelp, licorice, nettle, peppermint, seven-bark shrub, shepherd's purse, and yarrow

Impotence
Chickweed, ginseng, and licorice

Low blood pressure
Cayenne, cinnamon, dandelion, ginseng, goldenseal, hawthorn, licorice, kelp, and sarsaparilla

Menopause
Elecampane, black cohosh, cramp bark, feverfew, ginseng, hops, heal-all, licorice, rue, St. John's wort, sage, and wild yam

"Men's medicine"
Elm, ginger, and saw palmetto

Menstruation (flow of blood, cycles, and difficulties)
Alder tree, allspice or pimento tree, amaranth, black haw, blue cohosh, chamomile, elecampane, evening primrose, goldenseal, gold thread, heal-all, horehound, horse balm, Indian root, Indian tobacco, licorice, melissa balm, passionflower, periwinkle, piney weed, ragweed, raspberry, red clover, redroot, rhododendron, rosemary, rue, sampson snakeroot, shepherd's purse, St. John's wort, tansy, thyme, Virginia snakeroot, sunflower, wild cherry, witch hazel, and yellowroot

Morning sickness
Chamomile, ginger, and peppermint

Nervousness (menstrual cycle or chronic condition)
Catnip, lady's slipper, lobelia, melissa balm, motherwort, St. John's wort, sweet violet, and Venus looking glass

Pain and cramping
Balsam fir, black haw, black snakeroot, blue cohosh, Indian tobacco, rhododendron, skullcap, sunflower, wild lettuce, wild strawberry, wild yam, and willow bark

Sex (improve or enhance)
Ginseng, licorice, oats, saw palmetto, slippery elm, and wild yam

STD, or sexually transmitted disease
Dwarf bay, elecampane, heal-all, goldenseal, persimmon, pine, piney weed, prickly ash, strawberry bush or hearts-a-bustin', sweetgum, and wahoo

Sleep (insomnia)
Evening primrose, fennel, hops, lavender, skullcap, St. John's wort, and valerian

"Special Medicine"
Strawberries are mentioned in a Cherokee story for keeping love and commitment in a relationship. Venus flytrap and devil's shoestring were used by the earlier Cherokee in fishing by chewing the root and spitting it on the bait. Trillium, Indian balm, and balsam apple were used in a "love Medicine." Wild tobacco was offered to the sacred fire in ceremonies to send a message or give thanks to the Great One. Thistle root, bull nettle, and mother of corn are cut into small pieces and placed around a baby's neck for teething. Sunflower has a special place in Cherokee myths related to the Sun and cycles. Sweet William was used in ceremonies to protect babies and children. St. John's wort and broadleaf plantain were combined in a sacred formula for making a "root water" bath to provide strength to babies. Seven-bark shrub was used for women who had "bad dreams during their period." Red cardinal was used in an old Cherokee fishing formula; it was also used as rat poison. Ragweed, mistletoe, bear grass, longleaf pine, spring amaranth, sacred tobacco, wild tobacco, and sage were among those plants used in Green Corn Medicine and drink, which is considered sacred. Potato and pine were considered "moon Medicine" plants related to the "darkening land" or death, and used in ceremonies. Pitcher plant and Venus flytrap were considered sacred plants used only in formulas that are either no longer known or are held sacred. Easter lily as it is called today was considered a "West wind" or "West door" plant, used in ceremony "to open the West door from the East" for clearing and prayer. Mayapple was considered sacred in regard to females. Gourds were used for making ceremonial rattles, with corn and other objects inside, and were used as dippers for water and Medicine. Elecam-

pane, or cure-all, was used in most formulas as a "spirit Medicine" that had some special power, but none of the elders could remember where that idea came from. Button bush seeds were used to attract ducks, which were used for food and ceremonial feathers. Cardinal flower was used for the "bad disease"; the myth recounting its naming is based on an old Cherokee story. Blue ash was used for the blue dye used by one of the Cherokee clans; its use as a Medicine has been lost or is kept sacred. Amaranth was called "blood plant," and was given to a young woman at her first menstrual cycle with a ceremony; the fruit was used to attract certain birds, including the red tanager, for sacred and ceremonial feathers. Adam and Eve root was used in a special ceremony for joining a couple. Goldenrod is used as a dry kindle for starting the sacred fire. Black locust was used in ceremonial "clearing" formula for women, along with greenbrier, heartleaf, mistletoe, and ginseng root. The sacred fire was built with oak, locust, redbud, and wild plum. Special ceremonies used several woods for making the sacred fire, with bark being taken only from the east side of the tree; those woods included white oak, black oak, basswood, and chestnut. Partridge pea was used for clearing with females and to enhance fertility; red cardinal or Cherokee bean seeds were used for fishing. Rhododendron leaves were used in special dance around the fire, gifting a leaf and a prayer in each direction.

Tonic for the blood (male and female strength)
Agrimony, alder tree, alfalfa, anise, blackberries, burdock, elder, capsicum, Carolina spring beauty, dandelion, elderberry, ginger, ginseng, Indian poke, Indian root, licorice, melissa balm, moon root, parsley, red clover, sarsaparilla, sassafras, scurvy grass, senna, St. John's wort, strawberries, Virginia snakeroot, and yellow dock

Uterine and ovary health
Bayberry, black cohosh, black haw, burdock, button snakeroot, chamomile, cramp bark, dandelion, elecampane, feverfew, goldenseal, loosestrife, milk thistle, motherwort, Peruvian bark, poke root, red raspberry, valerian, wahoo, wild yam, willow, witch hazel, yarrow, yellow dock, and yellowroot

Vaginal (itching, fungal, and bacterial)
Elecampane, black birch, comfrey, garlic, goldenseal, horseweed, Indian poke, milk thistle, oak, plantain, purple coneflower, rosemary, sage, vervain, witch hazel, and yellowroot

Varicose veins
Elecampane, hawthorn, horse balm, and horse chestnut

"Weak males and females" (sexual strength)
Alfalfa, basswood, elecampane, ginseng, holly, moon root, red root, rosin weed, senna, sassafras, saw palmetto, St. John's wort, strawberries and blackberries, and Virginia snakeroot

SOUTH MEDICINE

Being the direction of innocence, in the South we celebrate childhood milestones, like rocks that cross the stream to the adult on the other side. Early behaviors and skills were observed as parents and extended family taught a child the way of right relationship with all things. South Medicine included the bull nettle necklace for teething and arrowwood for developing the skill of making arrows from stems.

Safety was taught through experiences rather than with "do's" and "don'ts." I remember my grandfather teaching me by example that when a stick falls into the water, the rushing water takes it down stream. That was a traditional means of teaching me to be careful and not be like the stick floating down the river. He taught me that rocks are slippery when they are wet with water, and even more slippery with green algae on it. Knives were used under supervision, and the bow and arrow was for hunting instead of play. Safety and protection were first and foremost in learning life-survival skills. South Medicine was about learning something for the first time, or relearning it again with the understanding of a child.

The South being connected with Mother Earth, choosing the right roots for cooking and the right greens for spring salad was an important lesson of the South and was learned by both boys and girls. Gathering food and Medicine was a learning opportunity rather than a chore. Children learned of the Indian "Band-aid," plantain leaf, for healing cuts and abrasions. Children learned about rashes, itch, and cough medicine from natural plants at an early age. We learned as children that catnip would be used as a salve or wash on us to repel insects and would be spread around the shoots of young plants with ashes to keep the little pests away from our future food products. We learned the old remedy of garlic as a "cure-all."

South Medicine includes plants for all of nature's environmental exposures that affect the skin and the external parts of the body. The majority of plant applications in the South were for wounds and infected areas of the skin, insects bites and stings, snakebites, and poisons or toxins in nature that caused irritation and rashes.

South Medicine included plant formulas and remedies for the bones, muscles, and joints. These were usually applied as poultices, oils, washes, and other topical pain relievers such as witch hazel that would be absorbed through the skin into the deeper tissue layers.

Ceremonial medicine in the South focused on children and nature, with plants being helpers and protectors prepared as "special Medicine," such as tobacco for offerings and sunflower as a sacred plant.

The South Medicine focuses on maintaining harmony and balance with nature and our environment. It is about whole-body health. South Medicine teaches us to play more like a young child as we enjoy the simple nature of all things around us.

Arthritis, neuritis, and neuralgia
American spikenard (Indian root), arnica, camphor, cayenne, chamomile, cloves, common phacelia, dog fennel, dog hobble, flaming azalea, lobelia, mullein, pine, rue, slippery elm, and wintergreen

Bursitis (tendons)
Cayenne, devil's claw, ginger, licorice, poke, and willow

Boils
Aloe, American spikenard (Indian root), arnica, beet, bloodroot, bouncing bet, corn, chamomile, dog fennel, dogwood, flax, four-o'clock, gourd, jimson weed, oats, pepper grass, pine, poplar, pretty-by-night, purple coneflower, Solomon's seal, speedwell, spikenard (spignet), sumac, thistle, turtlehead, violet, and yellowroot

Bruises
Aloe, arnica, basswood, bay tree, bilberry, comfrey, chamomile, dodder, jimson weed, leafcup, passionflower, St. John's wort, and witch hazel

Burns (and sunburn)
Aloe, alumroot, balm-of-Gilead, bamboo-brier, chamomile, Christmas fern, comfrey, elderberry, jimson weed, lavender, leafcup, oak, passionflower,

plantain, pumpkin, rosemary, spikenard (spignet), St. John's wort, sumac, and witch hazel

Dandruff, head or skin conditions, and lice
Birch tree, evening primrose, flaxseed, larkspur (for lice), marsh mallow, nettle, pawpaw, pine, poplar, sage, shinleaf, slippery elm, soapwort, sycamore tree, sweetgum tree, and willow

Foot (itch)
Aloe, American spikenard (Indian root), arnica, comfrey, chamomile, garlic, goldenrod, goldenseal, pepper, ragweed, richweed, staggerbush, wintergreen, and witch hazel, and yellowroot

Hair (condition and loss)
Arnica, nettle, onion, and soapwort

Hives
Aloe, arnica, burdock, comfrey, chamomile, ginger, licorice, marsh mallow, nettle, poplar, saffron, witch hazel, yarrow, and yellowroot

Insect bites and stings
Aloe, arnica, broom sedge, comfrey, chamomile, elm tree, forget-me-not, hemlock tree, houseleek, horehound, goat's beard, goldenrod, nettle, lavender, lobelia (Indian tobacco), marsh mallow, melissa balm, moss (reindeer moss), oak, plantain, pine, piney weed, poison ivy (special use), poplar, purple coneflower, saw palmetto, shinleaf, spiderwort (dayflower), valerian, wild or sacred tobacco, witch hazel, and yellowroot

Insect repellent
Garlic, pennyroyal, and narrow leaf plantain (hosta plantain)

Mouth (sores and herpes)
Alder tree, aloe, chamomile, crowfoot, goldenseal, horehound, lemon balm, licorice, oak, pine, poplar, purple coneflower, and St. John's wort

Muscles (soreness and twitching)
Aloe, American spikenard (Indian root), arnica, Carolina vetch, dogwood, hophornbeam, rosemary, rue, tickseed (devil's shoestring), wintergreen, witch hazel, and willow

Pain (external and with swelling)
Aloe, American spikenard (Indian root), arnica, cayenne, evening primrose, Indian physic, lady's thumb, rosemary, smartweed, St. John's wort, willow, wintergreen, and dogwood bark internally

Poison ivy, oak, sumac, and other
Aloe, arnica, alder tree, beech tree, comfrey, chamomile, cucumber, horse gentian, jewelweed, oats, pennyroyal, plantain, pine, poplar, self-heal, shinleaf, witch hazel, and yellowroot

Psoriasis
Aloe, arnica, chickweed, comfrey, chamomile, dandelion, goldenseal, marsh mallow, poplar, pine, sarsaparilla, sassafras, self-heal, sorrel, yellow dock, witch hazel, and yellowroot

Rheumatism (aches and pains)
Aloe, American holly, American spikenard (Indian root), arnica, bittersweet, Christmas fern, dog fennel, dog hobble, flaming azalea, Indian poke, horse gentian, mountain laurel, rheumatism root, turk's cap lily, and wood fern. See also arthritis entry, above.

Skin (aging and spots)
Aloe, American spikenard (Indian root), arnica, balm-of-Gilead, cucumber, comfrey, chamomile, and licorice

Skin (eczema, acne, and rash)
Aloe, arnica, black elder, bloodroot, broom sedge, burdock, chamomile, chickweed, comfrey, cucumber, dandelion, dock or curled dock, evening primrose, figwort, flax, garlic, golden glow, goldenseal, ivy, juniperberries licorice, marsh mallow, mountain laurel, oats, pansy, pine, plantain, poplar, purple coneflower, sorrel, self-heal, soapwort, sorrel, slippery elm, speedwell, witch grass, yellow dock, wintergreen, and yellowroot

Skin (cuts and wounds)
Aloe, alumroot, balm-of-Gilead, balsam fir, birch tree, blood leather, buckeye, comfrey, chamomile, dogwood, figwort, garlic, goldenseal, highland fern, horse gentian, geranium, goldenrod, horehound, horsetail, Indian plantain, jimson weed, leafcup, lizard's tail, maidenhair tree, melissa balm, mountain fern, pine, plantain, purple coneflower, rattlesnake fern, rosemary, rue, sage, self-heal, senega snakeroot, slippery elm, thyme, violet, Virginia snakeroot, water plantain, white oak, wild carrot, wild indigo, witch hazel, wood betony, woundwort, yarrow, and yellowroot

Skin (fungal, infections, and ringworm)
Aloe, arnica, bloodroot, cinnamon, comfrey, chamomile, garlic, geranium, goldenseal, laurel, lobelia (Indian tobacco), marigold, plantain, pine, poison ivy (for ringworm), poplar, ragweed, sarsaparilla, self-heal, slippery elm, soapwort, sorrel, wintergreen, witch hazel, yellow dock, and yellowroot

Skin (inflamed areas and sores)
Aloe, alumroot, arnica, bracken fern, buckeye, comfrey, crowfoot, dock (curled dock), chamomile, highland fern, horse chestnut, horse gentian, Indian fern, Indian root, poplar, swamp lily, twinleaf (rheumatism root), willow, and wintergreen

Skin (itch, irritation, and abrasion)
Aloe, alumroot, arnica, beech tree, broom sedge, buckeye, chickweed, comfrey, common sorrel, corn, chamomile, cucumber, devil's claw, elm, figwort, flax, garlic, goldenrod, maple, marigold, marsh mallow, nettle (bull nettle), ragweed, richweed, pennyroyal, pine, poison ivy (special use), poplar, self-heal, senega snakeroot, slippery elm, soapwort, sorrel, staggerbush, wintergreen, witch hazel, yellow dock, and yellowroot

Skin (sores and difficult or old sores)
Adam and Eve root (puttyroot), adder's tongue (dog's tooth violet), aloe, alumroot, arnica, balm-of-Gilead, balsam fir, basswood, bay tree, burdock, comfrey, coneflower, devil's walkingstick, dock (curled dock), dogwood, dutchman's breeches, elderberry, golden glow, goldenseal, goldthread, Indian fern, lady's thumb, laurel, mallow, masterwort, nightshade, oak, pepper grass, pansy, pumpkin, puffball or devil's snuffbox, purple coneflower, rattlesnake plantain (ratsbane), rhododendron, self-heal, senna, seven-bark shrub, shinleaf, Solomon's seal, sorrel, sycamore tree, vervain (self-heal), violet (bird's foot violet), walnut tree, water plantain, white oak, wild carrot, and willow

"Special Medicine"
"Sacred spirit water" was water from a creek where there was no blood shed. Sacred tobacco would be shared with a prayer-chant, then placed in a pottery bowl. Certain plant and bark juices associated with the Four Directions would be added, and the mixture would sit in the sun for four days. It would then be used on certain skin conditions and sores. Devil's shoestring would be used for ceremony with ball players after a "cold plunge." Wild or sacred tobacco was used for making offerings, gifting, and ceremony. Sage was used in ceremonial offerings; Indian tobacco would be used in old formulas for skin conditions, including joint pains.

Swelling (feet and legs)
Aloe, American spikenard (Indian root), arnica, couchgrass, devil's claw, dutchman's pipe, oak, wormwood, and yellowroot

Varicose veins
Aloe, bilberry, hawthorn berry, horse chestnut, nettle, thyme, sweet flag, wintergreen, and witch hazel

Warts (genital)
Arnica, bloodroot, black birch, dandelion, garlic, mayapple (Indian apple), milkweed, St. John's wort, and white cedar

WEST MEDICINE

The direction of West was traditionally considered the realm of challenge, competition, death, and all the things we have to deal with for physical survival. In essence, it is the direction of physical Medicine. The stories and myths tell of a time when the "Little People" met in council to decide how to revive the daughter of the Sun, who was bitten by a snake sent by the council to stop the Sun from bearing down so hard and hot on the people working in the planting fields. They were getting sick from the sun's tremendous heat, and the earth was drying without rain. Their efforts resulted in the death of the Sun's daughter. The decision was made in council to place the daughter in a pine box and take her to the "darkening land" where she could be revived if the spirit, or ghost, people touched sycamore rods that extended from the pine box. The belief was that the spirit people could give her life, thus appeasing the Sun.

The long trip to the West, or the darkening land, was made with the daughter inside the pine box. As they reached the circle of the darkening land, they could see the spirit people dancing in a circle. The Little People moved the box so the sycamore rods could touch the spirits. As they entered the energy circle of the "spirit ones," they heard some noise in the box. The Little People started their journey back to the direction of the Sun, which was slightly rising to take a peak at where the Little People were in their journey. As they continued their journey, they could hear some movement in the pine box, but they were told not to open the box until they were at their journey's end in the East.

The Little People carrying the pine box heard a voice, "Please let me out. I cannot breathe in here." They remembered what they were told, but they were also afraid the daughter of the Sun would die again from not being able to breathe. They continued their journey

East. Again, they heard the voice, "Please let me out, or just open the box enough so I can have a drink of water. I am very thirsty." This continued until they were very close to the East. Finally, the desperate voice sounded as though she was going to die, and they thought about having to make the long journey back to the darkening land of the West. They decided to open the box only slightly so she could breathe and have a drink of water. Suddenly, they heard a flutter, and a bird escaped from the pine box. All was well, because the special bird became the messenger between the people of Mother Earth and the Sun, who to this day continues the journey across the sky to visit with the grandmother who lives in the West. Some say the special bird is the ancestor of all birds, while others say it is the ancestor of the Great Eagle.

Some elders say the birds are manifestations of the spirit inside all of us that guide us to be care-free or not too grounded. They say we learn that internally we need air and water to live, but our spirit needs love and freedom to survive. The lesson teaches us to reach high and even to fly in spirit; otherwise, we look to the plant helpers on Mother Earth to maintain physical balance in our lives, called West Medicine.

The West Medicine, based on the myth or story with the plants as helpers for internal physical conditions and natural nutrition, related to physical health and wholeness. this was also a traditional guide to food as Medicine and a healthy balance of energy and internal harmony. One of the most important Medicine helpers that is not usually mentioned in the use of plants is water, which is considered a Medicine of the West. Tonics and drinks made from plant helpers became elixirs that were often called "Indian tonics" by non-Indians who were often called "snake-oil salesmen." The remedies were usually sold for snakebites and elixirs to cure backaches and all the conditions common at that time, including fevers and infections. Ironically, there was a respect in those early years for Indian remedies based on formulas made from natural plants. What was usually lost in the translation was the total concept of Medicine that included sweats, ceremonies, family and tribal support, song chants, and all the things used for total wellness, harmony, and balance. West Medicine helpers for the internal conditions to restore physical balance are as follows:

Arthritis
Angelica, black cohosh, devil's claw, evening primrose, feverfew, flaxseed, ginger, nettle, purple coneflower or echinacea, rue, valerian, willow, yellow gentian, and yucca

Appetite (improve for elders and "sick ones")
Anise, bilberry, blue-eyed grass, dogwood tree, fairywand or devil's bit or blazing star, flax, garlic, gentian, ginseng, goldenseal or yellowroot, horseradish, maple tree, milk thistle, nettle, juniperberries, mugwort, twayblade, watercress, and yarrow

Appetite (decrease appetite or weight loss)
Corn silk, chickweed, dandelion, fennel, ginger, goldenseal or yellowroot, kelp, sassafras, and Venus looking glass

Bladder
Aloe, agrimony, bittersweet, black cohosh, castor bean, chamomile, chickweed, comfrey, dandelion, goldenrod, goldenseal, gooseberry, hawkweed or rabbit's ear, Joe-pye weed or gravel root, oak tree, peppermint, purple coneflower or echinacea, and raspberry

"Cleansing" (including laxatives)
Aloe, alumroot, anise, asafoetida or ferula, asparagus, balsam tree, beans, beech tree, blackroot or culver's root, bloodroot, buckthorn tree, blue flag, cabbage, caraway, carrot, castor bean, chickweed, dandelion, false aloe, fennel, flax, garlic, goosegrass, horehound, hydrangea, hyssop, lamb's quarters, meadow rue, milk thistle, milkweed, pansy, purslane, ramps, rhubarb, sarsaparilla, sassafras, senna, Solomon's seal, sorrel, twayblade, and witch grass

Diabetes
Aloe, bilberry, birch, bitter weed, calamus, garlic, ginseng, huckleberry, milk thistle, pumpkin seeds, oats, valerian, and yucca

Diarrhea (including more severe cases of dysentery)
Adder's tongue or trout lily, alumroot, barberry, benne plant, birch, black cherry, black cohosh, blue-eyed grass, caraway, catnip, chicory, cinquefoil, columbine, false aloe, foxglove, fox grape, geranium or American cranesbill, ginger, hemlock, hog peanut, Indian mouse ear, physic, pansy,

parsley, pepper bush, peppermint, pipsissewa, raspberry, sage, self-heal, senna, shepherd's purse, sorrel, southern harebell, sweet flag, trillium or Indian balm, Turk's cap lily, white oak, wild rose, wild strawberry, wintergreen, witch hazel, and wood betony

Diuretic

Agrimony, angelica, beans, bearberry, blue flag, burdock, butterfly weed, celery, columbine, corn, cranberry or mountain cranberry, cucumber, dandelion, fairywand or devil's bit or blazing star, Dutchman's pipe, fennel, ginseng, goldenrod, hemlock, horsechestnut, horsetail, Joe-pye weed or gravel root, juniperberry, meadow rue or crowfoot, parsley, pipsissewa, poor robin's plantain, raspberry, sarsaparilla, sassafras, saw palmetto, sorrel, trumpet vine or wild potato vine, white snakeroot, yarrow, and yellowroot

Fever (related to internal problems and infections)

Arrowhead, ash tree, barberry, basil, bayberry or wax myrtle, black cohosh, boneset or Indian sage, dogwood, and purple coneflower or echinacea

Flatulence (carminative)

Angelica, anise, basil, calamus root or sweet flag, caraway, catnip, chamomile or yellowroot, fennel, ginger, goldenrod, melissa balm, prickly ash, rosemary, sassafras, self-heal, thyme, and valerian

Gallbladder (and stones)

Agrimony, apple tree, birch tree, comfrey (caution), crabapple, dandelion, peppermint, purple coneflower or echinacea, raspberry, and yellow bedstraw

Gastrointestinal

Aloe, alder tree, anise, ash tree, balsam tree, birch Tree, black cohosh, blackgum tree, black walnut tree, cabbage, caraway, capsicum, catnip, cayenne or capsicum, cinquefoil, false aloe, fennel, garlic, ginger, gentian, goldenseal, hornbean, horse chestnut or buckeye, juniper berries, knotweed, lavender, licorice, lousewort, meadowsweet, mulberry tree, onion, peppermint, persimmon tree, pine, potato vine or trumpet vine, purple coneflower or echinacea, red root, sage, savory, senna, slippery elm, sourwood, terrapin's foot, thyme, tickseed, watercress, wood betony, and wormwood

Gout

Adder's tongue or trout lily, American spikenard or Indian root, balsam tree, bearberry, birch tree, celery, cedar or white cedar, devil's claw, fleabane, horsetail, nettle, purple coneflower or echinacea, soapwort, witch-grass, and yucca

Indigestion
Angelica, arbutus or terrapin's foot, caraway, Carolina pinkroot, chamomile or goldenseal or yellowroot, chicory, colic root, fennel, ginger, lemon balm, licorice, marsh mallow, mugwort, parsley, peppermint, rosemary, savoy, white mustard, and wintergreen or teaberry

Kidney (gravel/stones, infection, and pain)
Aloe, arbutus or terrapin's foot, asparagus, balsam tree, bearberry, beggar lice, birch tree, black cohosh, blue devil, bracken fern, capsicum, chaparral, chicory, comfrey, corn silk, cucumber, fairywand or devil's bit or blazing star, fleabane, frostweed, galax, garlic, goldenrod, goldenseal, hops, horehound, hydrangea, loosestrife, marsh mallow, oak tree, parsley, persimmon tree, pipsissewa, pitcher plant, poke or pokeweed, poor Robin's plantain, poplar tree, purple coneflower or echinacea, queen of the meadow, raspberry, rhubarb, sarsaparilla, sassafras, shepherd's purse, skullcap, slippery elm, sorrel, speedwell, terrapin's foot, twayblade, valerian, watermelon, white snakeroot, wild plum, wild strawberry, wild yam, wintergreen, witchgrass, and wood betony, yarrow, yellow dock, and yellowroot

Laxative (see Cleansing)

Liver
Alumroot, ash tree, barberry, blackroot or culver's root, buckthorn tree, cabbage, comfrey (caution), dandelion, fairywand or devil's bit or blazing star, garlic, ginseng, milk thistle, purple coneflower or echinacea, and virginia creeper

Low Blood Sugar
Bilberry

Nausea
Catnip, ginger, and goldenseal

Pain
American spikenard or Indian root, angelica, birch tree, black birch tree, black cohosh, butterfly weed, button snakeroot or devil's bit or blazing star, catnip, celery, comfrey, dogwood, elder tree, garlic, gentian, hops, parsnip, purple coneflower or echinacea, skullcap, valerian, and willow

Prostate
Cayenne, ginseng, goldenseal, kelp, and pumpkin

"Special Medicine"
Indian pipe, lady's slipper, lobelia, purge root, stinging nettle, pitcher plant, tansy, yaupon, yellow-eyed grass, and yucca (Venus flytrap was included, but it is not mentioned in this text because it was considered sacred to the elders)

"Spring Tonic" (old Cherokee formula)
Ash tree, black elder, calamus or sweet flag, dandelion, ivy, nettle, sassafras, watercress, witchgrass, and others not included in text because they were considered sacred by the elders

STD or Sexually Transmitted Diseases
Black cohosh, blackgum tree, and purple coneflower or echinacea

Stimulate (metabolism and system)
Birch, blue flag, cayenne or capsicum, elder, garlic, ginger, ginseng, Joe-pye weed or gravel root, juniperberry, mullein, nettle, pricklyash, sassafras, sweet flag, white snakeroot, and wormwood

Stomach and Bowel (cramps and calming)
Agrimony, aloe, angelica, anise, asafoetida or ferula, belladonna, bittersweet, black cohosh, black snakeroot, blue cohosh, bracken fern, burdock, butterfly weed, calamus or sweet flag, Canadian snakeroot, caraway, capsicum, catnip, chamomile, comfrey (caution), cowslip, galax, gall-of-the-Earth or lion's foot, garlic, ginger, gentian, hairy beardtongue or broom sedge, hops, Indian turnip or Jack-in-the-pulpit, lady's slipper, lousewort, melissa balm, mint, oats, pipsissewa, purple coneflower or echinacea, sassafras, sedge, self-heal, senna, seven-bark shrub, skullcap, stinging nettle, thyme, watercress, wild potato or wild jalap, wood betony, and yellowroot

Thyroid
Black cohosh, kelp, and skullcap

"Tonic" (general health)
Alder tree, arnica, blackberry, chamomile, colic root, comfrey, dandelion, garlic, Joe-pye weed or gravel root, maple tree, masterwort, melissa balm, persimmon tree, ramps, raspberry, sarsaparilla, strawberry, thyme, walnut, wild black cherry tree, wild oats, and yellow gentian (there were others, but they were considered sacred by the elders)

"Tonic" (strength and endurance)

Angelica, carrot, ginger, ginseng, piney weed, sarsaparilla, St. John's wort, yellow gentian, and wild carrot (there were others not included in this text because they were considered sacred by the elders)

Ulcers

Capsicum, comfrey, goldenseal or yellowroot, knotgrass, nettle, oak, speedwell, and valerian

Urinary and Bladder (infection, "gravel," and pain)

Asparagus, barberry, bearberry, black cohosh, blue devil, corn, cranberry, cucumber, devil's shoestring, Dutchman's pipe, garlic, goat's beard, hearts-a-bustin', hops, hophornbean, Joe-pye weed or gravel root, juniper berry, ladies' tresses, parsley, persimmon tree, pipissewa, purple coneflower or echinacea, queen of the meadow, raspberry, red root, sage, shepherd's purse, smartweed, sorrel, trumpet vine or wild potato vine, twayblade, twinleaf or yellowroot, white snakeroot, wild cherry, wild oats, wild strawberry, sweet shrub, and yarrow

Worms (and parasites)

Agrimony, alder tree, alumroot, asafoetida or ferula, balsam fir, bayberry or wax myrtle, blackgum tree, blackroot or culver's root, bracken fern, broadleaf plantain, capsicum, Carolina pinkroot, castor bean, common rue, coralbread, devil's shoestring, false aloe, Fraser fir, garlic, ginger, Indian pink, lady's slipper, loblolly pine tree, male fern, maple tree, pine tree, pinkroot, pumpkin, purple coneflower or echinacea, rattlesnake plantain, purslane, ragweed, red root, senna, serviceberry tree, spleenwort, sweet fern, thyme, turtlehead, twinleaf or yellowroot, wild cherry, wild ginger, wild rose, wood betony, and wormseed

NORTH MEDICINE

The Medicine of the North is related to one of our basic needs for survival, which is air. Our relationship with the plants and trees is the focus of this Medicine with the balance of air associated with the exchange of air, or oxygen, breathed in by humans with the release of carbon dioxide. The trees and plants take in carbon dioxide and release oxygen, which we need to breathe and survive. While this was innately understood by earlier Indians, thanks was given for every plant and tree used for any purpose in ceremony and in daily life.

Formulas and remedies using plants in North Medicine relate to breathing and conditions affecting physical and mental balance. Conditions relating to the head such as headaches and calming were the focus of North Medicine. Cherokee elders shared with me stories and myths considered sacred for plant formulas used to influence others that included the senses such as smell and sight. This reminded me so much of mental conditioning, which could be considered positive or negative, depending on what you want to accomplish. As an example, a cold remedy using garlic can be a terrible-tasting liquid, or it can include wild cherry bark and honey that has a pleasant aroma and taste to it. If a child is to be conditioned to not like the elixir, but know it is "good Medicine," then the child will not want it unless he is really sick. Of course, the opposite can be true as well. Some of the old formulas are considered potions to bring about special powers for "keeping a clear head for hunting or for games of competition."

The use of natural plants by American Indians and Alaska Natives for North Medicine is still considered very effective for coughs, colds, and upper respiratory conditions. The same is true for fever remedies and conditions such as earache, eye irritation, and anxiety or depression problems. As an elder said, "Native Americans were once poked fun at for plant remedies, but just see how many of those plants are being synthesized today by non-Indians who have discovered something sold on the open market or as a prescription that is the same thing our ancestors used for survival."

The Medicine "helpers" for the North are as follows:

Anxiety
Catnip, celery, chamomile or yellowroot, clover, dandelion, gooseberry, heather, hops, Indian hemp or dropsy weed, jasmine, oats, periwinkle, lavender, motherwort, passionflower, skullcap, valerian, and vervain

Asthma
Anise, arrowroot, bitterweed, blackthorn, blue vervain, burdock, capsicum, coltsfoot, cotton, "co-we" (coffee), crested field fern, dandelion, evening primrose, eyebright, ferula, fireweed, foxglove, garlic, horehound, hyssop, licorice, lobelia or Indian tobacco, lungwort, ivy, maidenhair fern, mullein, rosemary, yarrow, and yellow dock

Bronchial/Bronchitis

Anise, coltsfoot, elecampane, echinacea, fennel, flax, horehound, hyssop, marsh mallow, mullein, peppermint, plantain, sundew, and thyme

Coughs

Anise, black cohosh, coltsfoot, comfrey, elecampane, ginseng, knotgrass, licorice, lobelia, lungwort, mullein, plantain, sage, spotted cranebill, thyme, wild cherry, and witchgrass

Colds

Boneset, coltsfoot, echinacea, elderberry, evening primrose, garlic, ginger, knotgrass, lemon balm, lungwort, mullein, peppermint, plantain, speedwell, St. Johns wort, witchgrass, and yarrow

Colds (children)

Coltsfoot, horehound, peppermint, and wild cherry

Colds (flu)

Anise, boneset, coltsfoot, comfrey, echinacea, elderberry, ginger, goldenseal (yellowroot), licorice, nettle, pleurisy root, slippery elm, spotted cranesbill, valerian, and willow bark or dogwood

Cold sores

Goldenseal (yellowroot), lemon balm, and licorice

Depression or "feeling low"

Lavender, oats, passionflower, and vervain

Earache

Echinacea, garlic, ginger, lemon balm, licorice, yellow dock, and yarrow

Eye soreness and irritation

Bilberry, eyebright, goldenseal (yellowroot), marigold, and rosemary

Eye (sties)

Berberine, eyebright, mullein, and yarrow

Fever

Ginseng, elderberry, feverfew, sassafras, vervain, wild ginger, willow bark, and yellow gentian

Gum soreness

Capsicum, dandelion, milk thistle, and willow

Headache

Capsicum, catnip, feverfew, ginger, passionflower, peppermint, thyme, valerian, willow bark or dogwood, and wood betony

Laryngitis
Coltsfoot, licorice, mullein, willow bark, and wild cherry

Motion sickness
Fennel, ginger, and peppermint

Mouthwash
Cloves, goldthread, oak, rosemary, spotted cranesbill, and sage

Nervousness
Hops, mistletoe, and passionflower

Respiratory complaints
Comfrey, mullein, marsh mallow, and saw palmetto

Rest and calm
Anise, catnip, dill, evening primrose, fennel, melissa balm, hops, lavender, passionflower, peppermint, skullcap, St. Johns wort, and valerian

Sinus conditions
Capsicum, echinacea, goldenseal, and willow

Sore throat
Capsicum, comfrey, echinacea, ginger, goldenseal (yellowroot), licorice, marsh mallow, mullein, plantain, wild cherry, and willow

Toothache
Blue flag (snake lily), clove, and garlic

Bibliography

Chiltoskey, Mary. Interviews from 1960–1966.

Coffey, Timothy. *The History and Folklore of North American Wildflowers.* New York: Facts on File, 1993.

Duke, James A. *The Green Pharmacy.* Emmaus, Pa.: Rodale Press, 1997.

———. *Handbook of Northeastern Indian Medicinal Plants.* Lincoln, Mass.: Quarterman Publications, 1986.

Doane, Nancy Locke. *Indian Doctor Book.* Charlotte, N.C.: Aerial Photography Services, 1983.

Elliott, Douglas B. *Wild Roots: A Forager's Guide to the Edible and Medicinal Roots, Tubers, Corms, and Rhizomes of North America.* Rochester, Vt.: Healing Arts Press, 1995.

Evans, E. Raymond, Clive Kileff, and Karen Shelly. *Herbal Medicine: A Living Force in the Appalachians.* Readings and Perspectives in Medicine, Booklet Number 4, 1982. Medical History Program and the Trent Collection, Duke University Medical Center, Durham, N.C.

Fetrow, Charles W., and Juan R. Avila. *The Complete Guide to Herbal Medicines.* Springhouse, Pa.: Springhouse Corp., 2000.

Foreman, Richard. *The Cherokee Physician: Indian Guide to Health.* 1857. Reprinted, Norman, Okla.: Hooper Printing Company, 1979.

Gabriel, Ingrid. *Herb Identifier and Handbook.* New York: Sterling Publishing Co., 1975.

Garrett, J. T., and Michael Garrett. *Medicine of the Cherokee: The Way of Right Relationship.* Santa Fe, N.M.: Bear & Company, 1996.

Hamel, Paul B., and Mary U. Chiltoskey. *Cherokee Plants*. Sylva, N.C.: Herald Publishing Co., 1975.

Hoffmann, David. *The New Holistic Herbal*. Rockport, Mass.: Element Books, 1992.

Hutchens, Alma R. *Indian Herbalogy of North America*. Boston: Shambhala, 1991.

Hutson, Robert W., William F. Hutson, and Aaron J. Sharp. *Great Smoky Mountains Wildflowers*. Northbrook, Ill.: Windy Pines Publishing, 1995.

Krochmal, Arnold, and Connie Krochmal. *A Guide to the Medicinal Plants of the United States*. New York: Quadrangle, 1973.

Lust, John. *The Herb Book*. New York: Bantam Books, 1974.

Meyer, Joseph E. *The Herbalist*. Glenwood, Ill.: Meyerbooks, 1981.

Mooney, James. *Myths of the Cherokee and Sacred Formulas of the Cherokee*. Nashville, Tenn.: Charles Elder, Bookseller, 1972.

PDR for Herbal Medicines. Montvale, N.J.: Medical Economics Company, 2001.

Reader's Digest. *Magic and Medicine of Plants*. Pleasantville, N.Y.: Reader's Digest Association, 1986.

Vogel, Virgil J. *American Indian Medicine*. Norman, Okla.: University of Oklahoma Press, 1970.

Join United Plant Savers

Become an Advocate for the Plants

United Plant Savers (UpS) is a nonprofit, grassroots organization dedicated to the conservation and cultivation of at-risk native medicinal plants. As an organization for herbalists and people who love plants, our purpose is to ensure the future of our rich diversity of medicinal species. Formed in the spirit of hope by a group of herbalists committed to protecting and preserving at-risk species and to raising public awareness, United Plant Savers reflects the great diversity of American herbalism. Our membership includes wildcrafters, seed collectors, herbal product manufacturers, growers, botanists, educators, practictioners, and plant lovers from all walks of life. We recognize that environmentally responsible cultivation, land stewardship, habitat protection, and sustainable wild harvesting are of critical imprortance to ensure an abundant renewable supply of medicinal plants for future generations. We invite you to join United Plant Savers. For more information, please write to UpS, P.O. Box 98, East Barre, VT, 05649.

Notes

Notes

Notes

Notes

BOOKS OF RELATED INTEREST

MEDICINE OF THE CHEROKEE
The Way of Right Relationship
by J. T. Garrett and Michael Tlanusta Garrett

WALKING ON THE WIND
Cherokee Teachings for Harmony and Balance
by Michael Garrett

THE CHEROKEE FULL CIRCLE
A Practical Guide to Ceremonies and Traditions
by J. T. Garrett and Michael Tlanusta Garrett

MEDITATIONS WITH THE CHEROKEE
Prayers, Songs, and Stories of Healing and Harmony
by J. T. Garrett

COYOTE HEALING
Miracles in Native Medicine
by Lewis Mehl-Madrona, M.D., Ph.D.

THE MAN WHO KNEW THE MEDICINE
The Teachings of Bill Eagle Feather
by Henry Niese

LEGENDS AND PROPHECIES OF THE QUERO APACHE
Tales for Healing and Renewal
by Maria Yracébûrû

SACRED EARTH
The Spiritual Landscape of Native America
by Arthur Versluis

Inner Traditions • Bear & Company
P.O. Box 388
Rochester, VT 05767
1-800-246-8648
www.InnerTraditions.com

Or contact your local bookseller